Global Health and Nursing

Global Health and Nursing

Global Health and Nursing

A NEW NARRATIVE FOR THE 21ST CENTURY

Edited by

BARBARA STILWELL, PHD, RN, RHV, FRCN, FAAN, FQNI

Consultant
Global Health Systems
Paddock Wood
United Kingdom

ELSEVIER

ISBN: 978-0-3238-7780-0

Content Strategist: Robert Edwards
Content Project Manager: Shubham Dixit
Cover Design: Bridget Hoette
Marketing Manager: Belinda Tudin

Printed in Poland

Last digit is the print number: 9 8 7 6 5 4 3 2

Working together to grow libraries in developing countries

www.elsevier.com • www.bookaid.org

CONTENTS

PREFACE

■ ■

Work on this book began in 2021 not long after the Nursing Now campaign ended. Nursing Now was an inspiration to me because it showed the power of nurses, who were connected across the world, to get the attention of both their governments and global institutions. It was inspiring to see nurses take part in international press conferences, to attract their Ministers of Health to Nursing Now launches and to speak at high-level meetings. The global pandemic propelled nurses into the spotlight in ways previously unimaginable and it demonstrated one reason why all of us need to be globally aware: there is much that crosses borders in our connected world, from people to goods to new programmes to microbes. Like it or not, we are a connected world in many ways – some good and some more of a challenge. This book sets out to show the landscape of globalisation that is especially relevant to nurses.

Looking back on those days from 2023 it is so apparent that the world moves quickly. In most countries, the coronavirus is almost forgotten and we are now more preoccupied with climate-related global disasters, such as wildfires and floods. There is an ongoing war in Ukraine and coups in West Africa. There are people displaced by all of these disasters in every region of the world, needing food, shelter and safety. It is now apparent that effects of the war in Ukraine have consequences that impact us globally, with rising oil prices, interruptions in the food chain and redeployment of funds from several countries to assist the war effort for Ukraine. Because of our technological sophistication and availability we can monitor what is happening on a daily basis on social media and old-fashioned television.

In nursing we continue to count the cost of the pandemic knowing that many of our colleagues died and others have succumbed to the stress they experienced, choosing to leave the profession and leaving the world with a global shortage of nurses. Migration is a commonplace now: in 2020 an estimated 281 million people lived in a country other than their country of birth, three times more than the estimated number in 1970. Now, one in 30 people in this world is a migrant (International Organization for Migration 2022).

This all seems like a challenging picture, but there are benefits to our global connectedness too. For example, we can share research and innovations, and this can bring disease prevention, treatments and cures to places where it might have taken years to reach only 10 years ago. Think of the rate at which the COVID-19 vaccines were developed and shared. We are now so much more aware of the need for cultural sensitivity and support for people who are different from us – surely a route to greater humanity for all of us. We have the potential to share wealth, but as you will see as you work through the book, this remains a potential and not a reality. Poverty remains the biggest underlying cause of disease and death in our world.

The book will take you on a journey, looking first at the big picture of global health: the Sustainable Development Goals are unpicked in Chapter 1, and then planetary health, with the effects of climate change and so much more, takes the stage in Chapter 2. Globalisation, economics and power are defined and discussed in Chapter 3, addressing issues of poverty and ways countries share knowledge and wealth. These first three chapters are the background to all of the other chapters, which provide us with the details of this landscape. Chapter 4 deals with the nurse's role in responding to global emergencies, while Chapter 5 looks at the impact of the COVID-19 pandemic on nursing around the world.

In Section 2 we take a deeper look at the issues of global relevance for nurses today: decolonising nursing, the challenges of a female-dominated profession and the changing roles of nursing. Section 3 shows ways in which the nursing voice has been raised and heard, through advocacy, leadership, the Nursing Now campaign and through global migration. In the final chapter we look to the future: what will the role of the nurse be in 10 years? And what about 50 years? This is a chapter of aspiration and I hope you might be inspired to write your own description of nurses of the future. The International Council of Nurses took the lead in creating this final chapter, which is appropriate as they have been, and continue to be, the internationally influential body for nurses everywhere. You will find their work much referenced in this book, including their *Caring for Courage* films which show so well the breadth and depth of nurses' work around the globe. I urge you to look at these films; you will be moved.

All of these chapters present best evidence but none of them can be conclusive. The world is changing rapidly and, to keep up, nursing must become adaptable and responsive. In editing this book in 2023 I have been amazed by the developments in nursing practice and research, and also by the pressure that global events put on nurses everywhere. Yet a look at Chapter 4 shows that throughout history nurses have responded to global emergencies and succeeded in continually developing the profession through what has been learned.

Throughout the book you will find Think Boxes. These can be used in a group or just to stimulate you to think further on the subject. There are extensive reference lists that can be used to help you find more information.

I have worked with a stellar team of authors to create this book – experts in their fields – and my profound thanks goes to all of them. We hope that you will find the book a valuable asset in learning about global health, that it will be well thumbed and that it will lead you to a greater understanding of the world we inhabit and care for.

In 2011 – more than a decade ago Ban Ki Moon, the then Secretary-General of the United Nations (UN), said this in his address to the UN Assembly:

> 'Saving our planet, lifting people out of poverty, advancing economic growth… these are one and the same fight. We must connect the dots between climate change, water scarcity, energy shortages, global health, food security and women's empowerment. Solutions to one problem must be solutions for all.'

I hope that this book will be a start for nurses to 'connect the dots' to see more clearly what our responsibilities are in finding solutions to the challenges to healthy flourishing in our world. Together, we *can* nurse the world to health.

Barbara Stilwell
September 2023

REFERENCE

International Organisation for Migration. (2022). *World Migration Report*. Online. https://worldmigrationreport.iom.int/wmr-2022-interactive/.

ABOUT THE EDITOR

Barbara Stilwell is a nurse, health visitor and primary care Family Nurse Practitioner with a decades-long interest in public health and in supporting health worker performance through a range of education and practice initiatives. She has worked for the World Health Organization and for non-profit organizations as a technical specialist in workforce development and education, and has lived in Switzerland, the United States, as well as countries in sub-Saharan Africa and the Eastern Mediterranean.

Barbara returned to the UK in 2018 to lead the global advocacy campaign Nursing Now from 2018, through the challenges of the pandemic, until it ended in 2021. She is now working as a consultant on a global research and implementation project on nurse leadership. In the UK, Barbara Stilwell is best known for introducing the nurse practitioner programme and role. She is a Fellow of the Royal College of Nursing, The Queens Nursing Institute and of the American Academy of Nursing.

CONTRIBUTORS

RADHA ADHIKARI, PhD, MSc, RN
Lecturer
School of Health and Life Science
University of the West of Scotland
Lanarkshire, United Kingdom

GILLIAN ADYNSKI, PhD, MHS, RN
Clinical Associate
School of Nursing
Duke University
Durham, NC, United States

THOMAS D. ÁLVAREZ, MS
Global Affairs Manager
CGFNS International, Inc.
Philadelphia, PA, United States

HOWARD CATTON, RN, MA, BS(ECON) (HONS)
Chief Executive Officer
International Council of Nurses

LYDIA DAVIDSON, PhD(CAND), MSc, RN
Clinical Research Fellow
London School of Hygiene and Tropical Medicine
London, United Kingdom

MARION ECKERT, PhD, MPH, MNS, GRADDIPLCARDNURS, DIPSC(NURSING)
Director
Professor of Health Innovation and Enterprise
Rosemary Bryant AO Research Centre
Clinical & Health Sciences
University of South Australia
Adelaide, South Australia, Australia

PANDORA HARDTMAN, DNP, CNM, RN, FACNM, FAAN
Chief Nursing and Midwifery Officer
Technical Leadership & Innovations Office Jhpiego
Baltimore, Maryland, United States

AISHA HOLLOWAY, BSc(HONS) NURSING, RGN, PhD, PGCHE, FHEA, FNMRCSI AD EUNDEM
Chair of Nursing Studies
Nursing Studies, School of Health in Social Science
The University of Edinburgh

ZIPPORAH IREGI
Registered nurse
Nursing Challenge champion and Youth champion
Africa CDC

CHERYL JONES, PhD, RN, FAAN
Interim Associate Dean for PhD and Postdoctoral
    Programs
Department of Nursing
University of North Carolina at Chapel Hill
Chapel Hill, NC, United States;
Director
Hillman Scholars Program in Nursing Innovation
Department of Nursing
UNC-Chapel Hill
Chapel Hill, NC, United States

SALLY KENDALL, MBE, PhD, RN, RHV, FQNI, FIHV, MFPH
Professor of Community Nursing and Public Health
Centre for Health Services Studies
University of Kent
Canterbury, CT2 7NZ, UK;
Adjunct Professor
Ngangk Yira Institute for Change
Murdoch University
Perth, WA

JUDY N. KHANYOLA, RN, MSC, DNP(CAND)
Chair, Center for Nursing and Midwifery
University of Global Health Equity
Kigali, Rwanda

TERESA LEWIS, PHD, M.E.C.M., POSTGRADDIPMID, RN
Sessional Academic
School of Health
UniSC
Sippy Downs, Queensland, Australia;
Sustainability Consultant
Sustainable Systems Proficiency Management
Noosaville, Queensland, Australia

ELIZABETH MADIGAN, PHD, RN, FAAN
CEO
Executive Services
Sigma Theta Tau International Honor Society of
  Nursing
Indianapolis, IN, United States

DIANA J. MASON, PHD, RN, FAAN
Senior Policy Service Professor
Center for Health Policy and Media Engagement
George Washington University School of Nursing
Washington, DC, United States;
Programme Director
Global Nursing Leadership Institute
International Council of Nurses
Geneva, Switzerland

EMILY MCWHIRTER, PHD, BSC(HONS), RN
Consultant
Hove, East Sussex
United Kingdom

CONSTANCE NEWMAN, MSW, MPH
Adjunct Associate Professor
Department of Maternal and Child Health
UNC Gillings School of Global Public Health
University of North Carolina at Chapel Hill
Chapel Hill, NC, United States

RUTH OSHIKANLU, BSC(HONS), PGDIP, PGDIP, MSC, REGISTERED NURSE, REGISTERED MIDWIFE, REGISTERED SPECIALIST COMMUNITY PUBLIC HEALTH NURSE – HEALTH VISITING, QUEEN'S NURSE, FIHV, FRCN, FAAN, FFNMRCSI, FRSPH
Independent Midwife and Health Visitor
Goal Mind
London, United Kingdom;
Director
Abule CIC
London, United Kingdom

TEDDIE POTTER, PHD, RN, FAAN, FNAP
Director of Planetary Health
Clinical Professor
School of Nursing
University of Minnesota
Minneapolis, MN, United States

IMOGEN RAMSEY, PHD, MPSYCH, BPSYCH(HONS), DIPLANG
Research Fellow
Rosemary Bryant AO Research Centre
Clinical & Health Sciences
University of South Australia
Adelaide, South Australia, Australia

JANET RODEN, BA(MACQ), MA(MACQ), PHD(UWS), RN, RM, FACN
Adjunct Appointment Senior Lecturer
School of Nursing & Midwifery
College of Health, Medicine & Wellbeing
University of Newcastle
New South Wales, Australia

WILLIAM ROSA, PHD, MBE, APRN, FAANP, FAAN
Assistant Attending Behavioral Scientist
Department of Psychiatry and Behavioral Sciences
Memorial Sloan Kettering Cancer Center
New York, NY, United States

FRANKLIN A. SHAFFER, EdD, RN, FAAN, FFNMRCSI
Advisor
Global Health Workforce
Philadelphia, PA, United States

GREG SHARPLIN, MSc(Epi), MPSYCH(Org&HF), BHSc(Hons), Bsc
Research and Strategy Manager
Senior Research Fellow
Rosemary Bryant AO Research Centre
Clinical & Health Sciences
University of South Australia
Adelaide, South Australia, Australia

PAM SMITH, PhD, MSc, BNurs, RN
Professor Emerita
Nursing Studies
University of Edinburgh
Edinburgh, Mid Lothian, United Kingdom

BARBARA STILWELL, PhD, MSoc, Sci, Bsc, RN, RHV, FRCN
Consultant
Global Health Systems
Paddock Wood, United Kingdom

GRETA WESTWOOD, CBE, PhD, MSc, RN
Professor
Florence Nightingale Foundation
London, United Kingdom

MARCUS WOOTTON, RN, MSc, PGCE, Bsc(Hons), BN(Hons), DTN
Senior Lecturer
Childrens Nursing
London Southbank University
London, United Kingdom

Section 1

SETTING THE SCENE. NURSES AND THE CURRENT GLOBAL CONTEXT

SECTION OUTLINE

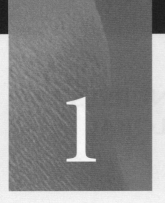

1

GLOBAL HEALTH GOALS: NURSING IN A RAPIDLY CHANGING WORLD

WILLIAM ROSA ■ DIANA J. MASON

INTRODUCTION

The world is confronting several urgent issues that require a renewed approach to nursing practice, scholarship, education and leadership (World Health Organization [WHO], 2021a). Among these pressing concerns are the evolving COVID-19 pandemic, an amplified social discourse on eradicating racism and other structural inequities, the climate crisis, poverty, food and housing insecurity, substance use disorders, a severe shortage of health care workers and substantive gaps in access to health care (United Nations [UN], 2021; UN Office on Drugs and Crime, 2019). The nurse of the future will need to understand these challenges in the context of their local roles and be able to identify and lead opportunities to make long-term, positive improvements to both individual and public health, in alignment with their professional responsibilities.

The idea of bedside nursing as an individual-level relationship confined to the point-of-care interaction is a notion of the past. The complex burden of health needs demands a holistic approach to sufficiently integrate the social and political determinants of health that directly predict nursing-related outcomes and the public's well-being (National Academies of Sciences, Engineering, and Medicine [NASEM], 2021a; Rosa et al., 2021c). Nurses in this new era of need must understand that when they care for a patient, they are caring for a family, a community and an entire social network that they might know little about—and that these contexts, in turn, affect the individual for whom the nurse is caring. Nurses must leverage their holistic, biopsychosocial training and education to inform nurse-driven innovation and foster nurse-led

academic-practice partnerships that will reduce duplicative efforts and advance the profession while improving health (All-Party Parliamentary Group [APPG], 2016; Crisp et al., 2018).

Global solidarity across settings and nations is needed now more than ever. Nurses—accounting for 59% of the health workforce globally—have a major part to play in service delivery, education, research and policy and advocacy arenas (World Health Organization [WHO], 2020). Nurses can no longer afford to adopt myopic views of their practice or define *nursing* in limited ways. Nursing, in its highest form, must include both a commitment to addressing local health needs and an awareness of global health priorities. In other words, a 21st-century future-facing nursing agenda must entail action-oriented items focused on local strategies with a global mindset (Rosa et al., 2019, 2021b).

COVID-19 has thoroughly unveiled the interdependence of humanity. Nurses will have to fully realise their potential across all practice domains to effectively ensure human dignity, health, well-being and environmental security and to alleviate suffering (International Council of Nurses [ICN], 2021a). The purpose of this chapter is to (1) understand the connection between local and global nursing and health actions; (2) identify the Sustainable Development Goals (SDGs) as a foundational blueprint to guide and connect nursing; (3) discuss the social determinants of health (SDOH) as a nursing directive to achieve health equity and (4) support readers in creating an action plan to link their local efforts with global multidisciplinary efforts to achieve high-quality universal health coverage (UHC). Working in isolation and in professional silos will prevent nurses from realising the highest possibilities of their contributions and careers. A key first step is to deepen an appreciation for the countless bridges between local and global nursing—a change in perspective that can transform the very nature of nursing practice.

THE LOCAL TO GLOBAL LANDSCAPE

Local is global and global is local. This is the mantra that nurses must embrace to understand their potential impact on the world around them. There is no 'us' and 'them'; there is only one global village—one community—one interconnected civilisation. Such an approach requires taking a global stance.

Rosa and Upvall (2019a, pp. 601–602) wrote:

There is power in taking a global stance in the challenges that face us as a profession, a people, a human race, and an international community of concerned citizens. Such power is created when we find solidarity in our goals and purpose and heal the fragmentation endemic to nursing and healthcare worldwide… A global stance assists nurses to find the global relevance in local issues and, conversely, to ensure global priorities are tended to at local levels… This global stance drives us to… [view] health as a human right, delivery of health as an equitable service, promotion of health as a global action item, and the experience of health as a social justice issue. It requires the dexterity to view the concept of 'health' through the lens of those we serve, and the flexibility and willingness to accommodate others' needs in a manner that is relevant and sustainable for them. The willingness to embrace a global stance on health is influenced by a host of questions that must be taken into consideration: what is needed, who is involved, when do we move forward, why is it important, where do we start, and how do we engage?… Ultimately, a global stance offers a rationale for nursing in a globalized world…

As nurses strive to adopt a global stance in their local work, clear definitions can help to identify the tenets and values inherent to global efforts. The Global Advisory Panel on the Future of Nursing and

THINK BOX 1.1

Reflect on the following questions using a video or written journal. Alternatively, use these questions to guide a discussion with colleagues or in a class. Consider how these questions relate to both your personal views and professional roles.

- Do I consider local health challenges through a global lens? Why or why not?
- Am I able to empathise with the patients, families and communities I serve and deliver care based on their unique needs, values and preferences?
- What are the barriers I anticipate in adopting a global stance in local efforts?
- How would taking a global stance inform and enhance my work as a nurse at a local level?
- In what ways would local- and/or system-level approaches to nursing care change if I were able to integrate a global stance into my work?

Midwifery (GAPFON) of Sigma Theta Tau International Honor Society of Nursing completed a comprehensive review of the definitions of *global health* and *global nursing* and synthesised major concepts to support nursing (Wilson et al., 2016; see Box 1.1). Concepts that arise in both definitions include collaboration, determinants of health, equity, population health and planetary health.

The major environmental changes, health threats and ecosystem impairment happening around the world call nurses everywhere to include planetary thinking into theory and knowledge development, educational frameworks and practice changes (Potter, 2021; Rosa, 2017a, 2020; Rosa & Upvall, 2019b; Schenk et al., 2021b). *Planetary health* refers to 'the health of human civilization and the state of the natural systems on which it depends' (Whitmee et al., 2015, p. 1978). A framework to guide planetary heath education (Guzmán et al., 2021) includes five interactive domains within the context of local learning priorities; local socioeconomic, cultural, and environmental conditions; global agenda and priorities and anthropogenic changes at a planetary scale (see Box 1.2). A collaborative and transdisciplinary commitment to 'One Health'—optimal health for people, planet, animals and ecosystems—in practice and policy and from local to global is, ultimately, what is needed to ensure future

BOX 1.1
DEFINITIONS OF 'GLOBAL HEALTH' AND 'GLOBAL NURSING' (WILSON ET AL., 2016, P. 1536).

Global Health

"...an area of practice, study, and research that places a priority on improving health, achieving equity in health for all people (Koplan et al., 2009) and ensuring health-promoting and sustainable sociocultural, political and economic systems (Janes & Corbett, 2009). Global health implies planetary health which equals human, animal, environmental and eco-system health (Kahn et al., 2014), and it emphasises trans-national health issues, determinants and solutions; involves many disciplines within and beyond the health sciences and promotes interdependence and interdisciplinary collabora-tion, and it is a synthesis of population-based prevention with individual holistic care"

(Koplan et al., 2009).

Global Nursing

"...the use of evidence-based nursing process to promote sustainable planetary health and equity for all people (Grootjans & Newman, 2013). Global nursing consid-ers SDOH, includes individual- and population-level care, research, education, leadership, advocacy and policy initia-tives (Upvall & Jeffers, 2014). Global nurses engage in ethical practice and demonstrate respect for human dignity, human rights and cultural diversity (Baumann, 2013). Global nurses engage in a spirit of deliberation and reflection in interdependent partnership with communities and other health care providers"

(Upvall & Jeffers, 2014).

BOX 1.2
PLANETARY EDUCATION FRAMEWORK DOMAINS WITH BRIEF DESCRIPTIONS (ADAPTED FROM GUZMÁN ET AL., 2021)

1. Interconnection with nature: fostering an approach that merges the cognitive (sense of connection), affective (caring component) and behavioural (com-mitment to act), as well as all ways of knowing (e.g., Indigenous, Western education/practice, diverse spir-itual traditions)
2. The Anthropocene and health: adopting a social and ecological approach to health promotion and disease prevention and control, including attention to indi-vidual- and population-level health factors of human, animal and ecosystem health
3. Systems thinking and complexity: cultivating a systems-based understanding that includes complex adaptive systems (e.g., tipping or leverage points, non-linear causal relationships) and acknowledges learner bias and worldview
4. Equity and justice: eradicating systemic disparities that cause some populations to disproportionately shoulder the burdens of environmental and health impacts while others thrive; rebuilding institutions that promote and perpetuate inequities and inform planetary living conditions
5. Movement building and systems change: developing inclusive relationships, thoughtful strategies, effective communication and transformational partnerships to reduce apathy, increase engagement and create much-needed momentum for change at a planetary level

survival (Leuddekke, 2016; World Health Organiza-tion [WHO], 2021b). Nurses can and should be at the forefront of this movement.

THE 17 SUSTAINABLE DEVELOPMENT GOALS

The United Nations (UN) 2030 Sustainable Develop-ment Agenda represents the boldest humanitarian and health agenda of our time and is comprised of 17 SDGs and 169 targets (United Nations [UN], 2016; see Fig. 1.1). The 17 SDGs aim to leave no one behind and build a safe, inclusive world and planet while erad-icating poverty and improving the lives of all people everywhere. Five major themes drive the SDGs: peo-ple, planet, peace, prosperity and partnership.

The SDGs were unanimously adopted by all UN member states in September 2015 and went into effect on January 1, 2016. The 2030 agenda grew out of the eight Millennium Development Goals (2000–2015) and member state discussions at the 2012 UN Conference on Sustainable Development in Rio de Janeiro (United Nations [UN], 2012). The SDGs are not legally binding for member states, and each is responsible for enacting policy and system changes that help to achieve targets at local and national levels, as well as at the global level, in partnership with other international stakeholders.

Two of the goals—SDG 3 (good health and well-being) and SDG 17 (partnerships for the goals)—serve as the main anchors of the overall 2030 agenda and are intimately connected to the success and status of all the others. Take SDG 3, for instance. All of the other goals

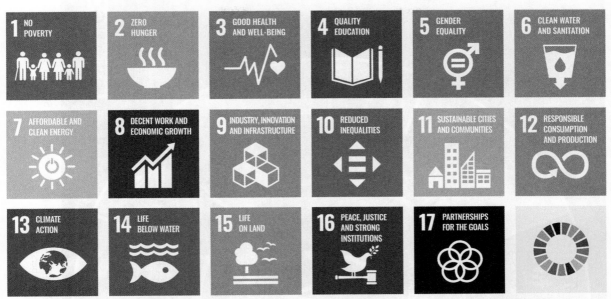

Fig. 1.1 ■ The 17 Sustainable Development Goals. Reprinted from the United Nations (UN). (n.d.). *Sustainable Development Goals communications materials.* https://www.un.org/sustainabledevelopment/news/communications-material/. (Retrieved on February 21, 2024.)

can be related to health issues, and over 50 SDG indicators measure health-related outcomes (World Health Organization [WHO], 2021c; see Fig. 1.2). Partnerships are the heart and soul of the SDGs. Whether directed at improvement of the economy, society or the biosphere, partnerships within and between nations, disciplines, sectors and communities are key to realising the SDGs (Upvall & Leffers, 2017; see Fig. 1.3).

THINK BOX 1.2

What local professional partnerships are key to success in your work? How do you maintain those partnerships? How do you identify stakeholders who are significant to your work?

Thinking about nursing globally, what partnerships would add strength to nursing interventions to achieve the SDGs?

There is more on partnerships later in this chapter and in Chapter 10.

The nursing profession plays a critical role in attainment of each of the 17 SDGs (Fields et al., 2021; Rosa, 2017b; Rosa & Iro, 2019; Squires et al., 2019). Nursing has a long history of leadership in UN initiatives and global health mandates that preempted the SDGs (Beck, 2017). Central to nursing involvement in the SDGs is the understanding that no single nurse or single organisation is responsible for achieving all 169 targets of the 17 SDGs. There is no need for heroics. Rather, it is incumbent upon each nurse and organisation to identify which targets are within the purview of local efforts and responsibilities and which can be improved upon at the local level, whether in acute, community-based, long-term care or environmental health settings (Dossey et al., 2019).

Scholars have articulated how nurses can integrate the SDGs throughout various domains of practice. For instance, nurse educators can adopt clinical and pedagogical approaches for implementing SDG content into already established nursing curricula by knowing

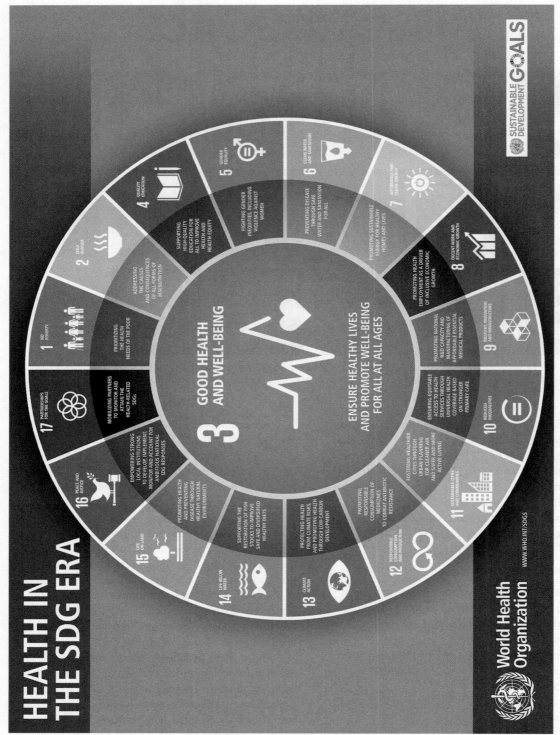

Fig. 1.2 ■ Health in the SDG era. Reprinted from World Health Organization (WHO). (n.d.). Health in the SDG era. Retrieved on February 21, 2024, from https://actionsdg.ctb.ku.edu/network-members/who/.

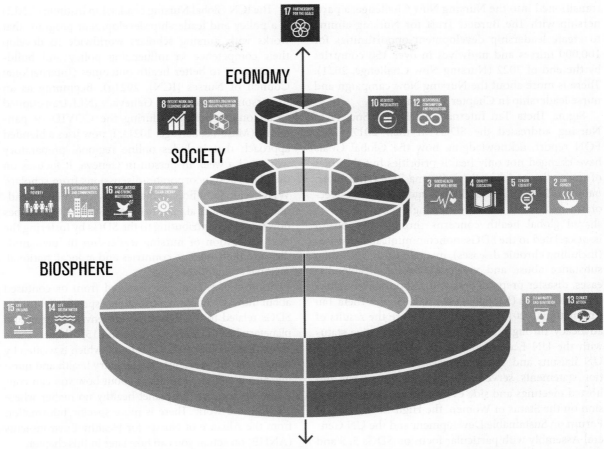

Fig. 1.3 ■ Partnerships: central to the SDGs. Reprinted from Stockholm Resilience Centre. (n.d.). *Partnerships are central to the SDGs*. https://www.stockholmresilience.org/images/18.36c25848153d54bdba33ec9b/1465905797608/sdgs-food-azote.jpg. (Retrieved on February 21, 2024.)

(understanding) the role of the SDGs in nursing, valuing (attitude) the SDGs in relation to nursing documents at the institutional level and taking action to promote necessary curricular adaptation (McKinnon & Fitzpatrick, 2017; Upvall & Luzincourt, 2019). Nurses in research must emphasise research capacity-building efforts that include the SDGs and foster the creation of new knowledge in the field. For example, all nurse leaders must strive to create consumers of research, develop language skills for nurses to become active in current academic initiatives, integrate research training into all professional development activities and promote sustained and mutually beneficial educational and research partnerships (Squires,

2019; Squires et al., 2017). In the policy realm, both micro- and macrolevel support is needed to advance the SDGs. Both the individual will of nurses and the collaborative efforts of professional organisations are needed to build momentum and achieve SDG targets (Miyamoto & Cook, 2019).

Multiple organisations have addressed the SDGs in nursing initiatives. Three SDGs—3, 5 and 8—formed the basis of the All-Party Parliamentary Group (APPG, 2016) report that called for leveraging the nursing workforce to achieve good health, gender equality and strong economies. That report created the theoretical and policy premises for the 2016–20 Nursing Now campaign (Holloway et al., 2021), which has now transitioned into the Nursing Now Challenge, a partnership with The Burdett Trust for Nursing aiming to create leadership development opportunities for 100,000 nurses and midwives in over 150 countries by the end of 2022 (Nursing Now Challenge, 2021). There is more about the Nursing Now campaign and nurse leadership in Chapter 10 of this book.

Sigma Theta Tau International Honor Society of Nursing addressed the SDGs in their 2017 GAPFON report, acknowledging how the Global Goals have changed not only health priorities but the roles of nurses in attaining them (Sigma Theta Tau International, 2017). The GAPFON model provides recommendations to advance nursing's contributions to shared global health concerns through five health issues related to the SDGs: noncommunicable diseases (including chronic diseases), mental health (including substance abuse and violence), communicable diseases, disaster preparedness and response and maternal-child health (Klopper et al., 2020; Sigma Theta Tau International, 2017). Other efforts were the results of advocacy through Sigma's special consultative status with the UN Economic and Social Council. Sigma's UN liaisons and youth representatives offered position statements, served as subject matter experts and hosted meetings and side events during the Commission on the Status of Women, the High-Level Political Forum on Sustainable Development and the UN General Assembly with particular focus on SDGs 5, 8 and 17 (Sensor et al., 2021).

The International Council of Nurses (ICN) has been a powerful organisational advocate for nursing's role in SDG attainment, dedicating their 2017 International Nurses Day theme as *Nurses: A Voice to Lead—Achieving the SDGs* (International Council of Nurses [ICN], 2017). Every International Nurse Day report since has focused on aspects of the SDGs, including attaining health as a human right and expanding nursing services to achieve high-quality UHC (International Council of Nurses [ICN], 2021b). The ICN's consistent participation in global policy forums to advocate on behalf of nurses' safety and well-being, particularly during the COVID-19 pandemic, has included a focus on strengthening the workforce and continuing to incorporate the SDGs into systems planning (International Council of Nurses [ICN], 2021c, 2021d, 2021e, 2021f).

The ICN Global Nursing Leadership Institute (GNLI) is a policy and leadership development program that works with nursing scholars worldwide to develop their competence in influencing policy and building capacity to better health outcomes (International Council of Nurses [ICN], 2021g). Beginning as an in-person experience in Geneva, GNLI transitioned to an online program during the COVID-19 pandemic (Mason & Salvage, 2021). It now uses a blended approach that includes online regional preparatory work and a week in person in Geneva. It focuses on the SDGs and incorporates discussions from scholars' WHO regional offices and a site visit to WHO headquarters (Rosa et al., 2021a). Case Study 1.1 describes how GNLI is contributing to the SDGs by fostering the next generation of nursing leadership in low-, middle- and high-income countries and at local, national, regional and global levels.

Some nurses may feel detached from or confused about how to make contributions specifically to the SDGs related to the biosphere and environmental and planetary health (SDGs 6, 13, 14 and 15). There is more about this in Chapter 2 of this book, which is written by nurses who are specialists in planetary health and nursing, and it will give you ideas about how you can contribute to keeping our planet healthy no matter where you live and work. There is more specific information from the Alliance of Nurses for Healthy Environments (ANHE) on action you can take later in this chapter.

When looking at the welfare of communities (SDG 11), it is vital to remember that health is prevented, created and/or sustained at the intersection of various social, environmental and political factors (e.g., COVID-19, systemic racism, climate change [Schenk et al., 2021b]). Organisations such as the ANHE have been spearheading efforts related to their mission since 2008: promoting health people and healthy environments by educating and leading the nursing profession, advancing research, incorporating evidence-based practice and influencing policy (Alliance of Nurses for Healthy Environments [ANHE], 2021a). Voluntary surveys, such as the Climate, Health, and Nursing Tool (CHANT), can help nurses evaluate how their climate awareness, perceptions and behaviours are evolving over time (Schenk et al., 2019; Schenk et al., 2021a). Case Study 1.2 describes several ANHE efforts that are creating a professional, social and global movement to

CASE STUDY 1.1
The Global Nursing Leadership Institute and the Sustainable Development Goals

The GNLI collaborates with nurse leaders to shape, develop, support and drive evidence-based health and social policy through skill development in stakeholder and political environment analyses; advocacy; stakeholder engagement and coalition building; framing the evidence base in various political, health and social contexts; communicating clear policy messages to appeal to decision-makers and the public and networking with regional and global nursing leaders in the policy realm. The COVID-19 pandemic posed barriers to conducting the program in person as had been the norm in the past. Despite challenges during the virtual platform transition, cross-regional participant connections were maintained through GNLI learning experiences. Preliminary evaluations of the online program support predominantly positive experiences of participants. GNLI is now a blended online and in-person program.

While considering the implications of the pandemic and the increased global discourse on health and social inequities, the SDGs provide the premise for GNLI Scholar projects as an expected outcome of the program. In the Pan American Health Organization (PAHO)/World Health Organization (WHO) region, the 2022 scholars focused their regional project on SDGs 3 (ensure healthy lives), 4 (quality education), and three other goals. Their project uses Brazil as a case study in understanding the barriers and facilitators to investing in nursing in South America. Scholars interviewed key informants and are conducting a thematic analysis of key factors and opportunities for such investments.

Case study is an adapted composite from the following references: ICN (2021g), Mason & Salvage (2021) and Rosa et al. (2021b).

take action on the environment-related SDGs through holistic and determined nursing efforts.

Importantly, integrating the SDGs into local efforts does not need to add to workload or burden. Conversely, consistently reflecting on the SDGs assists nurses in understanding how they are connecting to global initiatives within the scope of their current role, regardless of setting. This is an iterative process that ultimately expands the impact of nursing practice and increases the potential for making positive change. The journey connects each nurse to a global nursing community and multisector changemakers who are seeking to improve the health and life experiences of communities worldwide.

THE DETERMINANTS OF HEALTH

The 17 SDGs all recognise the myriad social, environmental and political determinants of health. The SDOH have become a significant focus in nursing policy and practice. According to the World Health Organization (WHO, 2021d), the SDOH are 'the non-medical factors that influence health outcomes. They are the conditions in which people are born, grow, work, live, and

THINK BOX 1.3

Consider how your everyday nursing practice contributes to improving the health and welfare of humanity and the planet in your local context and globally.

Does your answer show clear local to global implications? Could you be missing an opportunity to optimise your nursing practice? Do you think of your career as having global relevance?

age, and the wider set of forces and systems shaping the conditions of daily life... [including] economic policies and systems, development agendas, social norms, social policies, and political systems'. They can be positive or negative influences on health. Examples of the SDOH that impact health equity include income and social protection, education, unemployment and job security, food insecurity, housing, structural conflict, social inclusion and access to health and social care, among others (World Health Organization [WHO], 2021d).

SDOH are community-level factors that affect health, but they are expressed as 'social needs' in individual

CASE STUDY 1.2

Alliance of Nurses for Healthy Environments and the Sustainable Development Goals

A collaboration between ANHE and Project Drawdown, *Nurses Drawdown*, calls nurses from all specialties and practice settings to take action in key areas to directly mitigate the climate crisis. These areas include energy (supporting clean energy and advocating transitions to clean energy), food (commit to a plant-based diet, use of clean cookstoves, reduced food waste), mobility (bike infrastructure, walkable cities, mass transit), gender equity (educating girls, family planning) and nature-based solutions (planting trees, protecting forests and rainforests). The ANHE developed the Environmental Health Nurse Fellowship to train nurses to work with communities in addressing serious environmental health threats (e.g., toxic chemical pollution, water contamination, climate disruption). The fellowship pairs participants with expert environmental health nurse mentors to develop a project in their communities, support community-driven solutions and educate

health professionals and colleagues about environmental health issues and responses. In an effort to centre antiracism and health equity efforts while advancing leadership in environmental health initiatives, ANHE launched the Health Equity and Anti-Racism (HEAR) Leadership Institute. The goal of HEAR is to support participants to lead efforts that support environmental health and nursing practice outcomes that are beneficial to Black and Indigenous people and other people of colour. In partnership with Health Care Without Harm, ANHE coleads the Nurses Climate Challenge to educate health professionals about climate change, with a goal of educating 50,000 health professionals by 2022. The ANHE is developing a Global Nurse Action Agenda for Climate Justice to increase international collaboration and partnerships with nursing organisations to promote climate justice research, practice, and pedagogy.

Case study is an adapted composite from the following references: Alliance of Nurses for Healthy Environments (ANHE) (2021b), (2021c) and (2021d); Health Care Without Harm (2021); Nurses Drawdown (2021) and Schenk et al. (2021b).

---

patients (Castrucci & Auerbach, 2019). For example, housing is an SDOH within a community. The patient who has no home and is living on the streets presents with a social need for stable, safe housing. The nurse who is caring for this patient must consider this need when planning for discharge. Where will the discharged patient with a surgical wound be able to manage clean wound management if they don't have adequate housing? But addressing the individual patient's social need will not address the community-level SDOH. When the nurse sees a pattern of unhoused patients, the social need becomes an SDOH that the hospital, government, insurance company and others should address to improve the health of individuals and the community as a whole. And when one considers the rise in homelessness after natural disasters associated with climate change, the connection to the SDGs on a global scale becomes evident.

The National Academies of Sciences, Engineering, and Medicine (National Academies of Sciences,

Engineering, and Medicine [NASEM], 2021a) 'Future of Nursing 2020-2030' report emphasises the need for all nurses in all settings to directly address the SDOH in the journey toward health equity. In addition, a consensus paper from five expert panels of the American Academy of Nursing developed a conceptual framework grounded in evidence and health policy to clarify the meaning of SDOH for nurses across six key dimensions—economic stability, education access and quality, health care access and quality, neighbourhood and the built environment, social and community context and planetary conditions (Kuehnert et al., 2021). An international team of researchers and nurse leaders sponsored by the World Innovation Summit for Health (WISH) released a global policy report in 2021 entitled 'Nurses for Health Equity: Guidelines for Tackling the Social Determinants of Health' (Rosa et al., 2021c). With over 70 clinician-, national- and international-level guidelines across six domains of practice and expert input from nursing leaders worldwide, the

	TABLE 1.1		
	A Summary of Guidelines for Tackling the Social Determinants of Health		
Domain of Practice	**International Organisation-/ Association-Level Guidelines**	**National Organisation-/ Association-Level Guidelines**	**Nurse-Level Guidelines**
1. Understanding the issue and what to do about it: education and training	Cocreate a strategic nursing position statement on health equity led by the ICN.	Support curricular objectives that reflect health equity, social justice and structural inequalities as a core nursing focus.	Teach students to critically apply health equity concepts and evidence social determinants in care plans.
2. Building the evidence: monitoring and evaluation	Promote advanced health informatics knowledge and skills training for nursing supported by the WHO and ICN.	Call for access to national-level health and socioeconomic data to conduct health inequality monitoring at all levels.	Promote community coalitions to develop health equity interventions and translate evidence to improve policies and health outcomes.
3. The clinical setting: working with individuals and communities	Promote person-/community-centred care as a fundamental component of nursing to ensure informed action on the social determinants.	Call for local and national policymakers to allocate financial and clinical resources needed to decrease health inequalities.	Address explicit and implicit bias, prejudice and acts of discrimination within the profession and in the clinical setting.
4. Health care organisations as employers, managers and commissioners	Advocate to governments and professional associations for high-quality, safe and decent work conditions that support nurses' well-being.	Diversify the workforce by creating opportunities for training and employment for nurse candidates from historically disadvantaged and underrepresented backgrounds.	Cocreate budgets and initiatives while considering health equity and social status of the population being served and ensuring expert guidance from diverse groups.
5. Working in partnership: within the health sector and beyond	Drive globally for a 'health in all policies' approach that always includes and involves nurses as key stakeholders.	Include nurses in cocreating and commissioning services addressing the social determinants beyond information sharing to outcome-focused, measurable improvements.	Collect and collate community profiling and health needs assessment data to influence approaches to care and health promotion at individual and population levels.
6. Nurses as advocates	Collaborate with national nursing associations to advocate for strategic action on the social determinants globally.	Call for policy change to address the social determinants.	Use strong evidence to educate individuals, communities, partners and policy makers about why the social determinants matter.

Adapted from Rosa, W. E., Hannaway, C. J., McArdle, C., McManus, M. F., Alharahsheh, S. T., & Marmot, M. (2021). *Nurses for health equity: Guidelines for tackling the social determinants of health.* https://www.wish.org.qa/reports/nurses-for-health-equity/. (Retrieved on February 21, 2024).

WISH report garnered statements of support endorsing the recommendations from the WHO, the ICN, Sigma, the Commonwealth Nurses and Midwives Federation and international nongovernmental organisations such as Partners In Health and Jhpiego. Table 1.1 provides a snapshot of the guidelines across all domains of practice and at all levels of nursing and health.

Regardless of what health or social factors nurses are seeking to improve and address, it is vital that the collective nursing community is invested in recognising the moral determinants of health (Berwick, 2020). The moral determinants of health are characterised by social solidarity and the belief that individuals 'legitimately and properly can depend on each other for helping to secure the basic circumstances of healthy lives, no less than they depend legitimately on each other to secure the nation's defense' (Berwick, 2020, p. 225). Berwick (2020) goes on to suggest that if this social solidarity was the shared moral imperative, then governments—as an expression of society's moral values—would be invested to improve health with fervour through policy change and investments (e.g., acknowledgment of health as a human right, ending hunger and homelessness, demonstrating national-level commitment to reversing the climate crisis). The moral determinants of health and the accountability they inspire among nurses are in alignment with the global code of ethics for nurses to guide ethical practice and decision-making (International Council of Nurses [ICN], 2021h).

THINK BOX 1.4

If you were able to improve the critical SDOH indicators in your community or neighbourhood, what would be your priorities and why? What about the SDOH in your country? Are they the same or different? How can you track progress on SDOH in your neighbourhood and country?

THE WHO 'STATE OF THE WORLD'S NURSING' REPORT AND GLOBAL STRATEGIC DIRECTIONS

The first 'State of the World's Nursing' report in 2020 was developed in concert with the UN's Year of the Nurse and Midwife. It provided evidence, policy options and best practices for strengthening the global nursing workforce with substantive and pragmatic investments in nursing education, jobs and leadership (World Health Organization [WHO], 2020). The report uncovered the need to establish an internationally accepted minimum data set about the nursing profession with the national resources to gather the data. Nonetheless, it called for governments and other stakeholders globally to invest in a massive acceleration of nursing education, create at least 6 million new nursing jobs by 2030, primarily in low- and middle-income countries, and strengthen nursing leadership to ensure nurses' influential and active role in the health policy sphere and in decision-making to support effective health and social care systems. The report ultimately reminds nurses working in local contexts around the world that the nursing workforce requires community-based thinking and professional solidarity to realise nursing's greatest potentials. Finally, the report presented 10 key policy actions for multisector actors to consider at all levels (Box 1.3).

The WHO *Global Strategic Directions for Nursing and Midwifery 2021-2025* echo the emphasis on education, jobs and leadership and add a policy focus on service delivery (World Health Organization [WHO],

---

BOX 1.3
TEN KEY ACTIONS: FUTURE DIRECTIONS FOR NURSING WORKFORCE POLICY FROM THE WHO (2020) 'STATE OF THE WORLD'S NURSING' REPORT

1. Countries affected by shortages will need to increase funding to educate and employ at least 5.9 million additional nurses.
2. Countries should strengthen capacity for health workforce data collection, analysis and use.
3. Nurse mobility and migration must be effectively monitored and responsibly and ethically managed.
4. Nurse education and training programs must graduate nurses who drive progress in primary health care and UHC.
5. Nursing leadership and governance are critical to nursing workforce strengthening.
6. Planners and regulators should optimise the contributions of nursing practice.
7. Policymakers, employers and regulators should coordinate actions in support of decent work.
8. Countries should deliberately plan for gender-sensitive nursing workforce policies.
9. Professional nursing regulation must be modernised.
10. Collaboration (across sectors) is key.

Courtesy of the World Health Organization.

2021a). These policy priorities should be integrated into local, national and international nursing workforce planning to ensure alignment with global health agenda items and to reduce duplicative efforts across the profession (Fig. 1.4). Expressed through a health labour market lens, the *Global Strategic Directions* can guide nursing and cross-disciplinary partners to take pragmatic actions that can improve the effectiveness of health systems.

A second *State of the World's Nursing* report is to be prepared for 2025: this was announced by the WHO at the ICN's 2023 Congress. This is important news because the collection of data for the second report acts as a barometer for how far the recommendations of the *Global Strategic Directions* have successfully been implemented. Ministries of health can be held to account by nurses for their actions (or inactions). This is a significant opportunity for nurses to influence health systems' investment policies for the next 10 years.

EDUCATION

Strategic direction: Midwife and nurse graduates match or surpass health system demand and have the requisite knowledge, competencies and attitudes to meet national health priorities.

Policy priority: Align the levels of nursing and midwifery education with optimized roles within the health and academic systems.

Policy priority: Optimize the domestic production of midwives and nurses to meet or surpass health system demand.

Policy priority: Design education programmes to be competency-based, apply effective learning design, meet quality standards, and align with population health needs.

Policy priority: Ensure that faculty are properly trained in the best pedagogical methods and technologies, with demonstrated clinical expertise in content areas.

JOBS ➜

Strategic direction: Increase the availability of health workers by sustainably creating nursing and midwifery jobs, effectively recruiting and retaining midwives and nurses, and ethically managing international mobility and migration.

Policy priority: Conduct nursing and midwifery workforces planning and forecasting through a health labour market lens.

Policy priority: Ensure adequate demand (jobs) with respect to health service delivery for primary health care and other population health priorities.

Policy priority: Reinforce implementation of the WHO Global Code of Practice on the International Recruitment of Health Personnel.

Policy priority: Attract, recruit and retain midwives and nurses where they are most needed.

LEADERSHIP

Strategic direction: Increase the proportion and authority of midwives and nurses in senior health and academic positions and continually develop the next generation of nursing and midwifery leaders.

Policy priority: Establish and strengthen senior leadership positions for nursing and midwifery workforce governance and management and input into health policy.

Policy priority: Invest in leadership skills development for midwives and nurses.

SERVICE DELIVERY ➜

Strategic direction: Midwives and nurses work to the full extent of their education and training in safe and supportive service delivery environments.

Policy priority: Review and strengthen professional regulatory systems and support capacity building of regulators, where needed.

Policy priority: Adapt workplaces to enable midwives and nurses to maximally contribute to service delivery in interdisciplinary health care teams.

Fig. 1.4 ▪ Summary of Global Strategic Directions and Policy Priorities for Nursing and Midwifery 2021-2025. Reprinted from World Health Organization (WHO). (2021). *Global strategic directions for nursing and midwifery (2021-2025)*. https://www.who.int/publications/i/item/9789240033863. (Retrieved on February 21, 2024).

THINK BOX 1.5

Before you read on, jot down or discuss with colleagues what you think are the implications for nursing after what you have read in this chapter. There are no wrong or right answers—just a greater awareness of what nurses can contribute to human flourishing.

IMPLICATIONS

Nursing focuses on promoting health. But where and how is health created? An analysis of the research on multiple determinants of health by McGovern (2014) found that health care accounts for only 10%–25% of the variance in health despite many high-resource nations' high expenditures on health care. Cross-national studies have demonstrated that countries with higher spending on social needs have better health outcomes compared with countries that spend more on health care (Rubin et al., 2016). For example, the United States spends more than any other country on health care but ranks in the bottom of 17 peer countries on health outcomes (Schneider et al., 2017)—a finding associated with the fact that the United States spends only 9 cents on social services for every dollar it spends on health care, while nations with the best health outcomes spend $2 on social services for every health care dollar (Bradley et al., 2011; Rubin et al. 2016).

These findings have significant implications for the nursing profession and individual nurses. In most high-resource countries, a majority of nurses work in acute care, following the evolution of technological advances in medicine; however, low-resource nations that have emphasised public health and primary care may be using nurses more effectively to advance the health of their people. Nurses in high-resource countries can support and lead national efforts to shift resources to building healthier communities by building primary care capacity and public health efforts that address SDG 3. For example, primary care has a central role in improving the health of populations (National Academies of Sciences, Engineering, and Medicine [NASEM], 2021b). But even primary care needs to incorporate a view of health and health care that embraces people's social needs. Nurses can transform primary care in this direction by being care coordinators who address the physical, mental and social needs of patients as well as by working as primary care providers with this holistic

view (Bodenheimer & Mason, 2017). There is more on the role of nurses in driving forward primary health care in Chapter 7, along with case studies showing nurses' contribution to community health.

Acute care is an important component of health care, but even it must shift to embracing a holistic view of what affects the health of people. The cost of keeping social needs and services in a silo separate from health care is no longer viable. It is costly in terms of money, limited resources and human lives. While many hospital nurses have recognised that the patient without adequate housing is at high risk of being rehospitalised because of that social barrier to health, they have seldom had institutional support to advocate for addressing this social care need on some level. Nurses can advance their health care organisations' vision and approaches to addressing patients' social needs by raising health care administrators' and policymakers' awareness of the growing body of evidence on the financial and other costs of ignoring this reality. Indeed, one can argue that nurses have a moral imperative to do so (Mason, 2016).

The National Academies of Sciences, Engineering, and Medicine (NASEM, 2021a) 'Future of Nursing 2020-2030' report speaks to how nurses can foster health equity by addressing both the SDOH and social care needs of patients. The report replicated a model of action from a prior National Academies of Sciences, Engineering, and Medicine (NASEM, 2019) document, *Integrating Social Care into the Delivery of Health Care,* that identified five 'A's that can guide nurses' actions:

- *Awareness*—identifying patients' assets and risks, such as assessing whether a person has adequate housing or access to transportation.
- *Adjustment*—adapting a care plan to accommodate social barriers, for example, providing the patient with a wound dressing who does not require daily changes if they live in a shelter or, for someone without easy access to transportation, consolidating health care visits to multiple practitioners in 1 day instead of separate visits.
- *Assistance*—connecting the person with relevant resources, such as a housing agency or medical transport system.
- *Alignment*—health care organisations working with communities and others to address the SDOH. For example, the nurse's hospital could

invite community-based organisations, policy-makers, investors, payors and others to iden-tify opportunities for a community to provide transitional and permanent housing or develop a transportation fund for low-income people (Japsen, 2020).

■ *Advocacy*—promoting public policies that address the SDOH, such as advocating for a national or local housing policy that invests in low-income housing and housing supports or doing the same to build affordable public transportation.

This model links social needs with the SDOH and, when viewed on a global scale, with the SDGs.

THINK BOX 1.6

How would the five A's work in your practice? What are the opportunities and barriers to implementing them? What could change and who could make that happen?

On a global scale, nurses across the world can learn from each other about innovations and best practices in advocating for policies that address the SDOH, as well as paying for the integration of social care into health care delivery (Ewald et al., 2021). The ICN (International Council of Nurses [ICN], 2017) pro-vides exemplars of nurses addressing the SDGs. One is the Nurse-Family Partnership (NFP) that originated in the United States but is now established in the United Kingdom and the Netherlands. The NFP is a home vis-itation program that uses nurses to help the pregnant female develop her social support network, explore self-development options, engage in self-care, prepare for motherhood and more. Research over decades shows that it improves the short- and long-term out-comes for high-risk mothers and their newborns—and not just the usual health outcomes of maternal and infant morbidity and mortality. The program reduces child abuse, improves school performance, increases the mother's employment and economic self-suffi-ciency, reduces the child's contact with the criminal justice system as an adolescent and more. It illustrates nurses collaborating globally to adopt best practices in addressing SDGs and SDOH.

The opportunities for nurses to be involved in address-ing the SDOH and SDGs are endless, whether through

individual or collective action. 'Future of Nursing, 2020-2030' provides examples of mostly nurses in the United States who have developed approaches to promoting health equity through addressing the SDOH and social needs of patients (National Academies of Sciences, Engi-neering, and Medicine [NASEM], 2021a). These profiles range from advancing the education of people in disad-vantaged communities to improving access to healthy foods to addressing housing shortages. One exception is the profile of the work by the Royal College of Nursing (RCN) in the United Kingdom to address 'period pov-erty', the challenges that low-income girls and women face when they unable to access menstrual products and hygiene resources (Sommer & Mason, 2021). Nurses have been engaged in addressing this health disparity by advocating for the removal of taxes and charges on female hygiene products, making these products free and providing access to clean bathrooms for menstrual hygiene. But it is not just individual nurses who are addressing this issue. The RCN has taken on the issue with three aims (National Academies of Sciences, Engi-neering, and Medicine [NASEM], 2021a, p. 456):

■ Raise awareness of the problem among nurses and midwives, as well as the public.
■ Monitor the government's efforts to remove finan-cial barriers to sanitary products and end period poverty.
■ Encourage national discussion of the issue.

The RCN has been working towards these aims by engaging members in donating menstrual supplies to food banks and educating the public about this issue affects about one-fourth of the world's women and girls of reproductive age.

The UK campaign in which nurses took a prominent role has been successful. Since September 2022, the UK government has made a 'period product' scheme available to all state-maintained schools and educa-tional organisations for 16- to 19-year old females in England. It provides free period products to girls and adult females who need them in their place of study. In addition, tax on period products has been abolished. This shows the influence that nurse advocates, joining with others, can have on government policy. Imagine not being able to afford menstrual products or having no access to clean bathrooms. Then imagine if nurses worldwide collaborated on ending period poverty.

Addressing the SDOH cannot be done in isolation. It requires both cross-country collaborations among nurses and moving out of nursing's silo to partner with diverse stakeholders from the myriad sectors of any community, including the global one (Martsolf et al., 2018; National Academies of Sciences, Engineering, and Medicine [NASEM], 2021a). 'The Future of Nursing, 2020-2030' calls on nurses locally, regionally and nationally to partner with communities, community-based organisations and other stakeholders to address SDOH (National Academies of Sciences, Engineering, and Medicine [NASEM], 2021a). It is not for nurses to 'fix' communities but, rather, to determine what the community's priorities are for health care and to partner with the community to bring about the change that is wanted to promote health.

Cross-country collaborations strengthen the pressure within nations to address the SDGs and SDOH. While ICN was instrumental in leading the World Health Assembly's adoption of the WHO *Global Strategic Directions for Nursing and Midwifery*, that effort included nurses from various countries lobbying their ministers of health to support the document. The ICN Nurse Practitioner/Advanced Practice Network (International Council of Nurses [ICN], n.d.) provides a vehicle for advanced practice registered nurses to communicate about advanced practice issues and to support development of the role in countries that have not yet adopted it. There are also numerous international specialty nursing organisations, such as the International Nurses in Cancer Care and the International Society of Psychiatric-Mental Health Nurses, that can provide opportunities for individual nurses to engage in global conversations and actions around health.

The mandate for nurse educators to examine the curriculum of their schools of nursing is clear. Schools must revise the curriculum to reflect the global factors that affect health, including SDGs, along with their impact on the local level and how to influence them. Public and private sector policies are key to shaping the SDGs such that schools of nursing and continuing education programs for health professionals must incorporate policy analysis and political strategy competencies into their offerings (Mason et al., 2021). As universities and even health systems 'go global' with facilities all over the world, students and nurses should explore opportunities to study or work in another country. In addition, WHO collaborating centres (World Health Organization [WHO], 2022a) and regional offices (World Health Organization [WHO], 2022b) provide opportunities for cross-country experiences in addressing the SDGs.

CONCLUSION

'Think globally, act locally'. This adage encourages people to consider the health and well-being of the whole planet when taking local action. With the challenges of a pandemic, climate change, violent conflicts and other global issues, the phrase becomes a minimum of what global citizens must do. Today, addressing patients' social needs and a community's SDOH connects local action to the UN SDGs. But we need whole nations to adopt actions, including health-promoting policies, to ensure that the local health of individuals and communities is not undermined by global hazards and inadequacies. The SARS-CoV-2 pandemic illustrated this powerfully. In mid- to late 2021, the United States was getting booster vaccinations to its people, while other parts of the world had little or no vaccines, allowing the Omicron variant to emerge from outside of the United States and create another surge across the country that overwhelmed its health care system (Yong, 2022).

Nurses are in a key position to act locally, nationally and globally. The opportunities are endless. The United Nations and its World Health Organization have challenged all people to see the opportunities for improving the well-being of individuals, nations and the planet. 'The Future of Nursing 2020-2030' (National Academies of Sciences, Engineering, and Medicine [NASEM], 2021a) and the WHO *Global Strategic Directions for Nursing and Midwifery* (World Health Organization [WHO], 2021a) challenge nurses to lead in seizing the opportunities to address the SDGs, whether on a global or local scale. The time is now.

REFERENCES

All-Party Parliamentary Group (APPG). (2016). *Triple impact: How developing nursing will improve health, promote gender equality, and support economic growth*. Retrieved on February 21, 2024, from https://globalhealth.inparliament.uk/files/globalhealth/2020-12/DIGITAL%20APPG%20Triple%20Impact%20%283%29.pdf.

Alliance of Nurses for Healthy Environments (ANHE). (2021a). About. Retrieved on February 21, 2024, from https://envirn.org/about/.

Alliance of Nurses for Healthy Environments (ANHE). (2021b). ANHE environmental health nurse fellowship. Retrieved on February 21, 2024, from https://envirn.org/anhe-fellowship/.

Alliance of Nurses for Healthy Environments (ANHE). (2021c). Health Equity & Anti-Racism Leadership Institute. Retrieved on February 21, 2024, from https://envirn.org/hear-leadership-institute/.

Alliance of Nurses for Healthy Environments (ANHE). (2021d). The Global Nurse Agenda for Climate Justice is LIVE! Retrieved on February 21, 2024, from https://envirn.org/hear-institute/.

Baumann, S. L. (2013). Global health nursing: Toward a human science-based approach. *Nursing Science Quarterly, 26*, 365.

Beck, D. M. (2017). A brief history of the United Nations and nursing: A healthy world is our common future. In Rosa, W. (Ed.), *A new era in global health: Nursing and the United Nations 2030 Agenda for Sustainable Development* (pp. 57–84). New York, NY: Springer Publishing.

Berwick, D. M. (2020). The moral determinants of health. *JAMA, 324*(3), 225–226.

Bodenheimer, T., & Mason, D. (2017). Registered nurses: partners in transforming primary care. In, *Proceedings of a conference sponsored by the Josiah Macy Jr. Foundation in June 2016*. New York: Josiah Macy Jr. Foundation. Retrieved on February 21, 2024, from https://macyfoundation.org/assets/reports/publications/macy_monograph_nurses_2016_webpdf.pdf.

Bradley, E. H., Elkins, B. R., Herrin, J., et al. (2011). Health and social services expenditures: Associations with health outcomes. *BMJ Quality & Safety, 20*(10), 826–831.

Castrucci, B., & Auerbach, J. (2019). Meeting individual social needs falls short of addressing social determinants of health. *Health Affairs Blog*. doi:10.1377/hblog20190115.234942.

Crisp, N., Brownie, S., & Refsum, C. (2018). *Nursing and midwifery: The key to the rapid and cost-effective expansion of high-quality universal health coverage*. Qatar: World Innovation Summit for Health Retrieved on February 21, 2024, from https://www.researchgate.net/publication/329028272_NURSING_AND_MIDWIFERY_THE_KEY_TO_THE_RAPID_AND_COST-EFFECTIVE_EXPANSION_OF_HIGH-QUALITY_UNIVERSAL_HEALTH_COVERAGE_A_Report_of_the_WISH_Nursing_and_UHC_Forum_2018.

Dossey, B. M., Rosa, W. E., & Beck, D. M. (2019). Nursing and the Sustainable Development Goals: From Nightingale to now. *American Journal of Nursing, 119*(5), 44–49.

Ewald, B., Golden, R., & Mason, D. J. (2021). Promoting health equity by paying for social care. *JAMA Health Forum, 2*(12), e215023. Retrieved on February 21, 2024, from https://jamanetwork.com/journals/jama-health-forum/fullarticle/2787444.

Fields, L., Perkiss, S., Dean, B. A., & Moroney, T. (2021). Nursing and the Sustainable Development Goals: A scoping review. *Journal of Nursing Scholarship, 53*(5), 568–577.

Grootjans, J., & Newman, S. (2013). The relevance of globalization to nursing: A concept analysis. *International Nursing Review, 60*, 78–85.

Guzmán, C., Aguirre, A. A., Astle, B., Barros, E., Bayles, B., Chimbari, M., El-Abbadi, N., Evert, J., Hackett, F., Howard, C., Jennings, J., Krzyzek, A., LeClair, J., Maric, F., Martin, O., Osano, O., Patz, J., Potter, T., Redvers, N., Trienekens, N., … Zylstra, M. (2021). A framework to guide planetary health education. *The Lancet. Planetary Health, 5*(5), e253–e255.

Health Care Without Harm. (2021). Nurses climate challenge. Retrieved on February 21, 2024, from https://nursesclimatechallenge.org.

Holloway, A., Thomson, A., Stilwell, B., Finch, H., Irwin, K., & Crisp, N. (2021). Agents of Change: the story of the Nursing Now campaign. *Nursing Now/Burdett Trust for Nursing*. Retrieved on February 21, 2024, from https://www.nursingnow.org/nursing-now/.

International Council of Nurses (ICN). (2017). *Nurses: a voice to lead—achieving the SDGs*. Retrieved on February 21, 2024, from https://www.icnvoicetolead.com/home/.

International Council of Nurses (ICN). (2021a). Nursing definitions. Retrieved on February 21, 2024, from https://www.icn.ch/nursing-policy/nursing-definitions.

International Council of Nurses (ICN). (2021b). International nurses day. Retrieved on February 21, 2024, from https://www.icn.ch/international-nurses-day-2021.

International Council of Nurses (ICN). (2021c). *ICN report: 74thWorld Health Assembly*. Retrieved on February 21, 2024, from https://www.icn.ch/resources/publications-and-reports/icn-report-74th-world-health-assembly.

International Council of Nurses (ICN). (2021d). *2020 annual report: The global voice of nursing in the year of the nurse and the COVID-19 pandemic*. Retrieved on February 21, 2024, from https://www.icn.ch/node/1299.

International Council of Nurses (ICN). (2021e). *International Council of Nurses policy brief: The global nursing shortage and nursing retention*. Retrieved on February 21, 2024, from https://www.icn.ch/sites/default/files/inline-files/ICN%20Policy%20Brief_Nurse%20Shortage%20and%20Retention.pdf.

International Council of Nurses (ICN). (2021f). *ICN at the 73rd Worth Health Assembly, 2020 and the 148th WHO Executive Board, 2021*. Retrieved on February 21, 2024, from https://www.icn.ch/system/files/documents/2021-03/WHA%20%26%20EB%20Report_EN.pdf.

International Council of Nurses (ICN). (2021g). ICN leadership programmes: Global Nursing Leadership Institute. Retrieved on February 21, 2024, from https://www.icn.ch/how-we-do-it/nna-development-leadership-programmes/global-nursing-leadership-institutetm-gnli.

International Council of Nurses (ICN). (2021h). *The ICN code of ethics for nurses* (rev. 2021). Retrieved on February 21, 2024, from https://www.icn.ch/sites/default/files/inline-files/ICN_Code-of-Ethics_EN_Web.pdf..

International Council of Nurses (ICN). (n.d.). ICN Nurse Practitioner/Advanced Practice Network. Retrieved on February 21, 2024, from https://www.icn.ch/who-we-are/icn-nurse-practitioneradvanced-practice-network-npapn-network.

Janes, C. R., & Corbett, K. K. (2009). Anthropology and global health. *Annual Reviews of Anthropology, 38*, 167–183.

Japsen, B. (2020, June 4). UnitedHealth Group increases housing investments to $500M to address social determinants. *Forbes*. Retrieved on February 21, 2024, from https://www.forbes.com/sites/brucejapsen/2020/06/04/unitedhealth-group-boosts-housing-investments-to-500m-to-address-social-determinants/?sh=64515d022815.

Kahn, L. H., Kaplan, B., Monath, T., Woodall, L. J., & Conti, L. (2014). A manifesto for planetary health. *The Lancet, 383*, 1459.

Klopper, H. C., Madigan, E., Vlasich, C., Albien, A., Ricciardi, R., Catrambone, C., & Tigges, E. (2020). Advancement of global health: Recommendations from the Global Advisory Panel on the

Future of Nursing & Midwifery (GAPFON). *Journal of Advanced Nursing, 76*(2), 741–748.

Koplan, J. P., Bond, T. C., Merson, M. H., Reddy, K. S., Rodriguez, M. H., Sewankambo, N. K., & Wasserheit, J. N. (2009). Towards a common definition of global health. *Lancet, 373*, 1993–1995.

Kuehnert, P., Fawcett, J., DePriest, K., Chinn, P., Cousin, L., Ervin, N., Flanagan, J., Fry-Bowers, E., Killion, C., Maliski, S., Maughan, E. D., Meade, C., Murray, T., Schenk, B., & Waite, R. (2021). Defining the social determinants of health for nursing action to achieve health equity: A consensus paper from the American academy of nursing. *Nursing Outlook, S0029-6554*(21), 00201–00203. doi:10.1016/j.outlook.2021.08.003. Advance online publication.

Leuddekke, G. R. (2016). *Global population health and well-being in the 21st century: Toward new paradigms, policy, and practice.* New York, NY: Springer Publishing.

Martsolf, G., Sloan, J., Villarruel, A., Sullivan, C., & Mason, D. J. (2018). Promoting a culture of health through cross-sector collaborations. *Health Promotion Practice, 5*(19), 784–791. doi:10.1177/1524839918772284.

Mason, D. J. (2016). Promoting the health of families and communities: A moral imperative. *Hastings Center Report, 46*(Suppl 1), S48–S51.

Mason, D. J., Dickson, E., Perez, A., & McLemore, M. (2021). *Policy and politics in nursing and health care* (8th Ed.). St. Louise, Missouri: Elsevier.

Mason, D. J., & Salvage, J. (2021). International Council of Nurses' Global Nursing Leadership Institute: Responding to the pandemic. *International Nursing Review, 68*(4), 563–570.

McGovern, L. (2014, august 21). The relative contribution of multiple determinants to health. *Health Affairs Health Policy Brief.* doi:10.1377/hpb20140821.404487.

McKinnon, T. H., & Fitzpatrick, J. J. (2017). Nursing education imperatives and the United Nations 2030 Agenda. In Rosa, W. (Ed.), *A new era in global health: Nursing and the United Nations 2030 Agenda for Sustainable Development* (pp. 179–190). New York, NY: Springer Publishing.

Miyamoto, S., & Cook, E. (2019). The procurement of the UN sustainable development goals and the American national policy agenda of nurses. *Nursing Outlook, 67*(6), 658–663.

National Academies of Sciences, Engineering, and Medicine. (2019). *Integrating Social Care into the delivery of Health Care: Moving Upstream to Improve the Nation's Health.* Washington, DC: The National Academies Press. Retrieved from https://doi.org/10.17226/25467.

National Academies of Sciences, Engineering, and Medicine (NASEM). (2021). *The future of nursing 2020-2030: Charting a path to achieve health equity.* Washington, D.C.: The National Academies Press. Retrieved on February 21, 2024, from https://www.nap.edu/catalog/25982/the-future-of-nursing-2020-2030-charting-a-path-to.

National Academies of Sciences, Engineering, and Medicine. (2021). *Implementing high-quality primary care: rebuilding the foundation of health care.* Washington, DC: The National Academies Press. https://doi.org/10.17226/25983.

Nurses Drawdown. (2021). About. Retrieved on February 21, 2024, from https://nursesdrawdown.com/about.

Nursing Now Challenge. (2021). Home. Retrieved on February 21, 2024, from https://www.nursingnow.org.

Potter, T. M. (2021). Planetary health: An essential framework for nursing education and practice. *Creative Nursing, 27*(4), 226–230. https://doi.org/10.1891/cn-2021-0017.

Rosa, W. (2017a). A call for planetary thinking in theory and knowledge development. *Research and Theory for Nursing Practice, 31*(2), 93–95.

Rosa, W. (Ed.). (2017b). *A new era in global health: Nursing and the United Nations 2030 Agenda for Sustainable Development.* New York, NY: Springer Publishing.

Rosa, W. E. (2020). Nurses as global and planetary citizens. *American Journal of Nursing, 120*(4), 11.

Rosa, W. E., & Iro, E. (2019). The future of nursing and the advancement of the United Nations Sustainable Development Goals. *Nursing Outlook, 67*(6), 623–625.

Rosa, W. E., Burnett, C., Butler, C., Rolle, P., Salvage, J., Wignall, A., & Mason, D. J. (2021a). The ICN Global Nursing Leadership Institute: Integrating the SDGs into leadership and policy development. *American Journal of Nursing, 121*(12), 54–58.

Rosa, W. E., Catton, H., Davidson, P. M., Hannaway, C. J., Iro, E., Klopper, H. C., Madigan, E. A., McConville, F. E., Stilwell, B., & Kurth, A. E. (2021b). Nurses and midwives as global partners to achieve the Sustainable Development Goals in the Anthropocene. *Journal of Nursing Scholarship, 53*(5), 552–560.

Rosa, W. E., Hannaway, C. J., McArdle, C., McManus, M. F., Alharahsheh, S. T., & Marmot, M. (2021c). *Nurses for health equity: Guidelines for tackling the social determinants of health.* Qatar: World Innovation Summit for Health. Retrieved on February 21, 2024, from https://www.wish.org.qa/reports/nurses-for-health-equity/.

Rosa, W. E., Kurth, A. E., Sullivan-Marx, E., Shamian, J., Shaw, H. K., Wilson, L. L., & Crisp, N. (2019). Nursing and midwifery advocacy to lead the United Nations Sustainable Development Agenda. *Nursing Outlook, 67*(6), 628–641.

Rosa, W. E., & Upvall, M. J. (2019a). Integrative nursing and global health. In Kreitzer, M. J., & Koithan, M. (Eds.), *Integrative nursing* (2nd ed, pp. 601–611). New York, NY: Oxford University Press.

Rosa, W. E., & Upvall, M. J. (2019b). The case for a paradigm shift: from global to planetary nursing. *Nursing Forum, 54*(2), 165–170.

Rubin, J., Taylor, J., Krapels, J., Sutherland, A., Felician, M., Liu, J., Davis, L., & Rohr, C. (2016). *Are better health outcomes related to social expenditure? A cross-national empirical analysis of social expenditure and population health measures.* Santa Monica, CA: The RAND Corporation. Retrieved on February 21, 2024, from https://www.rand.org/content/dam/rand/pubs/research_reports/RR1200/RR1252/RAND_RR1252.pdf.

Schenk, E. C., Cook, C., Demorest, S., & Burduli, E. (2019). CHANT: Climate, Health, and Nursing Tool: Item development and exploratory factor analysis. *Annual Review of Nursing Research, 38*(1), 97–112.

Schenk, E. C., Cook, C., Demorest, S., & Burduli, E. (2021a). Climate, Health, and Nursing Tool (CHANT): Initial survey results. *Public Health Nursing, 38*(2), 152–159.

Schenk, E. C., Potter, T. M., Cook, C., Huffling, K., & Rosa, W. E. (2021b). Nurses promoting inclusive, safe, resilient, and sustainable cities and communities: Taking action on COVID-19, systemic racism, and climate change. *American Journal of Nursing, 121*(7), 66–69.

Schneider, E., et al. (2017). *Mirror, mirror 2017: International comparison reflects flaws and opportunities for better U.S. health care.* New York: Commonwealth Fund. Retrieved on February 21, 2024, from https://www.commonwealthfund.org/publications/fund-reports/2017/jul/mirror-mirror-2017-international-comparison-reflects-flaws-and.

Sensor, C. S., Branden, P. S., Clary-Muronda, V., Hawkins, J. E., Fitzgerald, D., Shimek, A. M., Al-Itani, D., Madigan, E. A., & Rosa, W. E. (2021). Nurses achieving the Sustainable Development Goals: The United Nations and Sigma. *American Journal of Nursing, 121*(4), 65–68.

Sigma Theta Tau International (2017). The Global Advisory Panel on the Future of Nursing & Midwifery (GAPFON) report. Retrieved on February 21, 2024, from https://sigma.nursingrepository.org/handle/10755/621599.

Sommer, M., & Mason, D. J. (2021, August 16). Period poverty and promoting menstrual equity. *JAMA Health Forum, 2*(8), e213089. doi:10.1001/jamahealthforum.2021.3089.

Squires, A. (2019). US nursing and midwifery research capacity building opportunities to achieve the United Nations Sustainable Development Goals. *Nursing Outlook, 67*(6), 642–648.

Squires, A. P., Abboud, S., Ojemeni, M. T., & Ridge, L. (2017). Creating new knowledge: Nursing- and midwifery-led research to drive the global goals. In Rosa, W. (Ed.), *A new era in global health: Nursing and the United Nations 2030 Agenda for Sustainable Development* (pp. 191–204). New York, NY: Springer Publishing.

Squires, A., Chavez, F. S., Hilfinger Messias, D. K., Narsavage, G. L., Oerther, D. B., Premji, S. S., Rosa, W. E., Ambani, Z., Castañeda-Hidalgo, H., Lee, H., Pallangyo, E. S., & Thumm, E. B. (2019). Sustainable development & the year of the nurse & midwife - 2020. *International Journal of Nursing Studies, 94*, A3–A4.

Stockholm Resilience Center. (n.d.). Partnerships are central to the SDGs. Azote Images for the Stockholm Resilience Center, Stockholm University. Retrieved on February 21, 2024, from https://www.stockholmresilience.org/images/18.36c25848153d54bdba33ec9b/1465905797608/sdgs-food-azote.jpg.

United Nations (UN). (n.d.). Sustainable Development Goals communications materials. Retrieved on February 21, 2024, from https://www.un.org/sustainabledevelopment/news/communications-material/.

United Nations (UN). (2012). United nations conference on sustainable development, 20-22 June 2012, Rio de Janeiro. Retrieved on February 21, 2024, from https://www.un.org/en/conferences/environment/rio2012.

United Nations (UN). (2016). *Transforming our world: The 2030 agenda for sustainable development.* Retrieved on February 21, 2024, from https://sustainabledevelopment.un.org/content/documents/21252030%20Agenda%20for%20Sustainable%20Development%20web.pdf.

United Nations (UN). (2021). *The Sustainable Development Goals Report 2021.* Retrieved on February 21, 2024, from: https://unstats.un.org/sdgs/report/2021/.

United Nations Office of Drugs and Crime. (2019). Understanding the global opioid crisis. Retrieved on February 21, 2024, from https://www.unodc.org/documents/scientific/Global_SMART_21_web_new.pdf.

Upvall, M. J., & Leffers, J. M. (eds.). (2014). *Global health nursing: Building and sustaining partnerships.* New York, NY: Springer Publishing.

Upvall, M. J., & Leffers, J. M. (2017). Raising consciousness through global nursing collaboration. In Rosa, W. (Ed.), *A new era in global health: Nursing and the United Nations 2030 Agenda for Sustainable Development* (pp. 489–510). New York, NY: Springer Publishing.

Upvall, M. J., & Luzincourt, G. (2019). Global citizens, healthy communities: Integrating the Sustainable Development Goals into the nursing curriculum. *Nursing Outlook, 67*(6), 649–657.

Whitmee, S., Haines, A., Beyrer, C., Boltz, F., Capon, A. G., de Souza Dias, B. F., Ezeh, A., Frumkin, H., Gong, P., Head, P., Horton, R., Mace, G. M., Marten, R., Myers, S. S., Nishtar, S., Osofsky, S. A., Pattanayak, S. K., Pongsiri, M. J., Romanelli, C., Soucat, A., ... Yach, D. (2015). Safeguarding human health in the Anthropocene epoch: report of The Rockefeller Foundation-Lancet Commission on planetary health. *Lancet, 386*(10007), 1973–2028.

Wilson, L., Mendes, I. A., Klopper, H., Catrambone, C., Al-Maaitah, R., Norton, M. E., & Hill, M. (2016). 'Global health' and 'global nursing': proposed definitions from The Global Advisory Panel on the Future of Nursing. *Journal of Advanced Nursing, 72*(7), 1529–1540.

World Health Organization (WHO). (n.d.). Monitoring health for the SDGs. Retrieved on February 21, 2024, from https://www.who.int/data/gho/data/themes/sustainable-development-goals.

World Health Organization (WHO). (2020). *State of the world's nursing: Investing in education, jobs and leadership.* Retrieved on February 21, 2024, from https://www.who.int/publications/i/item/9789240003279.

World Health Organization (WHO). (2021a). *Global strategic directions for nursing and midwifery (2021-2025).* Retrieved on February 21, 2024, from https://www.who.int/publications/i/item/9789240033863.

World Health Organization (WHO). (2021b). One Health High Level Expert Panel. Retrieved on February 21, 2024, from https://www.who.int/groups/one-health-high-level-expert-panel.

World Health Organization (WHO). (2021c). *World health statistics 2021: Monitoring health for the SDGs.* Retrieved on February 21, 2024, from https://www.who.int/publications/i/item/9789240027053.

World Health Organization (WHO). (2021d). Social determinants of health. Retrieved on February 21, 2024, from https://www.who.int/health-topics/social-determinants-of-health#tab=tab_1.

World Health Organization (WHO). (2022a). WHO collaborating centres. Retrieved on February 21, 2024, from https://www.who.int/about/collaboration/collaborating-centres.

World Health Organization (WHO). (2022b). WHO regional offices. Retrieved from https://www.who.int/about/who-we-are/regional-offices.

Yong, E. (2022, January 7). Hospitals are in serious trouble. *The Atlantic.* Retrieved on February 21, 2024, from https://www.theatlantic.com/health/archive/2022/01/omicron-mild-hospital-strain-health-care-workers/621193/.

2 PLANETARY HEALTH: ENSURING A VIABLE FUTURE FOR ALL

TERESA LEWIS ■ JANET RODEN ■ TEDDIE POTTER

INTRODUCTION

While the world continues to adapt to constant planetary change, health care education must modify its practices to a sustainable-centric systems process. This means moving beyond a medicalised-centric domain to include a more holistic approach to person/community-centric care, one that is all encompassing of planetary health (PH). In fact, PH promotes *kincentricity,* where all life is valued and protected. The contemporary Australian nursing education system is beginning to embrace concepts of PH, sustainability and climate change. The reason for addressing these concepts is because climate change is known to be a major challenge to human health and thus to the health care ecosystem (Hospedales, 2021; Luschkova, et al., 2022; Watts et al., 2018). Kalogirou et al. (2020) argue that climate change has extensive universal nursing implications, but nurses are more often focused on individual patient care rather than larger environmental concerns. Nevertheless, nurses have been keen to support institutional interventions to promote PH. The health effects of climate change are already growing as a topic of discourse within health care as they are being experienced globally, and increasing amounts of literature provide evidence of this (Alvarez-Nieto et al., 2022; Cruz et al., 2018; Watts et al., 2018). Despite climate change being recognised as a global challenge, there are other interruptions to PH that cause equally harmful outcomes, such as water management and mining. They continue to impede the symbiotic-like relationship we require with the planet in order to flourish because PH is not a core concern for many businesses or even for individuals.

THINK BOX 2.1

- In your country and region, what are you noticing about the effects of climate change on people?
- Who is concerned about this?
- Who is taking action?
- Are there other threats to PH where you live?

PLANETARY HEALTH

Planetary Health and Health Care

The Planetary Health Alliance (PHA) is a global consortium of universities, nongovernmental organisations, research institutes and government entities that are committed to understanding and addressing global environmental change and its health impacts (Planetary Health Alliance, n.d.-a). The PHA defines PH as 'a solutions-oriented, transdisciplinary field and social movement focused on analysing and addressing the impacts of human disruptions to Earth's natural systems on human health and all life on Earth' (Planetary Health Alliance, n.d.-b).

Asaduzzaman et al. (2022) and Hancock (2021) describe PH as a new discipline that is crucial for health care professionals and health promotion for 'one planet' communities. There are more courses now available for health workers in PH, sustainability and climate change, and Asaduzzaman et al. (2022) take a step further in recommending that a dedicated network of motivated health care professionals and regional hubs be formed with an agenda to ensure a comprehensive, uniform and inclusive PH education curriculum and practice.

Planetary Health Education

The PHA offers the resources and professional networks that Asaduzzaman et al. (2022) call for. Before discussing PH education, it is important to acknowledge that PH knowledge and practices are not new and can be traced historically as practices of Indigenous peoples all over the world. Later in this chapter, there is a larger discussion of the importance of acknowledging the contribution of Indigenous people to planetary knowledge. The PHA acknowledges that the source of human disruptions of the Earth's natural systems represents a rupture between humans and the rest of nature, caused by humans. 'To heal this rupture, we need different stories—a new fabric woven with threads from the world's faith traditions, Indigenous knowledge, with science, literature, and the arts to reassert our species' spiritual connection to the Earth' (Planetary Health Alliance, n.d.-c). Much of PH education views Indigenous ways of knowing as a key paradigm for healing this rupture between humans and the rest of nature: Indigenous science holds that there is no separation between each one of us, and the whole of nature and ways of knowing are diverse and holistic, based on history and accumulated experiences.

Creating a Shared Language and Shared Vision

Planetary Health Education Framework: A Shared Language

Creating a transdisciplinary movement requires a shared language and shared vision that permit us to move beyond disciplinary silos to cocreate effective mitigation and adaptation strategies and policies. We need to educate students in higher education who are just discovering their vocations, as well as professionals currently in practice. This education begins with the *Planetary Health Education Framework* (PHEF) (Faerron Guzman & Potter, 2021). Authored by over two dozen experts from around the world, the PHEF comprises the essential knowledge that all students should experience during their higher education.

There are five core PH domains, shown in Fig. 2.1. The domains are interconnected and not linear or hierarchical. In recognition of the importance of healing the human–nature rupture, the PHEF centres focus on 'interconnection within nature'. The choice of 'within' rather than 'with' is intentional and reflects the essential paradigm of Indigenous peoples. It is not a matter of reconnecting humans to nature. Humans *are* nature. We are absolutely interconnected and inseparable

from the rest of life on the planet. The belief that we are separate has allowed us to mine, extract, deforest, pollute and enslave without regard for the harms that these behaviours bring. Interconnection within nature, however, enhances our consciousness, informs our decisions and promotes a commitment to sustainability and the viability of future generations.

THINK BOX 2.2

- What do you think about this concept of interconnection *within* nature?
- Is this how you think of the human experience?
- Do you see it as separate?
- How might your ideas about this influence your style of life?

The other domains include 'the Anthropocene and health', which helps us recognise and acknowledge human culpability in the disruption of the Earth's natural systems, including planetary boundaries, which cannot be exceeded if humans are to continue to thrive as a species. The 'systems thinking and complexity-based approaches in planetary health' domain helps students recognise and value diverse ways and scales of knowing. It also promotes awareness of the risk of unintended consequences when complexity is ignored and sectors are marginalised. Chapter 1 also refers to the importance of systems thinking in managing the social determinants of health (SDOH): the diverse chapters of this book indicate the many systems involved in the big picture of health and well-being.

Transdisciplinary solutions to restore PH must be founded on principles of 'equity and social justice'. This fourth PHEF domain recognises the rights of humans as well as the rights of nature. 'Planetary health professionals must commit to imagining bold alternatives and implementing practices that address the root causes of injustice within and between societies' (Faerron Guzman & Potter, 2021, p. 34). To challenge social and structural norms and policies that impact health outcomes, students must be versed in 'movement building and systems change', the fifth PHEF domain. This domain prepares students to lead the many changes that are required locally to globally to restore PH. Many wrongly assume that movements 'just happen' when, in fact, they require strategy and

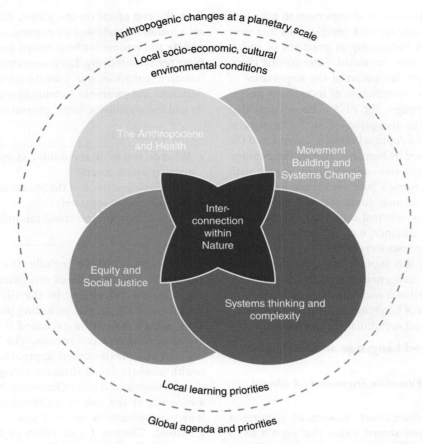

Anthropogenic changes at a planetary scale

Local socio-economic, cultural environmental conditions

The Anthropocene and Health

Movement Building and Systems Change

Inter-connection within Nature

Equity and Social Justice

Systems thinking and complexity

Local learning priorities

Global agenda and priorities

Fig. 2.1 ■ Planetary Health Education Framework. Courtesy of the Planetary Health Alliance.

relationship building over time. Chapter 10 discusses the power of social movements as explored in the Nursing Now campaign: building a social movement is an effective way to use power for change.

THINK BOX 2.3

- Have there been successful social movements in your country?
- How did you hear about them?
- What did they do to draw attention to their cause?

São Paulo Declaration on Planetary Health

Once people are educated to create change, a shared vision facilitates the work that needs to be done with a blueprint of the future we are trying to build. The

São Paulo Declaration on Planetary health (Planetary Health Alliance, 2021) provides this vision.

The declaration was agreed at the PH annual meeting in 2021. It represents a global vision for the future, including the unique work that each sector must do to bring about the great transition:

We need a fundamental shift in how we live on Earth, what we are calling the Great Transition. Achieving the Great Transition will require rapid and deep structural changes across most dimensions of human activity. This includes how we produce and consume food, energy, and manufacture goods; how we construct and live in our cities; and how we consider and measure growth, progress and development, and govern ourselves.

It will also require rethinking our values and relationships within Nature and to each other from human exceptionalism, domination, and scarcity to interdependence, equity, and regeneration.

(Planetary Health Alliance, 2021, p. 2).

The declaration then proceeds to envision changes that every sector can make to reach the great transition.

Nursing is one of the first sectors taking the next step to apply the PHEF domains to research, education, advocacy/policy and practice. 'Nursing for Planetary Health and Well-Being' (Astle et al., 2023) launches the nursing profession's commitment to the great transition and the unique ways that nursing can embody the five PHEF domains. Our hope is that 'Nursing for Planetary Health and Well-Being' will inspire other professions to follow suit.

A list of resources to help you remain up to date is shown in Box 2.1. Another way to remain up to date is to attend the PH annual meeting. The location varies, but the content always supports the dissemination of new knowledge and an opportunity to build a transdisciplinary network.

BOX 2.1
ADDITIONAL RESOURCES FOR PLANETARY HEALTH

The following print and online resources support curriculum development by offering foundational knowledge and emerging science.

- (Book) *Planetary health: Protecting Nature to Protect Ourselves*, by Samuel Myers and Howard Frumkin, published by Island Press in 2020.
- (Book) *Planetary health: Safeguarding Human Health and the Environment in the Anthropocene*, by Andy Haines and Howard Frumkin, published by Cambridge University Press in 2021.
- (Journal) *The Lancet Planetary Health*: https://www.thelancet.com/journals/lanplh/home.
- Planetary health support for educators: the PHA offers syllabi, videos, and course designs (https://www.planetaryhealthalliance.org/ph-education-materials). In addition, the PHA has produced global case studies complete with teaching guides on a variety of planetary health topics.

There are numerous ways to connect with other professionals in a PH community of practice. For example, Clinicians for Planetary Health is a global network of health professionals, and the Next Generation Network is a community of practice for students. Both are supported by the PHA.

Hubs bring people together to work on PH issues that impact a local or regional setting. For example, the Oceania Hub brings over 30 organisations from Australia, New Zealand, Fiji, Samoa and Papua New Guinea (https://www.planetaryhealthalliance.org/pha-regional-hubs). Small islands face particular problems with rising sea levels, and sharing solutions makes sense.

To be part of the solution to addressing PH, start by learning the shared language and transdisciplinary domains of the PHEF and then realise the unique contributions that you can make to the shared vision of the *São Paulo Declaration on Planetary Health*. Finally, join the movement by becoming a member of a hub or community of practice. There is plenty of work to be done, and all are welcome.

THINK BOX 2.4

- Think about a time when you felt connected within nature. Share your story with a friend or colleague.
- Which PH crisis do you feel personally called to address—loss of biodiversity; land, water and air pollution; changing land use and loss of forests and wilderness; climate change; or another issue?
- Are you hopeful that we will restore PH so future generations can thrive? If yes, what gives you hope?
- What is one small step you can take today in your nursing work to strengthen the PH movement?

Symbiosis Between Humans and Nature

This symbiotic-like relationship we have with the planet means nurses and midwives are being called upon to be knowledgeable about PH and how it can be embedded in nursing research, education, advocacy/policy and practice, addressed earlier. So, how does this symbiotic-like association between humans and the rest of nature work (Table 2.1)?

Consider a health care symbiotic-like relationship that humans have with the rest of nature; it is complex, interesting and so closely interlinked that one

TABLE 2.1		
The Symbiotic-Like Relationship Of Humans And Planetary Health From A Healthcare Perspective		
Relationship	Species A (humans)	Species B (other life form/element)
Commensalism	Receives benefit	Unaffected
Mutualism	Receives benefit	Receives benefit
Parasitism	Receives benefit	Harmed

Adapted from Knox, B., Ladiges, P., Evans, B., & Saint, R. (2006). *Biology: An Australian Focus* (3rd Ed.). McGraw-Hill and with permission from Roden, J. E., & Lewis, T. M. A. (2023, 7–9 June). *Sustainable-centric health care model for healthcare educators.*

really cannot exist happily without the other. Therefore this health care symbiotic-like relationship is paramount for existence. For example, commensalism is the way that species A (humans) and species B (other life form/element) can work together so that neither is harmed. One simple example is the practice of rainwater collection in tanks so that it can be used to water gardens, thus decreasing overuse of the Earth's natural water system. Mutualism is the action between humans and the Earth's natural ecosystems. Both rely on and live together in a process that is ideal for equity to both systems—that of humans and that of the planet, the result being better planetary and human health. However, the sinister side of parasitism is difficult to address: it's a process whereby species A (humans) violates species B (other life form/element) so that humans can benefit from its extensive, yet not inexhaustible, resources.

Interruptions in symbiosis, besides climate change, can occur where both species A and species B are so closely entwined that disastrous outcomes arise for both. Some examples of intolerable attacks on the planet and humans are often caused by anthropogenic (human-made) activities such as the careless discarding of industrial waste that is harmful in some way to other species as well as to humans. Think of oil pipeline disasters or sewage in the ocean—both widely reported in the news media.

THINK BOX 2.5

Thinking about the symbiotic-like relationship that humans have with the planet.
1. Which stage do you believe we are in now?
2. Is there a stage that you think can provide a better relationship for both humans and the planet?
3. Can you think of different ways in which you can aid human and PH viability?

Impacts on Planetary Health

The Council on Foreign Relations (2023) produced a timeline of global ecological disasters. Some of it is presented as follows, showing the causation that occurred, the country of environmental impact and the health aftermath (Table 2.2).

This snapshot of the global environmental and health impacts is just that, a snapshot in time. but on occasion, a kind of harmony is seen so that 'man and the biosphere' can work together for a result that gains a UNESCO world-class reputation. The community of Noosa, Queensland, Australia, is one such place that holds not one but three UNESCO biosphere reserves. The reserves are successful in bringing both the community and environment together through projects and research (Noosa Biosphere Reserve, n.d.). Even though there are small steps to gain positive results such as biosphere reserves, health care facilities are also trying to implement climate-friendly initiatives. However, many nurses and midwives within the Australian context still struggle to comprehend the necessity of such actions, and so, health care facilities are often unable to fully mitigate their carbon footprint (Lewis et al., 2018).

THINK BOX 2.6

Consider the many climate-related disasters worldwide.
1. How do these disasters make you feel?
2. Do you think these disasters are caused by global warming or have humans contributed to certain ones?
3. Is there anything going on in your community that you can be part of to aid planetary and human viability?

	TABLE 2.2		
	Snapshot of Environmental Disasters and Health Issues		
Year	Cause	Environmental	Health aftermath
1912	Dumping of cadmium	Japan: the Jinzu River	Itai-itai disease: painful condition of the skin and bones.
1956	Methylmercury poisoning	Japan: local water system; mercury was bioaccumulated and biomagnified into the muscle of fish.	Aftermath of consuming fish. The first well-documented case of a child with Minamata disease that causes neurological symptoms such as convulsions and difficulties in walking and speech.
1976	Dioxin cloud (known as the Seveso cloud)	Seveso, Italy: (atmosphere)	Two thousand people became unwell, and to prevent the poison from entering the food chain, 80,000 animals were required to be slaughtered.
1984	Cyanide gas leak (methyl isocyanate gas)	Airborne (atmosphere)	Bhopal, India: at least 4000 people killed, half a million unwell. Survivors battled with blindness, respiratory issues and birth defects.
2006	Toxic waste (caustic soda and petroleum)	Côte d'Ivoire: Waste was dumped into the Ivorian waste system	More than 100,000 people encountered nausea, headaches breathing difficulties. Approximately 15–17 people died.

Adapted from Council on Foreign Relations. (2023). *1912–2020 Ecological disasters*. https://www.cfr.org/timeline/ecological-disasters.

Dichotomy of Health Care Facilities: Another Interruption to a Mutualistic Sustainable-Centric System

Health care professionals are often not aware that certain environments in which they work (health care facilities) have an environmental dichotomy—one that harms and another that heals (Lewis et al., 2018). For example, on different levels, a hospital both harms and heals; on a micro level, it can promote personal health through diagnostic precision, yet on a macro level, medical technology also threatens the environment through using excessive energy (Topf, 2005). Beside the high energy consumption, hospitals generate considerable waste (Lewis et al., 2018) and use a massive amount of water which can also accentuate global warming through energy consumption required to move and/or treat water, contributing to increased carbon emissions that cause climate changes (Lewis et al., 2018; Ro, 2020). One reason why nurses do not understand the importance of PH is that their identity and practice have been historically entrenched within a medicalised domain and not challenged to understand or accept the difference between the medical model and a sustainable and planet-sensitive model.

Change of Identity and Practice

Many nurses and midwives within the Australian health care context fail to see the value in adopting a mutualistic sustainable-centric health care process. This process nurtures PH, and PH, in return, provides the necessary conditions that are vital for sustaining *kincentricity* without depleting its own resources. Sustainable health care moves beyond a medical-centric model of practice; it is more contemporary in approach and can be inclusive to a person/community model. It is the type of health care that has an awareness of the mutualistic symbiotic-like relationship between humans and the rest of the environment. Fig. 2.2 portrays how the change develops.

To begin to develop some of the processes in Fig. 2.2, health practitioners will need to think of how they will begin withdrawing from some of the traditional medical-centric methods; they will need to break down barriers to change and work toward more sustainable models of education and practice in nursing and health care. This will be a transformative change, but it can start if nurses and midwives begin to champion sustainable practices and show an awareness of the need for mutualistic health care—where no harm is done to other species or the

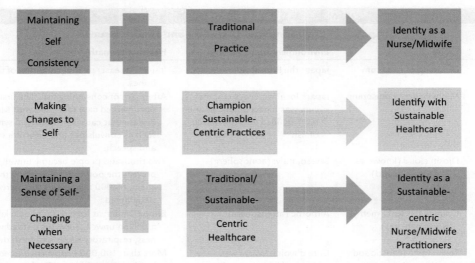

Fig. 2.2 ■ Sustainable-centric healthcare vs. traditional practice (Lewis, 2023) with permission. *Sustainable-centric health care model for healthcare educators.*

planet—that is, *kincentricity* (this word is discussed earlier; go back if you missed it). By going one step further and maintaining a nursing role and also championing and implementing more sustainable-centric models of practice, nurses* become change agents within health care.

Change Is a Challenge

Changing a systems process, such as a change to identity and practice as shown in Fig. 2.2, even when the end goal is perceived as positive, can be challenging, particularly if employers and colleagues are not familiar with the need for change. Despite there being many commissions and nongovernmental agencies stating a consistent message that climate change urgently needs to be addressed (Australian Nursing and Midwifery Federation, 2023; Whitmee et al., 2015; World Health Organization, 2023a), many health care professionals continue to ignore the need for such a transformation.

---

*We refer to nurses particularly, as they are the target audience for this book, but all other health workers can become more aware of the need for planetary health and sustainable-centric health care practices. All are welcome.

THINK BOX 2.7

- Would you find it difficult to change from the identity of a nurse/midwife in the traditional medical model (assuming that is how you identify) to become recognised as a sustainable-centric nurse/midwife practitioner?
- What would colleagues say if you were to be a PH champion?

Breaking Down the Barriers

Becoming an agent of change is not easy, and as Lewis et al.'s (2018) research on climate-friendly hospitals and the implications for health care practice showed, there was very little information for practitioners working in such environments to demonstrate that new practices being implemented were actually environmentally friendly. Longenecker & Longenecker (2014) point out that there are 10 reasons as to why organisational change can be difficult (Table 2.3).

Table 2.3 shows more reasons why health care professionals, although they work in a medicalised domain in health care, are unable to progress to an understanding about implementing mitigation strategies so that they aid in PH viability.

TABLE 2.3
Top 10 Barriers to Successful Hospital Change
1. Poor implementation planning and overly aggressive timelines
2. Failure to create buy-in/ownership of the initiative
3. Ineffective leadership and lack of trust in upper management
4. Failure to create a realistic plan or improvement process
5. Ineffective and top-down communication
6. A weak case for change, unclear focus and unclear desired outcomes
7. Little or no teamwork or cooperation
8. Failure to provide ongoing measurement, feedback and accountability
9. Unclear roles, goals and performance expectations
10. Lack of time, resources and upper management support

Adapted from Longenecker, C. O., & Longenecker, P. D. (2014). Why hospital improvement efforts fail: A view from the front line. *Journal of Healthcare Management, 59*(2), 147–157. https://pubmed.ncbi.nlm.nih.gov/24783373/.

Sustainable-Centric Education

The solutions by Longenecker & Longenecker (2014) (Table 2.3) are only a part of what is needed to initiate action from health care organisations and their employees to develop sustainable-centric health care that will ensure PH. Sustainable-centric education offers a powerful mechanism to unite health care professionals and hence health facilities.

Implementing sustainable-centric education for PH is paramount for a change in identity and behaviour among health professionals and has the potential to raise both awareness and performance of health workers, creating alignment to mitigate global warming and other planetary degradation. This is needed in Australia, but all countries should be examining their educational frameworks to address PH issues. Ways forward to achieve such a mutualistic and harmonious state is to embrace the three pillars of sustainability—social, environmental and economic—which work together to achieve planetary and therefore human viability (Roden & Lewis, 2023).

Sustainable development has evolved from decades of work from 1992 to 2023 by many countries through the United Nations (UN). We are now at the point where there are 17 Sustainable Development Goals (SDGs) with 169 targets (United Nations, 2023). It is not expected that we achieve all these goals individually; by tackling one goal, we can influence other goals, too. (For a fuller discussion on SDGs and nursing, see Chapter 1 of this book.) Educators who are knowledgeable within this field of the holistic view of health and well-being of the planet and of humans are needed to drive forward the comprehensive goals of the SDGs and explore with nurses how they apply to nursing practice.

THINK BOX 2.8

1. Do you think that as nurses/midwives we should be more environmentally friendly in practice? If so, how could this be achieved?
2. Can you identify within your workplace barriers to progression?
3. What is regarded as the 'master key' to unite organisations such as health care facilities and their health care professionals?

RODEN'S 2023 SUSTAINABLE-CENTRIC HEALTH CARE MAP FOR PLANETARY AND HUMAN HEALTH

Roden's (2023) example of a sustainable-centric health care map, shown in Fig. 2.3, demonstrates the importance of nurses working towards PH.

Not only can nurses work towards PH stability in their primary practice roles but they can also undertake mitigating actions which reduce resource consumption and promote a more stable environment. Fig. 2.3 depicts the relationships between sustainable-centric health care and nurses and nursing practice. In this map, concepts of sustainability and climate change are related to Australia and how they impact nursing

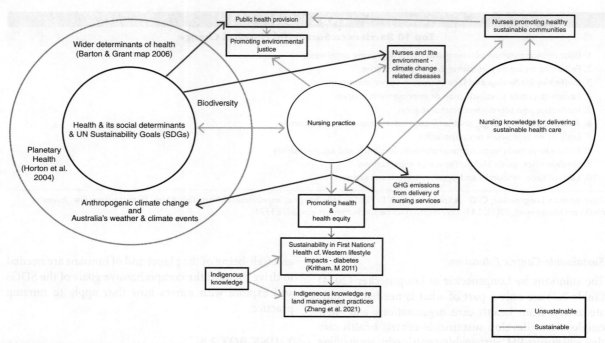

Fig. 2.3 ■ Australian nursing practice and its relationship with Planetary Health and sustainable healthcare knowledge (Roden, 2023) with permission.

practice there. You might like to consider if and how this mapping is relevant to your country.

In Fig. 2.3, the concentric circles on the far left of the map display:

Wider determinants of health: a diverse range of social, economic and environmental factors that impact people's health.

PH which refers to the need for us to live in harmony with our environment to ensure PH.

Biodiversity means changes over time to plants and animal life, both as extinction occurs and new species evolve.

Anthropogenic climate change and Australia's weather and climatic events refers to weather events caused through 'human-made' climate change such as higher temperatures, more extreme droughts, fire seasons, and floods and more extreme weather.

The SDOH are the conditions in which people are born, grow, live, work and age. They include factors like socioeconomic status, education, their neighbourhood and their physical environment, employment/unemployment and social support

networks, as well as access to health care, and are closely associated with the UN SDGs which are discussed in several places in this book, most fully in Chapter 1.

The central part of Fig. 2.3 portrays the actual and potential scopes of nursing practice and includes the following six aspects:

1. Working towards achieving the UN SDGs. Chapter 1 discusses in detail how nurses can contribute to the SDGs. To do this requires a whole system approach so that people who are seeking help with health are seen as a part of all the systems they belong to—for example, socioeconomic, environmental, social—all of which will impact their health and well-being. For nurses, taking account of these factors through actively seeking information that goes beyond clinical questions can elicit valuable information to guide treatment approaches and can also alert other team members to the importance of SDGs.

2. Health promotion and promoting health equity by providing access to health care for all, especially people from different cultures.
3. Relevant to Australia, but applicable to other countries and groups is acknowledgement of First Nations people through an Australian Referendum to recognise First Peoples voice in Parliament. 'The Bill' was passed on 19 June 2023. On 14 October 2023 Australians were able to vote in a referendum for a First Nations people representative to Parliament. This presence would have benefited a sustainable future for all Indigenous Australians (Parliament of Australia, 2023), the outcome was unsuccessful.
4. Environmental justice for all. The International Council of Nurses (ICN) Code of Ethics has a section on nurses and global health, which specifically calls for nurses to work towards attaining the Sustainable Development Goals (SDGs) as well as recognising the significance of the Social Determinants of Health (SDOH) (International Council of Nurses, 2021).
5. Promoting healthy, sustainable communities through community resilience. Community nurses are in a position to promote a wide range of events and activities that help communities to become more resilient. This is particularly important for people with mental health challenges or those who are anxious after COVID-19, as it provides connection with others. Activities may be the more conventional group approaches and can also involve outdoor activities that promote a greater awareness of the environment and opportunities for exercise.
6. Adhering to public health policies. Nurses working in public health are aware of public policies surrounding health, but for all nurses, they have taken on a new significance since the global pandemic. For example, the New South Wales Minister of Health introduced 70 public health orders over a 6-month period in 2020 because of COVID-19 (Ombudsman New South Wales, 2020; see 'hindsight: the first 12 months of the COVID-19 pandemic'). Do you know where to find public health policies for your country or region?

Fig. 2.3 developed in Australia and based on nursing roles there, indicates how nurses can support PH.

However, Australian hospitals and health facilities produce 7% of greenhouse gases (GHGs) per year (Charlesworth et al., 2018) compared to the global health care sector, which emits 4.4% of all GHGs according to Health Care Without Harm & Arup (2019). The red lines in Fig. 2.3 from nursing practice to anthropogenic climate change show that GHGs are produced by health care facilities, combine with other GHGs caused by other human activity and affect anthropogenic climate change, which is on the left side of Fig. 2.3. The world is beginning to experience the disastrous overall effect of GHGs in extreme weather events such as heat and flooding. Without rapid and effective interventions, these events will continue and are likely to worsen.

Through the effects of the weather events on the eastern coast of Australia (Hannam, 2022), nurses found that climate change conditions and resulting diseases impacted their patients (this is represented by the red line coming from anthropogenic climate change circle on the left to the climate change diseases box above nursing practice). There were challenges for hospital nurses with an increased case load. Conditions like respiratory infections for young and old patients in 2022–23, numbers of respiratory syncytial virus in young children and young childhood asthma cases increased with climate change and air pollution (Lloyd & Scott, 2022). In addition, serious conditions such as Japanese encephalitis, a mosquito-borne virus, have been seen in Australia for the first time since 1998 (Davey, 2022). Why this disease has reappeared is unclear, but the extended and heavy raining season may have been a contributory factor (World Health Organization, 2022). Melioidosis also occurred after the Queensland floods (Gassiep et al., 2022).

THINK BOX 2.9

Are you familiar with the condition of melioidosis? If not, check it out here: https://www.google.com/search?client=firefox-b-d&q=Melioidosis.

Lack of access to health care facilities due to a serious event related to the degradation of the environment has had devastating outcomes for people, including failure to get emergency treatment because of floods or fires, as widely experienced in recent years in Australia. Primary health care nurses were challenged, as they were unable to undertake their community patient role, as rural and regional areas were cut off for many weeks due to floodwaters. Telehealth services were vital in this situation, and sometimes nurse practitioners, as well as doctors, were flown into the affected areas.

THINK BOX 2.10

Thinking about your own health care facility's GHG emissions:

• What can be implemented in your area to help mitigate (reduce) these gasses?

  Discuss with colleagues to see if you can come up with a plan. Here is a link to a resource that will help you: https://jme.bmj.com/content/medethics/49/3/204.full.pdf.

NURSING EDUCATION

As we face increasing evidence of planetary degradation and its effects on human well-being, it is clear that nurses will have to understand much more about PH, the environment and the notions of *kincentricity*. Nurses are the largest component of the global health care workforce and together can be leaders and change agents in addressing PH. To do this requires that we educate ourselves as well as our communities, clients and patients and that we become more political and influential with policymakers in this arena.

Preservice and continuing education of nurses and midwives should by now include climate change and PH in curricula, and while this is increasingly being seen, it is far from common. The Global Consortium on Climate and Health Education (n.d.), a collaborative of nursing, public health and medical schools that was formed in 2017, is developing interprofessional curricula on climate change and health. Sorensen et al. (2023) have developed core competencies that support the Global Consortium efforts to prepare health professionals to deal with climate change and PH. The competences are organised into five domains, which are as follows:

■ Knowledge and analytical skills of the effects of climate on health and ways to mitigate them.
■ Collaboration and communication in interprofessional teams and with all stakeholders, such as

communities, families, patients and policymakers, to provide education and influence.
■ Policy influencers, which means being able to communicate messages effectively and also being familiar with the political discourse on PH, as well as its socioeconomic impacts.
■ Public health practice, which includes community health assessments to understand vulnerabilities and build resilience.
■ Clinical practice, including preparing for emergencies and helping patients to survive changing conditions, which may be caused by emergencies or occur more slowly through planetary degradation such as climate change. Examples might include helping older people cope with extremes of heat or ensuring that a facility has emergency drugs available.

The core domains can be integrated into health professional education in several ways, including into a degree program or as a foundation for postgraduate courses. If broadly adopted, they may also serve as a convening mechanism to 'facilitate the development of common knowledge, skills, ethics and rhetoric among health professionals globally, thereby enabling more coordinated transdisciplinary action' (Sorensen et al., 2023).

While the PHEF (Fig. 2.1) is comprehensive and appropriate, there are no guidelines on implementation, as it is assumed that all learning contexts will be different. There has already been anecdotal feedback from individuals working within traditional academic spaces that there are challenges in teaching the interconnection within the nature domain, as it is still so alien to traditional learning concepts and curricula, especially for health professionals (Redvers et al., 2023), yet understanding the significance of disconnection from nature is fundamental to understanding why we are at this stage of planetary ill health. Redvers et al. (2023) suggest that educational approaches will have to change to become more effective at teaching this new domain by building on the classic concept of praxis, which they define as 'reflection and action upon the world in order to transform it'. They further suggest that compassion, knowledge and reflection are three essential elements for praxis—and these elements are familiar to all nurses. Nurses could be leading the way in introducing a new style of education that values PH, social justice and *kincentricity*.

The science of PH changes quickly, with new concerns constantly arising. The formal and continuing education of nurses and midwives must keep pace with this rapidly changing picture to include climate change and health matters, especially as they relate to nursing practice (Kurth, 2017). We are all having to find new ways of learning to tackle the interconnected causes and effects of planetary degradation, and these new ways will be disruptive to traditional ways of thinking (Redvers et al., 2022). Such transformative changes in thinking and approaches will need powerful advocates to be adopted; as trusted members of the health team who are familiar with compassion, reflection and knowledge of a curriculum, nurses and midwives are well positioned to raise awareness and be champions for change.

Analysis of critical pathways, which encompass social contexts, SDGs and policy frameworks, to explain the causes of health inequalities is an important approach to address health equity and can be taught. This links with research, too, as learning about measuring and monitoring interventions for impact on determinants of health is vital. This might include consideration of a PH monitoring framework or frameworks to measure climate hazards and the disease conditions they are associated with (Valentine et al., 2022). Valentine et al. go on to suggest that learning pathways should also show how the life course of an individual shapes social determinants and health outcomes and how to find the best entry points and interventions to maintain or improve health and equity. For many nursing education programmes, this approach to considering human health against SDOH and the health of the planet will be disruptive and transformative, and yet, until nursing curricula incorporate much more of the social, economic and environmental aspects of health, nursing will be missing an opportunity to address what is perhaps the most critical issue facing the health of the world today.

PLANETARY HEALTH AND NURSING RESEARCH: WHAT SHOULD WE BE DOING?

Just as a PH perspective requires advancements in nurse education, it also encourages nurse researchers to develop this field further through the study of climate change and implications for nursing practice. Nurses and midwives can contribute to building resilient health care systems based on a PH perspective as part of multidisciplinary teams or within their own practice through investigating the risks inherent in their own practice and within their health facility.

The link between human health and PH is complex given the many interactions between family, community and individuals and between all of those systems and the health care system. Weber (2023) point out the importance of building possible scenarios to reflect the uncertainty in the future of PH, and this is a good way to include teams in considering the impact of practices on the environment. Scenario planning is a tool used in systems thinking and is especially useful when looking at an uncertain future. It can begin with the question 'what if?' which allows some imagination about future events. Ebi et al. used this method to explore the possible impact on health of climate change—which, of course, is uncertain. They used current evidence to look at possible futures, and though this is speculative, it is a valuable method to bring people together to look at the value of change. There are many courses available in systems thinking if you would like to learn more. It is becoming an essential skill for public health (Peters, 2014), and there is more on the benefits of systems thinking to PH later in this chapter.

Ebi et al. (2020) have identified four priority areas for research to promote PH and human well-being. These are:

- Risk identification and management (including that related to water, hygiene, sanitation and waste management; food production and consumption; oceans; and extreme weather events and climate change).
- Strengthening climate-resilient health systems.
- Monitoring, surveillance and evaluation.
- Risk communication.

There are PH risk assessment tools available online through several organisations, notably the national and regional alliances for nurses with an interest in the health of our planet. Some national nursing associations are also beginning to take a stance on PH following the position paper from ICN (International Council of Nurses, 2018), so it is worth asking your local nursing association or even a local university nursing department for help if you want to get involved in research.

THE ROLE OF INDIGENOUS PEOPLE AND PLANETARY HEALTH

In July 2023, the World Health Organization (WHO) held its first ever global workshop on biodiversity, traditional knowledge, health and well-being (World Health Organization, 2023b). Invited were representatives of Indigenous peoples, African descendants, ministries of health and civil society to discuss the traditional knowledge held by Indigenous people, especially as it applies to land management, climate mitigation and adaptation (Redvers et al., 2022).

This chapter has stressed the close links between healthy flourishing and PH, and Indigenous communities often have a deep understanding of their natural surroundings that includes the use of plants for medicine and food and how plant and animal life support nutrition, food security and livelihoods. Closer consideration of what we can learn from Indigenous knowledge and ways of living is therefore valuable (Wilson et al., 2018).

THINK BOX 2.11

- What do you understand by the term 'Indigenous peoples'?
- Where you live and work, are there communities of Indigenous people?
- What do you know about their cultures and knowledge?

Indigenous people are social and cultural groups that share strong ancestral ties to the land on which they live or from which they have been displaced. Their land and its natural resources are closely tied to their spiritual and physical well-being. Our planetary degradation has brought new and serious challenges for Indigenous communities. Think, for example, of deforestation, rising sea levels causing saltwater flooding or wildfires destroying he tracts of land and its biodiversity. The irony of this tragic situation is that Indigenous people contribute least to GHG emissions and other global environmental changes, having such well-established ways of land management.

The WHO inaugural workshop on traditional knowledge relating to improving PH heralds a new interest in the important knowledge held by Indigenous peoples. It should be acknowledged that Indigenous people are not one homogenous group. In fact, globally, 4000 Indigenous languages are spoken (United Nations, 2018) by Indigenous groups, even though they account for only 6% of the global population. It is therefore critically important to recognise each Indigenous community and its practices.

Sadly, what all Indigenous people have in common is a shorter life expectancy than the general population, and they account for 19% of the world's extreme poor (World Bank, 2023). This is often because they have been excluded from their lands through colonialism, and with this exclusion comes a rupture of their traditional ways of living. (See Chapter 6 for an in-depth discussion on decolonising nursing). The World Bank (2023) comments:

"Insecure land tenure is a driver of conflict, environmental degradation, and weak economic and social development. This threatens cultural survival and vital knowledge systems – loss in these areas increasing risks of fragility, biodiversity loss, and degraded One Health (or ecological and animal health) systems which threaten the ecosystem services upon which we all depend."

World Bank (2023)

Indigenous people are skilled managers of natural resources, and it is noted that currently 80% of the world's biodiversity is conserved by Indigenous people (World Bank, 2023). Further, it is now becoming more widely acknowledged that Indigenous communities hold vital ancestral knowledge and expertise on how to adapt, mitigate and reduce climate and disaster risks. The World Bank (Sobrevila, 2008) calls Indigenous people 'the natural but often forgotten partners' in biodiversity conservation.

There is much to learn from the ways of knowing and living practiced by Indigenous people. When, as nurses with a global interest, we think of systems in which people live, it is wise to add these systems to our thinking for the coming years, as we seek 'kincentricity'.

The development of a PH monitoring framework by Indigenous people has been led by Redvers et al. (2022), who used a global Indigenous-centric perspective to ascertain the determinants of PH, working with a diverse group of Indigenous people from many countries. This group identified 10 determinants of PH from their perspective that could be grouped under three domains which are as follows (Redvers et al., 2022, p. 158):

Mother Earth–level determinants

- respect of the feminine
- ancestral legal personhood designation

Interconnecting determinants

- human interconnectedness within nature
- self and community relationships
- the modern scientific paradigm
- governance and law

Indigenous peoples–level determinants

- indigenous land tenure rights
- indigenous languages
- indigenous peoples' health
- indigenous elders and children

The 'respect of the feminine' is of particular interest. It highlights the strength and resilience of the feminine and of females. It resonates with the idea of Mother Earth as the nourisher for all of us. Furthermore, it highlights that females are often discriminated against by patriarchal, political, economic, racial and gender-oppressive systems: there is a lot more about this in Chapter 8 of this book.

The interconnecting determinants speak to much of what we have addressed in this chapter in terms of the interlinking of humans and nature, while Indigenous people's rights are fundamental to equality in health, discussed in this chapter and in Chapter 1.

THINK BOX 2.12

- As we work through this chapter, can you see how so many elements of health, social justice, PH, colonialism and gender are interlinked?
- How does this apply to your country?

BENEFITS OF A SYSTEMS APPROACH TO PLANETARY HEALTH

A systems thinking approach to PH offers a framework in which key dynamic interactions, feedback and unintended consequences across sectors can be observed and understood (Pongsiri et al., 2017). Systems are defined as the set of subcomponents and their interrelationships that 'go together' and interact. In exploring PH in this chapter, we have seen that humans and nature are one system but have become divided into many systems as humans have moved away from close interaction with nature. It is also apparent that there are important feedback loops between system components, and it is critical to maintaining systems that feedback loops are functioning for systems to self-correct and adapt. Clearly, looking at the state of the planet currently, there has been a rupture in the feedback.

Using a systems-based framework to plan for a sustainable, healthy future is of benefit because, as mentioned earlier, scenarios can be modelled and tested to deal with uncertainty. A systems approach to PH involves understanding that human health outcomes emerge from complex interactions between natural and social systems and that there may be unexpected results on health from planetary degradation. A systems approach to PH allows for the identification of nonlinear changes and interactions between environmental stressors through pattern identification rather than simple cause-and-effect research.

WORLD HEALTH ORGANIZATION COMMITMENT FOR THE FUTURE

The World Health Organization Council on the Economics of Health for All, which was convened in 2020, aimed to reframe health for all as a public policy objective and ensure that national and global economies and finance are structured in such a way to deliver on this ambitious goal. The council have just produced their final report (World Health Organization, 2023a) and suggests that if health for all is truly valued, then we should be measuring human and planetary flourishing and investing in improving health systems. One of the recommendations in the report is to: 'restore and protect the environment by upholding international commitments to a regenerative economy which links planet and people' (Raworth, 2017; World Health Organization, 2023a, p. iv). It is clear from the report that the council considered that health, inequality and climate change are deeply connected and that tackling these three issues together is an imperative that should be driving a new focus on health for all economies. What the council said was:

> *The ultimate outcome must be that every person should be able to flourish physically, mentally and emotionally, endowed with the capabilities to lead a life of dignity, opportunity and community, as part of a healthy living planet. This is Health for All.*

Furthermore, the report suggests that we need to restore and protect the environment through a regenerative economy which links the planet and health. A healthy economy will be determined by using core metrics like the Sustainable Development Goals (SDGs) rather than GDP. The need to adopt a comprehensive, stable long-term approach to funding health for equity as well as ensuring an adequate crisis funding response is critical and can only be achieved if Health for All is at the heart of how we design our social and economic systems.

THINK BOX 2.13

- What are the questions that come to mind when considering this WHO Health for All people report?
- Do you think that an economic approach whereby we ensure every person is healthy, rather than using the GDP approach we now have, would be a viable way forward for developing a successful relationship between human health and our planet?
- Who would resist this approach?

There is more on the economics of PH as follows.

This WHO final report echoes the work of Raworth (2017), who provides an economic model for the pursuit of human well-being in the Anthropocene. She states that human well-being is dependent on PH. Raworth's doughnut model (Fig. 2.4) helps to focus attention on addressing inequalities when both theorising and pursuing human well-being, but it also implies the need for a deep renewal of economic theory and policymaking. She replaces the continued widespread political prioritisation of gross domestic product growth with an economic vision that seeks to transform economies, from local to global, so that they become regenerative and distributive by design. Raworth aims to create an effective map of the road ahead, leading us to understand and appreciate the complex interdependence of human well-being and PH (Raworth, 2017).

The doughnut in Fig. 2.4 depicts the two boundaries—social and ecological—that together encompass human well-being. The inner boundary is a social foundation around which 12 dimensions are shown which are necessary for human flourishing. They underpin the SDGs, too. The doughnut's outer boundary is an ecological ceiling of safety, and outside this lies the pressure on Earth's life-supporting systems that we are currently seeing. These include global warming and its sequelae such as climate change, ocean acidification and biodiversity loss. If balance can be sustained between these boundaries, then all of us—humans and all species—will be able to thrive in an ecologically safe and socially just space. Raworth hopes that the doughnut might offer a 21st-century compass to fully appreciate the interdependence of human well-being and PH.

Raworth has suggested elsewhere that doughnut economics (Raworth, 2012) represents economic complexity and, in the way it is pictured here, an attempt to nurture nature rather than dominate it, which, she argues, has been the past economic model. This has resulted in humans using planetary resources to increase income and GDP instead of seeking to care for nature. She strongly suggests that economics of 21st century should:

- Aim to meet the needs of all people within the means of the living planet.
- See the big picture.
- Nurture human nature.
- Think in systems.
- Be distributive in other words focus on social justice.
- Be regenerative, not destructive.
- Aim to thrive rather than to grow.

One example of new economics, such as suggested by Raworth, is using incentives to drive more sustainable choices. If biodiverse forests are lost, then human health and well-being are affected by climate change. Lost primary forests in tropical areas are difficult to recover. Preserving forests through payment to plant and maintain them could be a way forward in the short term, though in the longer term, it would be too expensive and requires great understanding of the

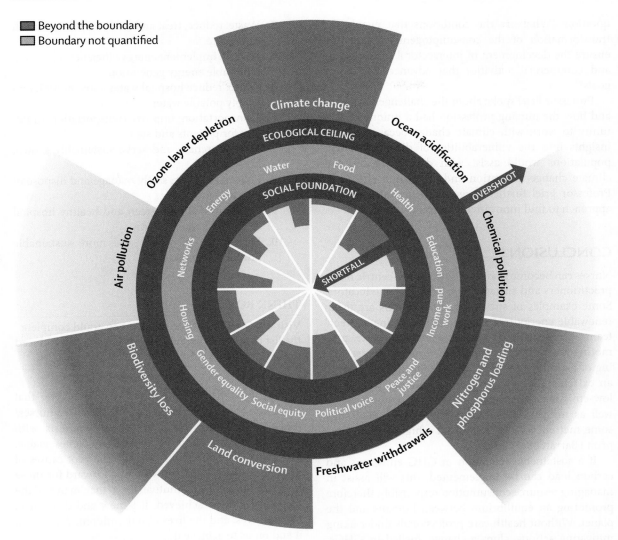

- Beyond the boundary
- Boundary not quantified

Fig. 2.4 ■ The doughnut model. From Raworth, K. A. (2017). Doughnut for the Anthropocene: Humanity's compass in the 21st century. *The Lancet, 1*(2), E48–E49. https://doi.org/10.1016/S2542-5196(17)30028-1.

social, cultural and economic incentives can be shaped to drive more sustainable systems and choices (The Lancet Planetary Health, 2023).

THINK BOX 2.14

Think of all the biodiverse forest land that has been lost in the Amazon.

- How do you think we should go about preserving forests?
- What would work in this global world?

PLANETARY HEALTH EQUITY IN AUSTRALIA

In 2022, Professor Sharon Friel from the Australian National University (ANU) launched Planetary Health Equity, an initiative of the Australian Research Council (ARC) called the Hothouse (Australian National University, 2023). This is an interdisciplinary initiative focusing on a rising public health burden, social inequality and climate change, and it aims to provide a roadmap to PH equity by looking for answers to the question: 'What are the conditions that enable the transformation of the consumptogenic system and ensure the development of intersectoral public policy and commercial activities that advance PH equity goals?'

Professor Friel spoke about the challenge for nurses and how the nursing profession had a unique opportunity to work with climate change because nurses' insights into the vulnerabilities of different patient populations would assist with developing targeted climate change mitigation and adaptation strategies. Professor Friel further suggested a multidisciplinary approach to find innovative solutions.

CONCLUSION

Nurses can become leaders as sustainable-centric nurse practitioners and sustainable-centric nurse educators. Some examples of such mitigating actions are using renewable energy (solar generated), starting a 'green' team and focusing on recycling hospital waste, promoting low carbon health care by limiting overservicing of pathology tests and MRI scans, which produce an extremely large carbon footprint, and promoting low-emissions alternative anaesthetic equipment as well as mitigating asthmatic medication agents like some metred-dose inhalers with a high carbon footprint (Barratt et al., 2022).

If a sustainable reduction in GHG emissions and carbon load can be implemented, this will assist in managing resource consumption responsibly, therefore promoting an equilibrium between humans and the planet. Without health care professionals undertaking mitigating actions, climate change, fuelled by GHGs, will continue to affect our global weather, creating further adverse events such as floods, fires, extreme heat and drought.

It is vital for PH that all nurses are knowledgeable about and practice sustainable-centric health care. There is much in this chapter to help you on your way, and you can learn more practical steps from the Global Green and Healthy Hospitals (GGHH) website (Global Green and Healthy Hospitals, n.d.).

GGHH promotes 10 goals for hospitals:
1. Leadership: prioritise environmental health
2. Chemicals: substitute harmful chemicals with safer alternatives
3. Waste: reduce, treat and safely dispose of health care waste
4. Energy: implement energy efficiency and clean, renewable energy generation
5. Water: reduce hospital water consumption and supply potable water
6. Transportation: improve transportation strategies for patients and staff
7. Food: purchase and serve sustainably grown, healthy food
8. Pharmaceuticals: safely manage and dispose of pharmaceuticals
9. Buildings: support green and healthy hospital design and construction
10. Purchasing: buy safer and more sustainable products and materials

THINK BOX 2.15

Visit the GGHH website to see if you could complete the list of goals. What documents have been produced to support these goals?

It is unequivocally portrayed in this chapter that education about, and practice of, PH will assist nurses/midwives to reach the state when symbiosis with nature is possible and *kincentricity* becomes viable. The chapter has discussed some of the root causes of disruptions to PH and shown a way forward for those interested in achieving mutualism so that 'man and the biosphere' can be achieved. It is new and disruptive, but our lives, and the lives of our children, depend on it and on us to achieve it.

ADDITIONAL READINGS

https://www.cfr.org/timeline/ecological-disasters.
https://www.healthandenvironment.org/our-work/publications/.
https://onlinelibrary.wiley.com/doi/10.1111/ddi.13265.
https://www.coursera.org/articles/health-economics.
https://www.bmj.com/content/314/7091/1409.full.
https://www.weforum.org/agenda/2016/04/five-measures-of-growth-that-are-better-than-gdp.
https://www.theworldcounts.com/stories/how-can-we-stop-deforestation.
https://www.aljazeera.com/opinions/2014/12/12/keep-the-forests-standing-for-people-and-the-planet.

FURTHER QUESTIONS FOR REFLECTION AND LINKS TO HELP STUDY

1. Does your health care organisation work in an interdisciplinary fashion?
https://www.ncbi.nlm.nih.gov/pmc/articles/PMC7261256/.
https://www.pnas.org/doi/10.1073/pnas.1803726115.
https://www.researchgate.net/publication/315541531_Interdisciplinarity_Practical_approach_to_advancing_education_for_sustainability_and_for_the_Sustainable_Development_Goals.
2. How easily can vulnerable patient populations be reached in the event of an emergency climate event?
https://www.hhs.gov/climate-change-health-equity-environmental-justice/climate-change-health-equity/health-sector-resource-hub/referral-guide/index.html.
https://www1.racgp.org.au/ajgp/2020/august/responding-to-the-climate-health-emergency.
https://www.google.com/search?client=firefox-b-d&q=How±easily±can±vulnerable±patient±populations±be±reached±in±the±event±of±an±emergency±climate±event.
3. Can we educate patients and their families on the negative health consequences of climate change?
https://www.health.vic.gov.au/health-strategies/tackling-climate-change-and-its-impact-on-health.
https://noharm-uscanada.org/content/us-canada/climate-and-health-patient-education.
4. How might climate change impact our practice and those we work with?
https://oxfordre.com/publichealth/display/10.1093/acrefore/9780190632366.001.0001/acrefore-9780190632366-e-39;jsessionid=2FB712477DFCD198E15073C7DA38451E.
https://www.ncbi.nlm.nih.gov/pmc/articles/PMC9564616/.

REFERENCES

Alvarez-Nieto, C., Richardson, J., Angeles Navarro-Peran, M., Tutticci, N., Huss, N., Elf, M., Anåker, A., Aronsson, J., Baid, H., & Lopez-Medina, I. M. (2022). Nursing students' attitudes towards climate change and sustainability: A cross-sectional multisite study. *Nurse Education Today, 108*, 105185. https://doi.org/10.1016/j.nedt.2021.105185.

Asaduzzaman, M., Ara, R., Afrin, S., Meiring, J. E., & Saif-Ur-Rahman, K. M. (2022). Planetary health education and capacity building for healthcare professionals in a global context: Current opportunities, gaps and future directions. *International Journal of Environmental Research and Public Health, 19*, 11786. https://doi.org/10.3390/ijerph1911811786.

Astle, B., Cipriano, P., LeClair, J., Luebke, J., Potter, T., Honegger Rogers, H., & Sheppard, D.-A. (2023, July 1-5). Nursing for planetary health and well-being. [Conference Symposium presentation]. *2023 Congress of the International Council of Nurses, Montreal, Canada.*

Australian National University. (2023). *Planetary health equity hothouse.* Retrieved from https://hothouse.anu.edu.au.

Australian Nursing and Midwifery Federation. (n.d.). *Climate Change.* Retrieved from https://www.anmf.org.au/professional/professional-issues/climate-change.

Barratt, A. L., Bell, K. J. L., Charlesworth, K., & McGain, F. (2022). High value health care is low carbon health care. *Medical Journal of Australia, 216*(2), 67–68. https://.org/10.5694/mja2.51331.

Charlesworth, K., Stewart, G., & Sainsbury, P. (2018). Addressing the carbon footprint of health organisations: Eight lessons for implementation. *Public Health Research and Practice, 28*(4), 1–5. https://doi.org/10.17061/phrp2841830.

Council on Foreign Relations. (2023). *1912-2020 Ecological Disasters.* Retrieved from https://www.cfr.org/timeline/ecological-disasters.

Cruz, J. P., Felicilda-Reynaldo, R. F. D., Alshammari, F., Alquwez, N., Alicante, J. G., Obaid, K. B., Rady, H. E. A. E. A., Qtait, M., & Silang, J. P. B. T. (2018). Factors influencing Arab Nursing Students' Attitudes toward climate change and environmental sustainability and their inclusion in nursing curricula. *Public Health Nursing, 35*(6), 598–605. https://doi.org/10.1111/phn.12516.

Davey, M. (2022). Floods and warm weather perfect storm for Japanese encephalitis outbreak, researchers warn. *The Guardian.* https://www.theguardian.com/australia-news/2022/oct/20/floods-and-warm-weather-perfect-storm-for-japanese-encephalitis-outbreak-in-australia-researchers-warn.

Ebi, K. L. & Hess, J. J. (2020). Health risks due to climate change: Inequity in causes and consequences. *Health Affairs, 39*(12), 2056–2062. https://doi.org/10.1377/hlthaff.2020.01125.

Editorial. (2023). Preserving forests means culture change. Retrieved from https://www.thelancet.com/planetaryhealth.

Faerron Guzman, C. A., & Potter, T. (Eds.). (2021). *The planetary health education framework.* Planetary health Alliance. https://drive.google.com/file/d/1mFCa7gvoH5ekijzc6ffAvwzi5walOl93/view.

Faerron Guzman, C. A., Aguirre, A. A., Astle, B., Barros, E., Bayles, B. F., Chimbari, M., El-Abbadi, N., Evert, J., Hackett, F., Howard, C., Jennings, J., Krzyzek, A., LeClair, J., Maric, F., Martin, O., Osano, O., Patz, J., Potter, T., Redvers, N., … Zylstra M. (2021). *A framework to guide planetary health education.* The Lancet Planetary Health, Elsevier.

Gassiep, I., Ganeshalingam, V., Chatfield, M. D., Harris, P. N. A., & Norton, R. E. (2022). The epidemiology of melioidosis in Townsville, Australia. *Transactions of the Royal Society of Tropical Medicine and Hygiene, 116*(4), 328–335. https://doi.org/10.1093/trstmh/trab125.

Global Consortium on Climate and Health Education. (n.d.). *Global Consortium on Climate and Health Education.* https://www.publichealth.columbia.edu/research/centers/global-consortium-climate-health-education.

Global Green and Healthy Hospitals (GGHH). (n.d.). A Comprehensive Environmental Health Agenda for Hospitals and Health. https://greenhospitals.org/sites/default/files/2021-09/Global-Green-and-Healthy-Hospitals-Agenda_3.pdf.

Hancock, T. (2021). The IUHPE's Global Working Group on Waiora Planetary health: Towards healthy One Planet cities and communities: planetary health promotion at the local level. *Health Promotion International, 36*(1), i53–i63. https://doi.org/10.1093/heapro/daab120.

Hannam, P. (2022). *Bureau of Meteorology declares third La Niña is officially under way for Australia.* Retrieved from https://www.theguardian.com/australia-news/2022/sep/13bureau-of-meteorology-to-declare-thrid-la-nina-is-under-way-for-australia.

Health Care Without Harm & Arup. (2019). Health care's climate footprint: How the health sector contributes. Retrieved from https://noharm-us-canada.org/ClimateFootprintReport

Hospedales, J. (2021). Caring for the earth for better health and well-being for all: Addressing climate change as a planetary health emergency. *Christian Journal for Global Health, 8*(1), 3–7. https://doi.org/10.15566/cjgh.v8i1.575.

International Council of Nurses. (2018). *Nurses, climate change and health position statement.* Retrieved from https://www.icn.ch/sites/default/files/PS_E_Nurses_climate%20change_health_0.pdf. (Accessed April19, 2022).

International Council of Nurses. (2021). International Council of Ethics for Nurses: Revised 2021. https://www.icn.ch/node/1401.

Kalogirou, M., Dahike, S., Davidson, S., & Yamamoto, S. (2020). Nurses' perspectives on climate change, health and nursing practice. *Journal of Clinical Nursing, 29*(23-24), 4759–4768. https://doi.org/10.1111/jocn.15519.

Knox, B., Ladiges, P., Evans, B., & Saint, R. (2006). *Biology: An Australian Focus* (3rd ed.). McGraw-Hill.

Kurth, A. E. (2017). Planetary health and the role of nursing: A call to action. *Journal of Nursing Scholarship, 49*(6), 598–605. https://doi.org/10.1111/jnu.12343.

Lancet Planetary Health Editorial. (2023). *Preserving forests means culture change, (7)*5, e346. https://doi.org/10.1016/S2542-5196(23)00085-2.

Lewis, T., Moxham, L., Broadbent, M., & Fleming, R. (2018). *Becoming a climate-friendly hospital: Implications for nursing practice within the Australian healthcare context.* [Doctoral thesis. University of Wollongong, NSW].

Lewis. (2023). Figure. Agents of change: Sustainable-centric healthcare vs. traditional practice. 19th National Nurse Education Conference, 7-9 June (2023). Gold Coast, Queensland. https://az659834.vo.msecnd.net/eventsairaueprod/production-dcconferences-public/5447ec181a1746c9aac9a6e4041b1e91.

Lloyd, M., & Scott, S. (2022). Doctors plead for help as respiratory infections rise in Australia, putting young children at risk. *ABC News.* Retrieved from https://www.abc.net.au/news/2022-07-12/respiratory-infections-rise-young-children/101210778.

Longenecker, C. O., & Longenecker, P. D. (2014). Why hospital improvement efforts fail: A view from the front line. *Journal of Healthcare Management, 59*(2), 147–157. Health Center for Biotechnology Information. Retrieved from. https://pubmed.ncbi.nlm.nih.gov/24783373/.

Luschkova, D., Traidl-Hoffmann, C., & Ludwig, A. (2022). Climate change and allergies. *Allergo Journal International, 31*, 114–120. https://doi.org/10.1007/s40629-022-00212-x.

Noosa Biosphere Reserve. (n.d.). *Noosa Biosphere Reserve – A celebration of community and environment.* Retrieved from https://noosabiosphere.org.au/.

Ombudsman New South Wales. (2022). *2020 Hindsight: the first 12 months of the COVID-19 pandemic. A special report under section 31 of the Ombudsman Act 1974,* (22 March 2021). Retrieved from https://www.ombo.nsw.gov.au/Find-a-publication/publications/reports-to-parliament/other-special-reports/2020-hindsight-the-first-12-months-of-the-covid-19-pandemic.

Parliament of Australia. (2023). *Constitution Alteration (Aboriginal and Torres Strait Islander Voice).* 2023. Retrieved from https://www.aph.gov.au/Parliamentary_Business/Bills_Legislation/Bills_Search_Results/Result?bId=r7019

Peters, D. H. (2014). The application of systems thinking in health: why use systems thinking? *Health Res Policy Sys, 12*, 51. https://doi.org/10.1186/1478-4505-12-51.

Planetary Health Alliance. (2021). *São Paulo Declaration on Planetary health.* Planetary health Alliance. Retrieved from https://www.planetaryhealthalliance.org/sao-paulo-declaration.

Planetary Health Alliance. (n.d.-a). Our health depends on our environment. Retrieved from https://www.planetaryhealthalliance.org/home-page.

Planetary Health Alliance. (n.d.-b). Planetary health. Retrieved from https://www.planetaryhealthalliance.org/planetary-health.

Planetary Health Alliance. (n.d.-c). The constellation project. Retrieved from https://www.planetaryhealthalliance.org/the-constellation-project.

Pongsiri, M. J., Gatzweiler, F. W., Bassi, A. M., Haines, A., & Demassieux, F. (2017). The need for a Systems Approach to Planetary health. *The Lancet, 1*(7), e257–e259. https://doi.org/10.1016/S2542-5196(17)30116-X.

Raworth K. A. (2012). A Safe and Just Space for Humanity. Can we live within the doughnut? Oxfam Discussion Paper. https://www-cdn.oxfam.org/s3fs-public/file_attachments/dp-a-safe-and-just-space-for-humanity-130212-en_5.pdf.

Raworth, K. A. (2017). Doughnut for the Anthropocene: humanity's compass in the 21st century. *The Lancet, 1*(2), E48–E49. https://doi.org/10.1016/S2542-5196(17)30028-1.

Redvers, N., Celiwen, Y., Schultz, C., Horn, O., Githaiga, C., Vera, M., Perdrisat, M., Mad Plume, L., Kobei, D., Cunningham Kain, M., Poelina, A., Rojas, J. N., & Blondin, B. (2022). The determinants of planetary health: An Indigenous consensus perspective. *The Lancet, 6*, e156–e163. https://www.thelancet.com/planetary-health.

Redvers, N., Guzman, C. A. F., & Parkes, M. W. (2023). Towards an educational praxis for planetary health: A call for transformative, inclusive, and integrative approaches for learning and relearning in the Anthropocene. *The Lancet. Planetary Health, 7*(1), e77–e85. https://doi.org/10.1016/S2542-5196(22)00332-1.

Richardson, J. (2017). NurSus TOOLKIT: A teaching and learning resource for sustainability in nursing and healthcare. https://www.plymouth.ac.uk.

Ro, C. (2020). *The hidden impact of your daily water use.* Retrieved from https://www.bbc.com/future/article/20200326-the-hidden-impact-of-your-daily-wateruse#:~:text=The%20energy%20needed%20to%20move,the%20nation's%20overall%20carbon%20emissions.

Roden. (2023). Figure. Australian nursing practice and its relationship with planetary health and sustainable healthcare knowledge. Presented at the 19th National Nurse Education Conference, 7-9 June 2023. Gold Coast, Queensland. https://az659834.vo.msecnd.net/eventsairaueprod/production-dcconferences-public/5447ec181a1746c9aac9a6e4041b1e91.

Roden, J. E., & Lewis, T. M. A. (2023). Sustainable-centric health care model for healthcare educators. 19th National Nurse Education Conference, 7-9 June 2023. The exhibition centre, Gold Coast, Queensland Retrieved from https://az659834.vo.msecnd.net/eventsairaueprod/production-dcconferences-public/5447ec181a1746c9aac9a6e4041b1e91.

Sobrevila, C. (2008). *The role of indigenous peoples in biodiversity conservation: the natural but often forgotten partners (English).*

Washington, D.C.: World Bank Group. http://documents. worldbank.org/curated/en/995271468177530126/The-role-of-indigenous-peoples-in-biodiversity-conservation-the-natural-but-often-forgotten-partners.

Sorenson, C., Campbell, H., Depoux, A., Finkel, M., Gilden, R., Hadley, K., Haine, D., Mantilla, G., McDermott-Levy, R., Potter, T. M., Sack, T. L., Tun, S., & Wellbery, C. (2023). Core competencies to prepare health professionals to respond to the climate crisis. *PLOS CLIMATE*. https://doi.org/10.1371/journal.pclm.0000230.

Systems Around the World https://greenhospitals.org/sites/default/files/2021-09/Global-Green-and-Healthy-Hospitals-Agenda_3.pdf.

The Lancet Planetary Health. (2023). Preserving forests means culture change. Vol. 7 May. https://www.thelancet.com/journals/lan-plh/article/PIIS2542-5196(23)00085-2/fulltext.

Topf, M. (2005). Psychological explanations and interventions for indifference to greening hospitals. *Health Care Management Review*, *30*(1), 2–8. https://doi.org/10.1097/00004010-200501-00002.

United Nations. (2018). United Nations permanent forum on indigenous issues. Indigenous Languages. https://www.un.org/development/desa/indigenouspeoples/wp-content/uploads/sites/19/2018/04/Indigenous-Languages.pdf.

United Nations. (2023). The 17 Goals. Retrieved from https://sdgs.un.org/goals.

Valentine, N., Ajuebor, O., Fisher, J., Bodenmann, P., Baum, F., & Rasanathan, K. (2022). Planetary health benefits from strengthening health workforce education on the social determinants of health. *Health Promotion International*, *37*, 1–7. https://doi.org/10.1093/heapro/daac086.

Watts, N., Amann, M., Arnell, N. A., Aveb-Karlsson, S., Belesova, K., Berry, H, & Costello, A. (2018). The 2018 report of the Lancet Countdown on health and climate change: Shaping the health of nations for centuries to come. *The Lancet, 392*, 2479–2514. https://dx.doi.org/10.1016/S0140-6736(18)32594-7.

Weber, E., Downward, G. S., Ebi, K.l., Lucas, P. L. & van Vuuren, D. (2023). The use of environmental scenarios to project future health effects: a scoping review. *The Lancet. Planetary Health, 7*(7), e611–e621. https://doi.org/10.1016/S2542-5196(23)00110-9.

Whitmee, S., Haines, A., Beyrer, C., et al. (2015). Safeguarding human health in the Anthropocene epoch: report of The Rockefeller Foundation–*Lancet* Commission on planetary health. *The Lancet, 386*(10007), 1973–2028. Retrieved from https://www.thelancet.com/journals/lancet/article/PIIS0140-6736(15)60901-1/fulltext.

Wilson, M., Gathorne-Hardy, A., Alexander, P., & Boden, L. (2018). Why "Culture" matters for Planetary health. Comment. *The Lancet, 2*(11), E467–E468. https://doi.org/10.1016/S2542-5196(18)30205-5.

World Bank. (2023). Indigenous Peoples. Understanding Poverty. https://www.worldbank.org/en/topic/indigenouspeoples#:~:text=There%20are%20an%20estimated%20476%20million%20Indigenous%20Peoples%20worldwide.

World Health Organization. (2022). *Global Competency Framework for Universal Health Coverage*. Retrieved from https://apps.who.int/iris/rest/bitstreams/1415843/retrieve.

World Health Organization. (2023a). *Health for All: Transforming economies to deliver what matters. Final Report*. Retrieved from https://cdn.who.int/media/docs/default-source/council-on-the-economics-of-health-for-all/council-eh4a_finalreport_web.pdf?sfvrsn=a6505c22_5&download=true.

World Health Organization. (2023b). *WHO to host first global workshop on biodiversity, traditional knowledge, health and well-being*. https://www.who.int/news/item/25-07-2023-who-to-host-first-global-workshop-on-biodiversity–traditional-knowledge–health-and-well-being.

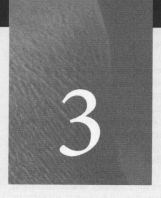

3

GLOBALISATION AND NURSING

CHERYL JONES ■ GILLIAN ADYNSKI ■ BARBARA STILWELL

INTRODUCTION

Globalisation is a word that might scare you. It is rightly associated with economics, finance, trade and development as well as politics and policies. But do consider engaging with this chapter because at no other time in recent memory has the nursing workforce been more affected by globalisation than now. Since late 2019 and early 2020, COVID-19 has changed our world, including health care, as it spread globally and mutated into different variants (five at the time of this writing) that impacted the health of countries and societies. Governments and health care organisations rushed to develop treatment options and vaccines and to secure essential supplies such as protective personal equipment, drugs and health workers. There were dramatic shifts in care delivery and work environments for the health workforce, and nurses, in particular, were thrust into the spotlight as they responded to the global pandemic. Of course, the pandemic was a particular and extreme example of how our connected world impacts health and health systems and thus nursing. However, anyone with an interest in global health must seek to understand globalisation because, although less dramatic, its effects are important for the development of our profession. In this chapter, we explore factors inherent in globalisation that shape not only our health and health systems but also the nursing workforce.

THINK BOX 3.1

- How did the COVID-19 pandemic make you more aware of global issues related to health care?
- How did you make new global connections during that time (for example, through webinars, Nursing Now or joining online communities)?

DEFINING GLOBALISATION

Globalisation is the process through which people and nations become increasingly interconnected and interdependent through the integration of economies, global communication and a variety of mechanisms for cultural exchange (Azevedo & Johnson, 2011). Globalisation comes about through the opening of borders to increase flows of goods, services, finance, people and ideas across borders and the institutional and policy regimes that support such flows, leading to our modern interconnected world (Kavinya, 2014). The term 'globalisation' became more common in the 1980s following the Cold War[1] through narratives that urged greater connectivity between nations, rather than a focus on ideological difference. The term 'global village' (Öncü, 2018) became popular at around the same time, reflecting the realisation that there is interconnection and interdependence between countries and, without this understanding, global and national systems will not function. Today, the flow of goods, capital and services across borders totals USD $1.5 trillion worth of transactions daily (Azevedo & Johnson, 2011). However, globalisation is more than just the formation of a global economy. It also involves integration of transnational structures of culture, economies, environment, politics, religion, morals, art, education and social aspects of the world (Öncü, 2018; Rennen & Martens, 2003), and all of these factors impact health (Öncü, 2018). Globalisation has pros and cons for the well-being of global citizens (Kavinya, 2014). For example, globalisation

---

[1] The Cold War commonly refers to the American-Soviet Cold War of 1947–1991, where there was no physical conflict but a lack of collaboration and cooperation between the countries.

can be a mechanism for disseminating best practices and technologies that could help to eradicate diseases and build knowledge in health care and for health care professions, which are knowledge driven in their development (Azevedo & Johnson, 2011). But globalisation can also be blamed for increasing inequalities between the global north and south, exacerbating global warming, increasing consumption trends, decreasing biodiversity and impacting wars and conflicts, all of which threaten global health (Öncü, 2018).

THINK BOX 3.2

- Is this definition of globalisation what you expected?
- Why or why not?
- How have you been affected positively or negatively by globalisation?

WHY NURSES SHOULD BE INFORMED ABOUT GLOBALISATION

Nursing, in all its aspects—nursing practice, health care delivery, nursing knowledge development and nursing education—is not exempt from the impacts of globalisation (Ergin & Akin, 2017; Salvage & White, 2020). Nurses are the largest group of health workers worldwide, making them integral components of all health and welfare systems that are strongly impacted by globalisation today (Zarshenas et al., 2017). For this reason, it is imperative that nurses appreciate their roles and actual or potential impact in the modern globalised world (Lee et al., 2018). To be effective leaders in health care, nurses must understand not only patient care but the wider issues that have an impact on global lives: environmental changes and policies, especially the effect on diseases; human migration as it relates to the health of all people and the need for health professionals; economics as it pertains to the allocation of scarce resources; health policy, global health governance and their health effects worldwide; information technology and artificial intelligence as the sharing of information (despite the degree of accuracy) spreads quickly; and social justice and health equity as individuals and groups attempt to bring parity to our world (Lee et al., 2018). These are vast areas to understand, yet unless nurses are willing to become involved with global issues, the profession is likely to be blindsided by the increasingly rapid pace of change in our globalised world.

This chapter lays the groundwork for this book, which seeks to address all of these issues related to globalisation. Each subject may not be dealt with exhaustively, but all are introduced for further consideration and with pointers to the ways in which nurses and nursing are likely to be affected.

THINK BOX 3.3

As you use this book, start discussions with colleagues, friends and family about their thoughts on our world.
- What has been impacting the people you talk to?
- Climate?
- The rapid spread of diseases?
- Migration?
  Be sure to talk to older people and find out how life has changed for them over the last decades.

GLOBALISATION AND ECONOMICS

Economic news can be bewildering as interest and exchange rates change, banks crash, share prices fluctuate and the economic effects of the pandemic play out in shortages from interrupted supply chains, higher prices for food and medicines and closures of many businesses. The global interconnectedness of systems means that economics must also have a global perspective. The word 'economics' comes from an ancient Greek word meaning 'household management'. Now, in our 'global village', it encompasses much more, although the building blocks of household and individual spending and choices remain influential. Economics is about the allocation of scarce resources and the science of making choices; it is built on the notion that individuals, groups and societies make choices using rational human behaviour. That is, people make choices based on the decision that offers the best payoff for them—the item, activity and purchase that best meets their needs at an acceptable quality and price.

THINK BOX 3.4

- Consider the last time you bought something significant—a car, house, holiday, coat, large food order—how did you decide what to buy?
- Were you entirely rational in your choice?

Of course, not all choices are based on a cold reality check. People are capricious and emotional, and the science of behavioural economics, which integrates behavioural science with economics, has proliferated in the last decade (Geiger, 2017). Behavioural economics assumes irrationality in decision-making and acknowledges that people make poor decisions at times. For example, people may live for the moment and discount (or care less about) the future, and so, instead of saving for a pension, they will spend everything they earn on great holidays. Most pertinent to nursing work is the way that people seeking health care make health choices. Some people choose to continue smoking or taking drugs even though there is much evidence that these behaviours are unhealthy. Consider how hard it is for people to lose weight and choose healthy eating options. Sometimes this is related to cost, but not always; emotions, habits, availability, culture and peer pressure may all play a role in the health choices people make (Carminati, 2020). Behavioural economics has identified a phenomenon called 'present-biased preference', which describes a failure to take into account future rewards, preferring to look only at the present. This bias helps to explain many health behaviours, including those that impact planetary health, such as driving or flying. For most people, thinking of the distant future impact of current decisions or behaviours is difficult.

Opportunity Cost

Most of us think of the cost of buying or doing something as the resources we spend on it. For example, the cost of going to university could be the tuition, plus expenses—accommodation, food, books and so on. Economists also consider what is called opportunity cost, which means the costs or resources given up by choosing one course of action over another. For example, when thinking about going to university, the other choice given up might be getting a job. The opportunity cost of this choice is foregoing the earnings from a job instead of investing resources in becoming a student. Choosing one option usually means not choosing another. In health care, we see this play out in how governments allocate funding. For example, there is an opportunity cost associated with investing predominantly in acute care rather than improving primary health care. What is the opportunity cost associated with this decision?

The concept of opportunity cost helps to determine if resources are being put to best use, particularly when aligned to the value put on choices. If the goal of a national health system is to provide access to equitable, high-quality care and responsiveness to environment changes, then choosing investment options that move towards this goal would seem to make sense, yet this is a situation where choices are not always made rationally. For example, political interests may dominate so that high-visibility results, such as number of surgeries done, are seen as more important than long-term but less immediate or visible goals, such as improving equity of access to care. This is where economics links to power and politics: resources are not evenly distributed among a population, nor among nations, and neither is power. Individuals may be powerful because they were born to a powerful family (for example, royalty), or they may have access to better education or simply be wealthy. Some occupations are seen as more powerful than others and being of a certain race, family background, religion or ethnic group can either positively or negatively impact one's ability to succeed. Those with power have advantages that perpetuate their power, so receiving a good school education might make it more likely that the individual will be accepted into a good university educational program and then get a good job (Espinoza & Speckesser, 2022).

Richer nations—that is, those that have more resources—are more powerful than poorer nations, even in the allocation of their own resources (through aid programmes) to poorer nations, and nations that have a wealth of resources, such as oil or diamonds, may not distribute their wealth to their people. This all plays out in inequalities in health among people within and between countries. It is important to note in a book on global health that poverty affects the social determinants of health which then affect every aspect of our lives and our health. There is more on the social determinants of health later in this chapter and in several other chapters in this book; this is a thread that links many aspects of global health.

VALUE-BASED HEALTH CARE

Like it or not, economics has become the dominant language of our times. We all want value—that is, the best quality for the money spent—in every aspect of our lives. Everywhere, even in—and some would say, especially in—health care, we now have customers and service providers as well as competition for resources. There is pressure on managers in health systems to use resources efficiently as health care becomes ever more costly to deliver. We want value for money in health care, and yet decisions related to caring for people cannot always be based solely on clinical evidence nor on the most efficient way of using resources. There are always opportunity costs associated with making choices, even in health care.

The term 'value-based health care' is commonly in use now, although definitions vary. Value in health care means improving the patient's health outcomes measured against the cost of doing so (Teisberg et al., 2020), but focusing only on funds spent on each patient's care does not take into account how the available resources are allocated across the whole population, which, in some health systems, like that in the United Kingdom, is important for social justice, as the system is funded through taxation (Hurst et al., 2019). Teisberg et al. suggested that value should encompass what matters most to patients rather than solely the technical aspects of treatment, and this certainly aligns more closely with the goals of nursing practice.

THINK BOX 3.5

- Why do you think it is important for nurses to understand value-based health care?
- How might nurses be involved in providing and ensuring value-based health care?

The demand for health care is driven by changing population demographics, with ageing populations in many countries, new treatments and technologies that become available, changing patient expectations as people become better informed about health care by using internet-based information and an increase in multimorbidity (Hurst et al., 2019). The challenges in funding health systems are ubiquitous, with all countries, no matter their wealth, struggling to keep up with demand. In addition, there are enormous variations in health outcomes between countries, populations and even neighbourhoods, some explained by poverty and underlying social determinants.

The imperative to seek value in health care by looking not only at inputs but, more significantly, at what those inputs produce is justified by the variations in health outcomes that are seen globally, as well as the amount of national funding that goes into health systems in every country, often with little attention paid to what outcomes are produced because outcomes are difficult to measure (Veillard et al., 2015). In health care, what has traditionally been funded is the volume of patients or operations, and fees are paid for procedures and prescriptions rather than good outcomes. Health care is expensive everywhere, but what gets paid for is, in fact, curing sickness rather than creating healthy communities, families and individuals. It is important, of course, that a society can offer treatment for illness, but there is so much that could be invested in for health: good housing, green spaces, a healthier environment, food that keeps us active, safe exercise like walking and biking, access to a gym, early education opportunities—the list is long (Crisp, 2020). This is why nurses everywhere should know about opportunity costs and promoting value-based health care—there are costs and quality outcomes at the societal level associated with what we do and do not choose at a policy level.

An important reason for nurses to learn about health economics, cost savings and value inherent in having a healthier, happier society (and the choices that must be made for different investments in health) is that nurses are pivotal to the changes that need to happen to achieve these goals. Like it or not, nurses are part of the politics of health: we must be informed and understand where our power lies, and we must use our power to bring about change in our world.

POWER AND GLOBAL HEALTH GOVERNANCE

In a modern globalised world, political, economic and social power at an international level affects the health, well-being and daily lives of people everywhere. This happens because the forces that drive globalisation, such as technology, economies and politics, also impact nations and individuals, sometimes directly and sometimes as a downstream effect. One recent example from the United Kingdom concerned the flow of nurses from the European Economic Area (EEA) to the United Kingdom, which was interrupted when the United Kingdom signalled it would leave the EEA—the so-called Brexit referendum, which was held in 2016. A year after the referendum, the number of EEA nurses joining the Nursing and Midwifery Council register had dropped from 6400 in 2016–2017 to 800 in 2017–2018 (Carvalho, 2021; The Health Foundation, 2023). In 2019, nearly 5000 EEA-trained nurses and midwives had left the NHS over a period of 2 years, with 51% claiming that Brexit was the contributing factor. The political alliances that had forged an economic and political link between the United Kingdom and the EEA had profoundly affected the NHS workforce, and the delinking of the two also had a profound effect.

Now, the United Kingdom is a less attractive destination for EEA health professionals, so the United Kingdom is recruiting from other countries. Buchan (2023) has pointed out that in the 6 months to September 2022, more than 2200 (20%) of new international nurses came to the United Kingdom from Nigeria and Ghana. Both Nigeria and Ghana are at risk of damage to the functioning of their health systems if their workforces are depleted too heavily—even though there might be considerable benefit to migrant nurses from these countries in terms of better pay or educational opportunities.

Migration of nurses is not new (see Chapter 9 for more detailed information), but it results in winners and losers, and, in an attempt to manage migration, the World Health Organization (WHO) (World Health Organization, 2021) has developed a code of practice that seeks to strengthen the understanding and ethical management of international health personnel recruitment through improved data, information and international cooperation. But the code of practice is not legally binding, and individuals are still free to move around the world, constrained by the availability of visas to work and health systems to recognise qualifications from other countries.

Nursing has become a globally sourced profession, with nurses recruited from many countries, and it is managed by the demands of health systems (recruitment), the inability of some health systems to keep nurses in the workforce (retention) and the issuing of visas, which is how many countries control who can enter and who can stay. Migration is one example

of global border flows and, to some extent, trade, as money follows the migrant worker in terms of contributing to another economy and, for nursing, to the health of the nation, and money flows from the migrant worker back to their family at home. It shows how individual behaviour may be shaped by global policies on trade (ease of workforce flows across borders) and how national policies on investment in health systems will affect the nature of the nursing workforce by encouraging retention or relying on overseas recruitment. It is clear, looking at the example of migration, that richer countries have an advantage in these flows, and this advantage continues beyond migration into purchasing power in world markets. Richer countries can usually buy more and better commodities—so that will include drugs and equipment for the health sector.

We include this section on power and global heath governance to highlight how international powerplays may affect nursing—which is something nurses often do not realise or acknowledge (Salvage & White, 2020). Migration is one obvious example where local health systems may be impacted by global negotiations and decisions, but so, too, is planetary health, already causing climate-related emergencies. The impact of global policies is felt in food and fuel prices, as the world has recently experienced, and even in the supply of affordable drugs and vaccines—all heavily influenced by powerful vested commercial interests (Salvage & White, 2020).

Social determinants of health are the conditions in which all of us are born, grow up, live, work and age, and their considerable impact on health and well-being is now well described (Azevedo & Johnson, 2011; World Health Organization, 2023a). These conditions are shaped by the availability of resources and wealth worldwide and the influence of the policymakers who hold the power to distribute the resources between and within countries. This holds true at global, national and local levels (Azevedo & Johnson, 2011). Countries and societies across the globe have made decisions—individually and collectively—that have both created and affected inequities in wealth between and within nations and created imbalances in power.

Salvage & White (2020) point out that much more attention has been given to the links between health and poverty in the last two decades, with high-level acknowledgement that global collaboration is required to eradicate poverty. The United Nations (UN) has adopted the 17 Sustainable Development Goals (SDGs) for 2016–2030 which were fully discussed in Chapter 1. You may have noticed that health is linked to all of them—wealth, decent work, gender equality, education—all of these, and other goals, too, are essential foundations for health. These are the goals that currently drive the work of the WHO.

THINK BOX 3.6

- Where do you think power lies in global health?
- How about in regulating nursing?
- What powers are held nationally, and what are held globally?
- How does power affect determinants of health?

The next section gives some answers to these questions that you might want to discuss with colleagues—the idea of power in health and nursing.

The Role of the World Health Organization

Global health governance is centralised at the WHO which, since 1948, has been the lead international multilateral organisation that can influence global health policy (World Health Organization, 2017). The WHO is part of the UN, a multilateral organisation comprising 193 member states and founded in 1945, which is split into many funds and programmes. The WHO focuses on three roles to promote health and wellbeing: (1) to take regulative steps to introduce health standards worldwide; (2) to create the global health agenda in order to create incentives for concerted actions across nations; and (3) to promote national and global health policies and the distribution of health resources (Ergin & Akin, 2017). Earlier in this chapter, we mentioned that the WHO established an international code of practice for migration of health workers to protect poorer nations from the effects of losing their health workforce. This is a good example of international collaboration that can be shepherded by WHO, though not enforced. WHO is as powerful as its ability to bring its member nations together to negotiate and agree on actions that will sometimes benefit the weakest of nations. If you have never been to a WHO meeting, it is worth considering how you might attend one—maybe virtually during the World Health Assembly, held in May every year, or ask your

chief nurse to support you in joining the delegation as an onlooker. It provides an opportunity to understand how politics plays out in health affairs.

As well as monitoring the state of global health and health systems, the WHO establishes International Health Regulations that are legally binding for member states and provide a legal framework defining countries' rights and obligations in handling public health events and emergencies that have the potential to cross borders (World Health Organization, 2023b). The important role of the WHO became clear during the recent pandemic, with its monitoring of the pandemic reported in daily press briefings to keep the world updated. The WHO declared the outbreak to be first a 'public health emergency of international concern' and, later, a global pandemic. These declarations are based on parameters set by International Health Regulations and showcase the power that WHO has, even though the measures taken to protect people from the pandemic were created and implemented nationally.

THINK BOX 3.7

What other activities or actions can you think of in health care that are implemented nationally but based on global knowledge and guidelines?

Consider vaccines regimes, child development guidelines, laboratory standards of care, disease monitoring—there are more, but these will get you started.

The World Health Organization and Nursing

Nursing has been a key player in the WHO since its foundation, seeking to address challenges faced by nurses and midwives such as nursing shortages, need for training of nurses, and recruitment and employment standards (World Health Organization, 2017). In the 1970s, the WHO had an increased focus on primary health care and delivering people-centred care, and so, it also increased its focus on nurses and the nursing workforce, as they were key players in making primary health care a reality. There is much more about the WHO and nursing in Chapter 7 of this book. Today, the WHO engages with ministries of health, government chief nurses and other stakeholders to monitor the nursing and midwifery workforces (World Health Organization, 2020).

In 2020, WHO published the first ever 'State of the World's Nursing Report', and it has recently (2023) been announced that a second report will be prepared in 2024. This is an important acknowledgement by the WHO of the global critical inputs of the nursing workforce, and though it came a disappointing 70 years after the WHO's founding, it is a welcome and strong basis for all of us to hold our governments accountable for investing in nursing. It is also an opportunity to ensure that good data about the nursing workforce are collected in all member states. These data should include information on nurse education, scope of practice, regulation, employment and distribution in the workforce.

THINK BOX 3.8

Looking at globalisation and global health, why do you think good data on the nursing workforce might be significant to all of us?

Data enable us to have a better idea of the ways that nursing is developing as a profession in different countries—for example, advanced practice is not found everywhere and has the potential to change care pathways, especially in remote and impoverished places (Hassmiller & Pulcini, 2020; World Health Organization, 2021). We should, as a profession, all be concerned that the next state of the world's nursing report has comprehensive, accurate and timely information about the nursing workforce.

The Global Network of WHO Collaborating Centres for Nursing and Midwifery is an independent, voluntary organisation (though linked to the WHO) which includes centres across all six WHO regions which are focused on nursing and midwifery development. The primary goals of the network include promoting health for all through collaboration and advocating for the nursing and midwifery role, leadership and contribution to the WHO Health For All platforms. An annual report on the work and achievements of these centres is compiled every year. In global terms, this network has enormous potential to influence policies and to be an international voice for nursing. Do you know where the collaborating centre is in your WHO region?

NONGOVERNMENTAL ORGANISATIONS

If you have an interest in global health, you will by now have encountered the term 'NGO' and sometimes 'INGO'—which is an international NGO. NGOs may also be called civil society organisations, nonprofits, voluntary organisations or charities. They are known for ensuring that services and supplies get to people most in need (e.g. Red Cross or Oxfam) and for public campaigns for social transformation (e.g. Greenpeace or Stop Oil). They also take part in advocating for policy changes with governments and multilateral organisations, such as the WHO (Lewis, 2010). There are many definitions of NGOs: the World Bank (1995) definition is:

private organizations that pursue activities to relieve suffering, promote the interests of the poor, protect the environment, provide basic social services or undertake community development.

The key points about NGOs, national and international, are that they (Lewis, 2010; Sidiropoulos et al., 2021):

- Are largely or completely independent of governments
- Are generally not for profit and have charitable status in many countries
- Collaborate with international organisations such as the WHO, the World Bank and UN entities
- Typically are value driven with altruism and volunteerism as defining characteristics

NGOs have existed in various forms for centuries, but their numbers increased dramatically throughout the 1990s, probably reflecting the end of the Cold War and the drive towards more global cooperation. While it is difficult to estimate how many NGOs there are globally because data are not available, the UN put the estimate at 35,000 'large established NGOs' in 2000. Others have estimated that the number may be as high as 1 million (Lewis, 2010). In any case, what is clear is that NGOs are often funded by donor aid, such as that from governments, large private organisations or foundations such as the Gates Foundation. While there are no accurate figures available for the number of resources that NGOs receive from aid, contracts and private donations, it has been estimated that in 2004, NGOs were responsible for disbursing somewhere between US $23 and US $78 billion of total aid money (Lewis, 2010).

In many countries, NGOs fill the gaps that government sectors are unable to, especially in health care. In practical terms, this may be delivering services to hard-to-reach areas or providing more health facilities that can offer services to the poorest people (Sidiropoulos et al., 2021).

Lewis (2010) has suggested that NGOs work in three main ways. First, NGOs are implementers of contracts with governments and other donors, and implementers of the work specified by those contracts, which is often to provide goods and services to those in need. NGOs are often critical as humanitarian responders in natural disasters such as earthquakes. NGOs usually take a percentage overhead fee in these contracts, which pays for their core costs. The second role of NGOs that Lewis identifies is that of catalyst, which refers to the NGOs' role in influencing social change. Think of the work of Save the Children in raising awareness of the need for education for children everywhere. The third role for NGOs is that of partner, working in collaboration with other actors on joint activities, such as developing the capacity of health systems to function.

In recent years, NGOs have faced criticism on many fronts (McGann & Johnstone, 2006). Their credibility and transparency have been called into question, with allegations that the goals of NGOs' programmes are more likely to be those of their donors—often a government—and may therefore be political. As mentioned earlier in this chapter, their presence in a country may lead to wage distortions, which attract health workers away from the public sector, thus weakening it. It is not possible within the confines of this chapter to do a full analysis of NGO work and effectiveness, but what is worth noting is that the NGO sector remains strong and can bring a different perspective to global work. Confirming this, the WHO recently (August 2023) held their first meeting of the WHO Civil Society Commission to bring civil society organisations from different backgrounds together to advise the WHO.

THINK BOX 3.9

Consider the work of an NGO with which you are familiar.
- How is the NGO funded?
- What have been its greatest successes?
- What do you think the WHO Civil Society Commission should set as their priority for the work of NGOs?

Global Financial Power and Health

Following World War II, delegates representing 44 countries met in Bretton Woods, New Hampshire, with the goal of rebuilding global cooperation and promoting international economic growth. Global currencies were pegged to the value of the dollar to create an efficient foreign exchange system. The International Monetary Fund (IMF) and the World Bank were set up at that time to assist governments with financing and economic development. The Bretton Woods system lasted until the 1970s, though both the IMF and World Bank have remained strong pillars for the exchange of international currencies and, indeed, for international work in health.

It is worth knowing what the IMF and the World Bank do in the realm of international health; you will see these institutions cited frequently. They both enable concerted action towards addressing common global problems, such as health and well-being (Ergin & Akin, 2017). The IMF is funded by its 190 member states (World Economic Forum, 2022) through a quota system that is based on a country's relative size in the global economy. In other words, richer countries pay more, as they do throughout the UN system, including for the WHO. Arguably, the richer countries may see themselves as having more power in these large UN entities. The IMF provides funding to stabilise debt-ridden countries and support development projects (World Economic Forum, 2022). IMF loans are often accompanied by mandated economic reforms which may include adjustments such as fiscal austerity measures, privatisation and interest rate hikes. Many such reforms have been criticised because the conditions that are set may disadvantage the public and are more difficult for low-income countries to implement and sustain. One stark example of what can happen comes from an Oxfam analysis (Oxfam, 2022). Kenya and the IMF agreed to a US $2.3 billion loan program in 2021, which included a 3-year public sector pay freeze and increased taxes on cooking gas and food. More than 3 million Kenyans are now facing acute hunger, as the driest conditions in decades spread a devastating drought across the country. Nearly half of all households in Kenya are having to borrow food or buy it on credit (Oxfam, 2022). This is one example of unanticipated outcomes as a result of imposed macroeconomic policies. As well as loans, the IMF provides technical assistance to countries which includes the sharing of best practices for finance ministries, central banks and tax authorities (World Economic Forum, 2022).

The World Bank provides specific technical support and loans to help countries implement particular projects or reforms. Goals may be health related—for example, building health facilities or supporting growth of the workforce. World Bank loans are usually long term. The World Bank also has member states that fund its work, and it cooperates closely with the IMF to ensure coordination in its similar programmes. The IMF and the World Bank work together to support countries achieving the SDGs.

The IMF and the World Bank have attracted criticism for the conditions that have been imposed on their loans, which have, at times, called for structural adjustments. This means that the country is asked to put in place mechanisms that will supposedly help it to repay its loans, such as privatisation or reductions in government spending (Thomson et al., 2017). Such conditions may result in decreased government funding to public health and health system–strengthening efforts, and furthermore, aid funds may be siphoned from health and social sectors to repay these loans (Thomson et al., 2017). Several studies have found that these structural adjustment programs worsened child and maternal health outcomes (Thomson et al., 2017).

The Complexity of Power, Governance, Financing and Health Systems

This chapter has so far tried to give a fairly simple overview of all of these elements that feed into and emanate from globalisation. It is beyond the scope of this chapter to delve deeply into these areas, but this overview shows how these complex global elements interplay to influence population-level health. One example that is especially relevant to nursing is the funding, planning and regulation of the health workforce. Earlier in

this chapter, we discussed migration and how it can be affected by international agreements and financial inequalities; if government expenditures must be cut because of the structural adjustment required by the World Bank and IMF, this can significantly affect the level of local wages in the most challenged countries.

Low wages in the public sector make it difficult to produce and retain a skilled and motivated health workforce, and health workers may search for a better professional and economic environment, often outside a country and sometimes within it, by going to larger urban facilities or the private sector. The whole system is further weakened by their loss, while other perverse developments may include unlicensed providers stepping in to offer services or health workers demanding payments from providers (Mitchell & Bossert, 2013). Similarly, international donor interventions can affect health labour markets when salaries are higher than in the public sector and the health workforce loses staff to project-based work, which is almost always short term.

It is a complex picture, but it is important to understand how even big global institutions can adversely affect local health. The migrant nurse on your team might have ended up there because of wage distortions in their country. Most significantly, understanding global health also means recognising our global interdependence and our health care.

As Salvage and White (2020, p. 2) say,

> [W]hat happens in distant places affects the health and health care of our communities, our loved ones, and ourselves - just as what happens in our backyard affects people we will never meet.

Globalisation and Nursing

In this landscape of global players in health care, where do nurses find their power to be influencers and participants? The International Council of Nurses (ICN) has been the leading international nursing policy influencer since its foundation in 1899, with the goal of uniting nurses worldwide through its confederation of national nursing organisations. The ICN was founded in 1899—50 years before the WHO—by a British nurse and suffragist Ethel Gordon Fenwick, who was a leader in the British Nurses Association. Williamson (2023) has compiled a comprehensive history of the ICN which brings together previous works and summarises the major events in the ICN's developments.

The ICN unites nurses worldwide through efforts to improve the welfare of nurses, promote the interests of women and promote societal health (Boschma, 2014). The founding members of the ICN were deeply engaged in an international women's movement that sought improved rights for women, including the right to vote (Williamson, 2023). The development of professional work for women aligned with the larger global women's rights movement, and nursing education and regulation were central to the early discussions in the ICN. Reading about the early years of the ICN highlights the pioneering spirit and work of these early nurse leaders. Their first ICN 'Grand Council' meeting was held in Buffalo, New York, in 1901, with reports about nursing discussed from 15 countries (Williamson, 2023). Simply travelling to the United States must have been arduous in those days, and collecting national data posed a significant challenge. Each ICN president has a watchword, and it is little wonder that Susan Bell McGahey, the Australian president from 1904 to 1909, chose 'courage' as hers. These early nurse leaders were pioneers.

While the ICN was founded through the ideals of nursing in western Europe and North America, the first 15 countries to submit reports on their nursing workforce included Brazil, Egypt, Cuba and South Africa, thus establishing from the start that the ICN was global and concerned with nursing beyond borders. By the end of the 20th century, the ICN had become a large organisation of 124 national nurse association members, holding regular Congress meetings, which, in 2023, attracted 6000 nurses to Canada. This demonstrates the powerful growth of the ICN which continues to influence nursing policies worldwide, provide leadership and assistance to its members and work closely with the WHO to integrate nursing into all global health work. Without doubt, it is—and always has been —the global powerhouse for nurses to influence policies and address issues of health equity worldwide.

Globalisation has inevitably affected nursing through migration of nurses; ongoing challenges in demography and epidemiology, disease outbreaks and infections, including the coronavirus pandemic, and nurses' working environments and well-being.

Although the effects of the unmanaged migration of nurses were discussed earlier in this chapter and more fully in Chapter 9, they appear also in Chapter 10 on leadership, as nurses seek to support colleagues who migrate to their countries and face the challenges of relocating to a new country. Chapter 5 highlights the effects of the COVID pandemic on the nursing workforce, as the impact of the pandemic was devastating for nursing, resulting in deaths, high stress levels and ongoing mental health issues for many.

The ICN's role in all of these global challenges has been to raise awareness about the impact on the nursing workforce and to champion nurses' rights for decent work, including a fair salary, safety at work and freedom from all forms of harassment (Williamson, 2023). As the world faces a growing shortage of nurses, increases in industrial actions by nurses, disruptions and disasters because of climate-related events, and the ongoing threat of epidemics and pandemics, the ICN has a critical role, with its member national nursing associations, to ensure that the essential contribution of nursing to global health remains highly visible to global partners.

Global Spread of Knowledge and Technology

A key part of globalisation is the flow of innovations and ideas across borders, which has the potential to manage and possibly end epidemics and pandemics through more advanced and shared surveillance systems, more knowledge-based treatments and stronger disease prevention (Azevedo & Johnson, 2011). This spread of knowledge can lead to more rapid scientific discovery, creation of virtual communities of support, strengthening of diasporic communities and increased advocacy within global governance.

As an evidence-based profession, nursing may be highly impacted by more accessible research knowledge of best practices facilitated by information communication technologies (ICT) (Abbott & Coenen, 2008. Abbott and Coenen (2008) say this:

Where is the opportunity for nurses to make a difference in regards to health care in a digital world? When one considers that 50–90% of all health care provided "in country" is delivered by non-physician providers and the accessibility of ICT is accelerating, the opportunities for nurses and midwives are vast. As those who most often stand at the interface of the patient and the healthcare system, there is a growing awareness of the need for nursing leadership, nursing innovation, and the nursing voice in global health ICT. (p. 242)

The global dissemination of knowledge and technology would ideally lead to a global standardisation of education, research and practice in nursing (Zarshenas et al., 2017). Indeed, there is some evidence that this is the case, with reports of advances in education and collaborative learning in nursing, the use of telenursing/telehealth, the use of electronic health records and the sharing of nursing knowledge and knowledge generation (Abbott & Coenen, 2008; Öncü, 2018). Significantly, online availability of information and clinical support can make 'just-in-time' information available wherever there is mobile phone or internet connection. McGowan et al. (2008), in a formative study, carried out a randomised controlled trial to evaluate whether information offered to primary care providers by librarians in response to the clinical questions raised while seeing patients would impact their decision-making by rapidly providing information when it was needed. They showed that providing timely information to clinical questions had a highly positive impact on decision-making. The implications of this work are significant for nurses and other clinicians working in isolated areas and delivering primary care.

The global spread of knowledge means that nursing education could become standardised, which, given the global migration of nurses, would make global qualifications a possibility. The Global Alliance for Nursing Education and Sciences undertook a rigorous multinational study to develop global educational guidelines for preservice baccalaureate nursing education, reported in Baker et al. (2021). Their work has resulted in a framework for action that can be used by educators and educational institutions worldwide, along with recommendations for nursing and health policy which highlight the critical importance of country-level investments in nursing and nurse education if they are to achieve their health goals and the SDGs (Baker et al., 2021).

Nursing education has become increasingly globalised through the establishment of exchange programs, the spread of international research, the increase in global educational experiences for students and nurse migration (Zarshenas et al., 2017). Many students now seek education outside of their country of citizenship due to the increased access of higher education globally and a reduction in the costs of travel (Rizwan et al., 2018). But these developments are not the same as a globally standardised and acceptable curriculum; Chapter 6 on decolonising nursing provides additional insights into how the development of a globally standardised and acceptable nursing curriculum might actually impose inappropriate cultural frameworks on others through our education systems. Instead, nursing education must adapt and evolve for a globalised world, with nurses having global cultural knowledge to enhance their abilities to deliver care to increasingly diverse populations as well as being able to use changing technologies to deliver evidence-based care (Ergin & Akin, 2017).

There is now significant interest in global nursing research, with networks and centres established in Japan, Edinburgh, India and Africa (Global Health Network, 2023; Global Nursing Research Centre, 2023; Global Research Nurses, 2023). These networks have opened up new opportunities for nurses everywhere to collaborate on research and to connect with each other to share their findings and thus advance nursing practice. Such opportunities could not have been envisaged even 20 years ago, and the potential of what may be achieved in terms of knowledge generation and sharing is great. While much nursing research has, in the past, been centred on high-income settings, research resources, training and lessons can now be shared with nurses in low- and middle-income countries. Access to research-based knowledge, as well as knowledge of research methods and generation, allows for the development of new contexts appropriate for knowledge generation based on specific populations and needs. It offers the opportunity to increase alignment of research-generated nursing knowledge with local circumstances. Perhaps most significantly, it opens up a world where information can be available to all, rather than limited to high-income countries, thus addressing persistent asymmetries and inequities in knowledge (Abbott & Coenen, 2008).

Medical Tourism

As globalisation brings about the spread of goods across borders, it also brings about the increasingly more common spread of services across borders. In the context of health care, these services have been 'commercialised' and often focus on helping individuals to improve their access to health as people have the ability and financing to not only purchase the care they need but also travel more quickly and cheaply to seek more affordable and immediate care packages. Medical tourism is regarded as one of the most lucrative businesses in the hospitality industry of many countries, particularly in developing countries, and is also becoming more competitive because of cost awareness and quality of services (Nasurdin et al., 2018). Medical tourism can be used to receive necessary care that cannot be obtained in-country, described as obligatory care, or to receive optional, or elective, care, which is care that is scheduled based on convenience and may or may not be available in-country (Zhong et al., 2021).

THINK BOX 3.10

What do you think are the implications for nursing of increasing medical tourism? Jot down your ideas before you read the next section.

Nurses may have a number of roles in medical tourism in the future. The first may be to help clients find appropriate sites in which to obtain the desired care in other countries, and this role might include warning clients of possible risks associated with providers or geographic areas. To be effective in this role will require nurses to be familiar with medical tourism destinations and with possible risks. It will also be incumbent on nurses to understand ethical and legal issues pertaining to such a role—for example, does the risk assessment provided have legal consequences (Ben-Natan et al., 2009)? Secondly, serving as a care coordinator for medical tourists may become a more common nursing role, though there is scant information currently available. The third area of great relevance to nursing is the need to provide culturally sensitive care to promote safe communications in local areas and between clinicians and patients and to promote the delivery of safe care to patients who are medical tourists. Hamzehpour et al. (2023) point out that medical tourism requires cultural competence in care providers so that patients are both properly understood and therefore safely treated. They further suggest that the attitude and behaviour of nurses are important factors for international patients in reducing stress and promoting comfort (Hamzehpour et al., 2023).

Educational programs that train nurses in these skills are needed to better prepare nurses for the many responsibilities involved in the growing medical tourism industry. Such a course of study could include strong transcultural elements, as well as business, management and leadership studies, and ethical and legal discussions that relate to the care of patients in such circumstances (Ben-Natan et al., 2009).

Perhaps the primary concern in some of the most popular destinations for complex procedures, such as India or the Philippines, is the possibility that medical tourism means that international patients benefit from sophisticated, well-equipped and well-staffed private hospitals, whereas the local population only has access to basic, underresourced health facilities where there are staff shortages (Hazarika, 2010). Research is needed to look at the impact of this growing international market on patients and families, understand how it impacts countries and local economies, health systems, and providers and examine the barriers and facilitators to equitable and accessible medical tourism.

Impact of Globalisation on Health Outcomes

This chapter has explored some of the results of globalisation and its effects on health care delivery, especially with regard to nursing. We have seen how international decisions and policies can have an impact on the lives of individuals and families and on local communities. Globalisation, in itself, is neither good nor bad, but the evidence that it results in wealthier nations and people overall is not yet convincing (Labonté & Schrecker, 2011). In the global context, 'the most devastating problems that plague the daily lives of billions of people…emerge from a single, fundamental source: the consequences of poverty and inequality' (Labonté & Schrecker, 2011). So far, there is no convincing research that shows that globalisation makes poorer countries richer and that any wealth created actually trickles down to the poorest people.

Undoubtedly, there have also been positive outcomes, including the potential of connectedness through new technologies to share knowledge. There are new global social movements to promote human rights and planetary health, and while diseases can now spread rapidly with human travellers as their vectors, there is also increased collaboration between nations to report and contain infections.

CONCLUSION

Globalisation will continue to have an impact on the challenges in health care for nurses, and it is an issue that is literally as big as our world. Nurses have to be ready to face these new challenges. This book is about global health, and that means being willing to explore the structural and political conditions that lead to poverty and inequality, as well as to conflict. This chapter has made a start in introducing the myriad factors associated with globalisation and its impact on nursing and nurses. However, there is still much work that is needed to understand the impacts of globalisation on individual countries, the health care sector and nursing. Nurses are needed who are willing to step up and take bold actions to bring education, innovations, service and research to the field so that we can begin to, collectively, address some of the concerns that face societies, patients and the health care and nursing workforces. We hope we have demonstrated the need for nurses everywhere to think globally and piqued your interests in becoming more knowledgeable of globalisation and health and active in helping to harness the power of nursing to bring about substantive changes in health and health care worldwide.

CASE STUDIES

Two case studies are presented here by nurses who discuss what it means to have a global perspective in their work. One represents the voice of an advanced nursing leader, while the other represents the voice of an emerging nursing leader. We hope their perspectives will inspire you to act to bring global understanding, sensitivity and awareness to nursing and health care.

CASE STUDY 3.1

Nursing and Midwifery Enterprise: Investing to Empower Women and Strengthen Health Systems:
Voice of an Advanced Nurse Leader

By *Marla Salmon, PhD, RN, FAAN*
Professor, Global Health
Professor, Child, Family, and Population Health Nursing
Adjunct Professor, Evans School

The reach of nursing and midwifery has extended to encompass every country and community, resulting in increasing opportunities for global innovation and development involving these disciplines. Although long recognised as foundations for better health care, nurses and midwives are often the workers who make health innovations happen but are seldom those who lead, own and direct health enterprises.

In 2015, the Institute of Medicine released its workgroup report on investing in nursing and midwifery enterprise as a means for women empowerment and health system strengthening (Perez et al., 2015). This report focused on innovation that is taking place in lower-income countries and what higher-income countries might learn from this work. A series of articles, published in *Nursing Outlook* (Fairman, 2016; Krubiner et al., 2016; Pittman & Salmon, 2016; Salmon & Maeda, 2016), explored the body of work underpinning this report—and laid the groundwork for additional innovation. Also during this time, the Sasakawa Health Foundation in Japan launched its extraordinarily successful investment in training and launching more than 90 nurse entrepreneurs in a series of very successful nursing clinics serving remote and underserved populations (Samarasekera, 2022; Sasakawa, n.d.). Others have subsequently reported innovative strategies for nurse-led work, though continued evidence from these developments is crucial to inform nursing development globally.

When thinking about ways to advance nursing and midwifery leadership enterprise, there is much to learn from the field of global development financing. Decades-long investment in women's enterprise has had important impact on both the empowerment of women and improvement of social and economic well-being for them, their communities and their families. While much is known about these investments and their lessons, the enterprises have been confined to the agricultural and commercial sectors of lower-income countries.

It is important to note that while there have been important investments in the health sector aimed at services advancing women's health and empowerment, little has been done in support of women who make these services possible. In fact, not only are women working in the health sector left out of leading health innovation, but they are also frequently underpaid or even expected to provide services on a voluntary basis (Samarasekera, 2022).

The arguments for investment in nursing and midwifery are compelling and include the following:

1. Investment in Nursing and Midwifery Enterprise (NME) is investment not only in services to women, families and communities but in the development, status, economic well-being and societal engagement of those who own and/or lead these enterprises.
2. The NME investments also provide platforms for development of women who are not nurses and midwives. Nurses and midwives can engage in uplifting and improving the lives of these individuals, whether through providing training, mentorship or even inspiration to women and children in the community.
3. Entrepreneurship is complex, particularly in the health sector. Investment and long-term management of entrepreneurial practice arrangements

are complex and run far afield from the training and education received by nurses and midwives. Training and wraparound supports are crucial to the success of NME.

4. Individual, free-standing nursing and midwifery enterprises have vulnerabilities associated with 'going it alone' and having to learn it all, do it all, maintain it all, finance it all and ensure success in services, scaling and sustainability. Engagement in organisational arrangements and affiliations that provide financing, shared services, quality assurance, training and peer support are important potential avenues for the success of these enterprises. Collectives, cooperatives and social franchises are examples of this type of cooperation and have. Interestingly, some of these arrangements have grown from national nursing and midwifery organisations.

The recognition of the value of NME to women empowerment, health services and society at large is well aligned with the goals of impact investors and development finance, as well as global development goals, including those of the United Nations (United Nations, n.d.). Gender-lens investors are a particularly well-suited target group for engagement in advancing NMEs. Gaining footing in this and all aspects of launching, scaling and sustaining NME calls for nurses and midwives to strategically cross the boundaries between health, social finance and business. Success in this regard will be instrumental in moving NME's forward globally within individual countries and in our most remote and underserved communities.

CASE STUDY 3.2

Globalisation and Nursing—Voice of an Emerging Nurse Leader

By *Sinhye Kim, PhD, RN*
Nurse Scientist and Postdoctoral Researcher
School of Nursing at the University of North Carolina at Chapel Hill

Globalisation is a phenomenon that can no longer be ignored. On a small scale, the diversity of friends we meet, colleagues we work with and patients we care for is gradually expanding. On a larger scale, the world is becoming more interconnected and intertwined, as seen by the widespread impact of COVID-19 from one country to global society, economy and politics (Bickley et al., 2021). Nurses should recognise their roles and responsibilities in the era of globalisation and actively respond to this new world challenge. As I am a nurse scientist with international experience who

Continued

works in the nursing profession, I wish to speak for nursing students and colleagues who are beginning to learn about global health.

First, many nurses think that being a global nurse implies working beyond their own country. However, being a nurse in one's own community can also influence global health. For example, the cumulative efforts to provide better nursing care and improve nursing work environments in a community can be evidence of new nursing knowledge development. This new knowledge can contribute to improving nursing fields in other countries. Therefore we should recognise that having a broader perspective and realising global connections are the first steps to responding to globalisation as a nurse.

Second, future nurses must also be competent as cooperators within their community and worldwide. Globalisation of the health care workforce increases the proportion of internationally educated nurses and other health care professionals in our workplace (Jones & Sherwood, 2014). Current global health issues are more complicated and require interprofessional and interagency cooperation to find solutions. Nurses are in a unique position to lead and cooperate with teams that provide health services across the continuum of care (Sensor et al., 2021). Nurses should be able to increase their cultural acceptance of diversity and collaborate both internally and externally.

Throughout the COVID-19 pandemic, we have experienced how socio-economic and political differences between countries affect people's health inequities. In the future, the rapid development of information and technology may lead to another gap in digital literacy, further exacerbating this health inequity (Lyles et al., 2021). Nurses, who have long been health advocates (Selanders & Crane, 2012), must understand various social determinants that can influence population health outcomes and try to eliminate health disparities. To this end, nurses must respond quickly to rapidly changing environments and maintain an enthusiastic attitude toward learning new skills and knowledge.

Finally, nursing leaders, educators and policymakers should pay more attention to globalisation issues and policies in order to facilitate the active exchange of nurses in the global era. The COVID-19 pandemic has exacerbated the existing global shortage of nurses, and more nurses are moving between countries than ever before for work or education (Buchan et al., 2022). However, rigid regulations and policies hinder or delay the migration of nurses. Ensuring the flexibility of nurse mobility through mutual recognition agreements and deregulation of migration governance processes between nations will help to alleviate the current severe nursing workforce shortage. Nursing educators and researchers should also work to enhance and standardise the nursing education system so that nurses can provide quality care anywhere in the world.

This chapter helps us to better understand the concepts of globalisation, types of global governance, impacts of globalisation on society and health, and key issues nurses face. Nurses will need to act with broader perspectives in their roles as practitioners, educators, researchers and policymakers to improve global health. We should remember that when we are knowledgeable and prepared, we have the power to make an enormous, positive impact on our world as nurses.

REFERENCES

Abbott, P., & Coenen, A. (2008). Globalization and advances in information and communication technologies: The impact on nursing and health. *Nursing Outlook, 56*, 238–246.

Azevedo, M. J., & Johnson, B. H. (2011). *The impact of globalization determinants and the health of the world's population. New knowledge in a new era of globalization* (pp. 165–182). London: InTech.

Baker, C., Cary, A., & Bento, M. da C. (2021). Global standards for professional nursing education: The time is now. *Journal of Professional Nursing, 37*, 86–92. Global standards for professional nursing education: The time is now – ScienceDirect.

Ben-Natan, M., Ben-Sefer, E., & Ehrenfeld, M. (2009). "Medical Tourism: A New Role for Nursing?" *OJIN: The Online Journal of Issues in Nursing, 14*(3), B1.

Bickley, S. J., Chan, H. F., Skali, A., Stadelmann, D., & Torgler, B. (2021). How does globalization affect COVID-19 responses? *Global Health, 17*(1), 57. doi:10.1186/s12992-021-00677-5.

Boschma, G. (2014). International nursing history: the International Council of Nurses history collective and beyond. *Nursing History Review, 22*(1), 114–118.

Buchan, J., Catton, H., & Shaffer, F. (2022). Sustain and Retain in 2022 and Beyond: The Global Nursing Workforce and the COVID-19

Pandemic. *International Centre on Nurse Migration.* https://www.icn.ch/system/files/2022-01/Sustain%20and%20Retain%20in%202022%20and%20Beyond-%20The%20global%20nursing%20workforce%20and%20the%20COVID-19%20pandemic.pdf. (Accessed October 14, 2022).

Buchan, J. (2023). Brexit, Covid and the UK's reliance on international recruitment. *Blog for Nuffield Trust Evidence for Better Health Care.* https://www.nuffieldtrust.org.uk/news-item/brexit-covid-and-the-uk-s-reliance-on-international-recruitment. (Accessed February 2024).

Carminati, L. (2020). Behavioural Economics and Human Decision Making: Instances from the Health Care System, *Health Policy, 124*(6), 659–664.

Carvalho, F. (2021). The impact of Brexit and COVID-19 on nursing in the UK. *British Journal of Nursing, 30*(13), 822–823. https://doi.org/10.12968/bjon.2021.30.13.822.

Crisp, N. (2020). *Health is made at home. Hospitals are for repairs.* Billericay, UK: Salus.

Ergin, E., & Akin, B. (2017). Globalization and its Reflections for Health and Nursing. *International Journal of Caring Sciences, 10*(1), 607.

Espinoza, H., & Speckesser, S. (2022). A comparison of earnings related to higher technical and academic education. *Education Economics, 30*(6), 644–659. doi:10.1080/09645292.2022.2035321.

Fairman, J. A. (2016). Investing in nursing and midwifery enterprise to empower women and strengthen health services and systems: Commentary and context. *Nursing Outlook, 64*(1), 33–36.

Geiger, N. (2017). The Rise of Behavioral Economics: A Quantitative Assessment. *Social Science History, 41*(3), 555–583. doi:10.1017/ssh.2017.17. ISSN 0145-5532. S2CID 56373713.

Global Research Nurses. (2023). https://globalresearchnurses.tghn.org/.

Global Health Network. (2023). https://tghn.org/.

Global Nursing Research Centre. (2023). https://gnrc.m.u-tokyo.ac.jp/en/.

Hamzehpour, H., Ashktorab, T., & Esmaeili, M. (2023). Safe acceptance in the nurses' cultural care of medical tourists in Iran: a qualitative study. *BMC Health Services Research, 23*, 399. https://doi.org/10.1186/s12913-023-09378-8.

Hassmiller, S. B., & Pulcini, J. (Eds.). (2020). *Advanced Practice Nursing Leadership: A Global Perspective.* Switzerland: Springer Nature.

Hazarika, I. (2010). Medical tourism: its potential impact on the health workforce and health systems in India. *Health Policy and Planning, 25*(3), 248–251. https://doi.org/10.1093/heapol/czp050.

Hurst, L., Mahtani, K., Pluddemann, A., Lewis, S., Harvey, K., Briggs, A., Boylan, A.-M., Bajwa, R., Haire, K., Entwistle, A., Handa, A., & Heneghan, C. Defining Value-based Healthcare in the NHS: CEBM report 2019. https://www.cebm.net/2019/04/defining-value-based-healthcare-in-the-nhs/.

Institute of Medicine. (2015). Empowering Women and Strengthening Health Systems through Nursing and Midwifery: Implications of Innovative International Models for the United States. *Institute of Medicine Workshop Report.* https://www.nationalacademies.org/our-work/empowering-women-and-strengthening-health-systems-through-nursing-and-midwifery-implications-of-innovative-international-models-for-the-united-states-a-workshop.

Jones, C. B., & Sherwood, G. (2014). The globalization of the nursing workforce: Pulling the pieces together. *Nursing Outlook, 62*(1), 59–63.

Kavinya, T. (2014). Globalization and its effects on the overall health situation of Malawi. *Malawi Medical Journal, 26*(1), 27.

Krubiner, C., Salmon, M., Synowiec, C., & Lagomarsino, G. (2016). Investing in nursing and midwifery enterprise: empowering women and strengthening health systems—summary of a landscaping study of innovations in low- and middle-income countries. *Nursing Outlook, 64*, 7–23.

Labonté, R., & Schrecker, T. (2011). Globalization and social determinants of health: Introduction and methodological background (part 1 of 3). *Globalization and Health, 3*(1), 1–10.

Lee, E., Hamelin, T., & Daugherty, J. (2018). Globalization of health service: sharing of best practices in perianesthesia nursing care, a case study of cross-border institutional collaboration. *Journal of PeriAnesthesia Nursing, 33*(2), 209–219.

Lewis, D. (2010). Nongovernmental Organizations, Definition and History. In Anheier, H. K., & Toepler, S. (Eds.), *International Encyclopedia of Civil Society.* New York, NY: Springer. https://doi.org/10.1007/978-0-387-93996-4_3.

Lyles, C. R., Wachter, R. M., & Sarkar, U. (2021). Focusing on digital health equity. *JAMA, 326*(18), 1795–1796. doi:10.1001/jama.2021.18459.

McGann, J., & Johnstone, M. (2006). The Power Shift and the NGO Credibility Crisis. Global Policy Forum. Available at: https://archive.globalpolicy.org/component/content/article/176-general/31423.html.

McGowan, J., Hogg, W., Campbell, C., & Rowan, M. (2008). Just-in-Time Information Improved Decision-Making in Primary Care: A Randomized Controlled Trial. *PLoS ONE, 3*(11), e3785. doi:10.1371/journal.pone.0003785.

Mitchell, A., & Bossert, T. J. with Tedros Adhanom Ghebreyesus (2013). *Politics and Governance in Human Resources for Health in The Labor Market for Health Workers in Africa a New Look at the Crisis.* In Soucat, A., & Scheffler, R. (Eds.). Washington DC: World Bank.

Nasurdin, A. M., Ling, T. C., & Khan, S. N. (2018). The role of psychological capital on nursing performance in the context of medical tourism in Malaysia. *International Journal of Business and Society, 19*(3), 748–761.

Öncü, E. (2018). Globalization and changing nursing workforce within the framework of flexibility model. *Journal of Human Sciences, 15*(2), 1185–1192. Retrieved from https://www.j-human-sciences.com/ojs/index.php/IJHS/article/view/4842.

Oxfam. (2022). https://www.oxfam.org/en/press-releases/imf-must-abandon-demands-austerity-cost-living-crisis-drives-hunger-and-poverty.

Perez, M. M., Patel, D. M., & Cuff, P. A. (Eds.). (2015). *Empowering women and strengthening health systems and services through investing in nursing and midwifery enterprise: Lessons from lower-income countries: workshop summary.* National Academies Press.

Pittman, P., & Salmon, M. (2016). Advancing nursing enterprises: a cross-country comparison. *Nursing Outlook, 64*, 24–32.

Rennen, W., & Martens, P. (2003). The globalisation timeline. *Integrated Assessment, 4*(3), 137–144.

Rizwan, M., Rosson, N. J., Tackett, S., & Hassoun, H. T. (2018). Globalization of medical education: Current trends and opportunities for medical students. *Journal of Medical Education and Training, 2*(1), 1–7.

Salmon, M., & Maeda, A. (2016). Investing in nursing and midwifery enterprise to empower women and strengthen health services and systems: an emerging global body of work. *Nursing Outlook, 64*, 7–16.

Salvage, J., & White, J. (2020). Our future is global: nursing leadership and global health. *Revista Latino-Americana de Enfermagem, 28*, e3339. doi:10.1590/1518-8345.4542.3339.

Samarasekera, U. (2022). 6 Million female health workers are unpaid or underpaid. *Lancet, 400*(10346), 87.

Sasakawa Global Nursing website: https://www.shf.or.jp/en/community_health/.

Selanders, L. C., & Crane, P. C. (2012). The Voice of Florence Nightingale on Advocacy. *OJIN: The Online Journal of Issues in Nursing, 17*(1). https://doi.org/10.3912/OJIN.Vol17No01Man01. (Accessed October 27, 2022).

Sensor, C. S., Branden, P. S., Clary-Muronda, V., et al. (2021). Nurses achieving the sustainable development goals: the United Nations and sigma. *American Journal of Nursing, 121*(4), 65–68. doi:10.1097/01.NAJ.0000742544.07615.db.

Sidiropoulos, S., Emmanouil-Kalos, A., Kanakaki, M. E., & Vozikis, A. (2021). The Rise of NGOs in Global Health Governance and Credibility Issues in the 21st Century. *HAPSc Policy Briefs Series, 2*(2). doi:10.12681/hapscpbs.29516.

Teisberg, E., Wallace, S., & O'Hara, S. (2020). Defining and implementing value-based health care: a strategic framework. *Academic Medicine, 95*, 682–685. doi:10.1097/ACM.0000000000003122 First published online December 10, 2019.

The Health Foundation. (2023). Migration and the health care workforce. Online Evidence Paper. https://migrationobservatory.ox.ac.uk/resources/briefings/migration-and-the-health-and-care-workforce/.

Thomson, M., Kentikelenis, A., & Stubbs, T. (2017). Structural adjustment programmes adversely affect vulnerable populations: a systematic-narrative review of their effect on child and maternal health. *Public Health Reviews, 38*(1), 1–18.

United Nations, *Sustainable Development Goals*. https://sdgs.un.org/goals.

Veillard, J., Dhalla, I., Fekri, O., & Klazinga, N. (2015). Measuring Outcomes in the Canadian Health Sector: *Driving Better Value from Healthcare*. C.D. Howe Institute Commentary 438, Available at SSRN: https://ssrn.com/abstract=2689797 or http://dx.doi.org/10.2139/ssrn.2689797. (Accessed November 12, 2015).

Williamson, L. (2023). *The Global Voice of Nursing. A history of the International Council of Nurses from 1899-2022*. Switzerland. Geneva: International Council of Nurses.

World Bank. (1995). *Working with NGOs: a practical guide to operational collaboration between the World Bank and nongovernmental organizations (English)*. Washington, D.C.: World Bank Group. http://documents.worldbank.org/curated/en/814581468739240860/Working-with-NGOs-a-practical-guide-to-operational-collaboration-between-the-World-Bank-and-nongovernmental-organizations.

World Economic Forum. (2022). Online https://www.weforum.org/organizations/international-monetary-fund-imf#:~:text=It%20seeks%20to%20foster%20economic,ease%20balance%20of%20payments%20adjustment.

World Health Organization. (2017). Nursing and midwifery in the history of the World Health Organization 1948–2017. https://www.who.int/publications/i/item/nursing-and-midwifery-in-the-history-of-the-world-health-organization. (Accessed February 2024)

World Health Organization. (2020). *State of the World's Nursing 2020*. Geneva: World Health Organization. https://www.who.int/publications/i/item/9789240003279.

World Health Organization. (2021). *Global strategic directions for nursing and midwifery 2021–2025*. World Health Organization. https://www.who.int/publications/i/item/9789240033863.

World Health Organization. (2023a). Social Determinants of Health. https://www.who.int/health-topics/social-determinants-of-health#tab=tab_1.

World Health Organization. (2023b). International Health Regulations. https://www.who.int/health-topics/international-health-regulations#tab=tab_1.

World Health Organization. (2017). Nursing and midwifery in the history of the World Health Organization 1948–2017. https://www.who.int/publications/i/item/nursing-and-midwifery-in-the-history-of-the-world-health-organization-(1948%E2%80%932017). (Last Accessed December 2022).

Zarshenas, L., Sarvestani, R. S., Molazem, Z., & Moattari, M. (2017). Globalization in Nursing: A concept analysis. *Asian Journal of Nursing Education and Research, 7*(1), 115–119.

Zhong, L., Deng, B., Morrison, A. M., Coca-Stefaniak, J. A., & Yang, L. (2021 Oct 16). Medical, Health and Wellness Tourism Research-A Review of the Literature (1970-2020) and Research Agenda. *International Journal of Environmental Research and Public Health, 18*(20), 10875. doi:10.3390/ijerph182010875. PMID: 34682622; PMCID: PMC8536053.

4

RESPONDING TO GLOBAL EMERGENCIES: WHAT HAS THE ROLE OF NURSES BEEN AND WHAT CAN IT BE IN THE FUTURE?

MARCUS WOOTTON ■ LYDIA DAVIDSON

INTRODUCTION

Modern nursing was forged in response to emergencies and crises. Conflict and disaster have shaped and moulded the profession, as those who practice nursing are often forced to adapt to the changing health landscape and the world around them. The need for health professionals to innovate and respond to health emergencies runs like a seam throughout the professionalisation and development of nursing (Fletcher et al., 2022) from wars and conflict, through pandemics and into a modern unstable world grappling with global and political upheaval and the climate emergency. What cannot be disputed is that nurses have an unparalleled role to play in the response to global health emergencies, and developing their skills and role in this area of work will be fundamental to improving the profession and humanity's response to such events in the future (Veenema, 2018).

Global health emergencies place care quality, standardisation, regulation, advocacy and humanity, the central pillars of modern nursing, under enormous pressure. The chaotic nature of a sudden disaster or the slow deterioration of a health system can leave those who work in them struggling to rationalise care and provide effective treatment. We also know that the best humanitarian response to these events are the guiding principles of effective nursing: empathy, advocacy and compassion supported by an effective and evidence-based approach. This should place nurses at the very apex of the modern humanitarian response, and yet, often this is not the case. The nursing role in global health emergencies has frequently been mischaracterised, marginalised and, in some cases, diminished.

It is a mistake to view nursing's contribution to broader humanitarianism as a one-way street. Nurses have, and will always, play a significant part in health emergencies. But what is sometimes not appreciated is the role that innovations made by nurses responding to the crisis have had in shaping the practice of the modern nurse. Many of the advances in modern nursing practice stem from the reforms of Florence Nightingale and have continued to change and grow through the pandemics and wars of the 20th and 21st centuries, driven by nurses working in crisis and emergency.

This chapter sets out how nurses have responded to health emergencies, past and present, describes the challenges that they have faced, and explores possible pathways to the future. We discuss the historical context of nurses' work in emergencies and some of the developments in the profession that this work has led to. We also look at some notable examples of nursing in the context of natural and human-made disasters against the wider backdrop of international development, politics and aid. Finally, we discuss the challenges for nurses in the 21st century and beyond.

THINK BOX 4.1

- What do you know about the history of nursing in the country where you trained?
- Where could you find out more about it?
- Do you think the history of nursing is important?

CRISIS AND WAR—THE BIRTHPLACE OF THE MODERN NURSE

Nursing and its principles have their roots in the earliest human civilisations, with evidence of a form of semiorganised health care in Europe stretching from at least the Reformation, which lasted from 1517 to

1648 (Laurent, 2019). Early nursing was entwined with organised religion. Echoes of this history, such as the title of 'sister', remain in the nursing lexicon to this day (Helmstadter & Godden, 2016). In Europe and beyond, the modern nurse, certainly within political and public consciousness, was informed by the seminal work of Nightingale, who responded to the health emergency resulting from the Crimean War (a conflict between the Russian Empire and an alliance of Britain, France and the Ottoman Empire in the mid-1800s) and championed many of the components of modern nursing practice (Bostridge, 2015). The Crimean War was a pivotal point in the career, not only of Nightingale, a true daughter of the British wealthy middle class, but also of Mary Seacole, a self-styled 'doctress' whose mother was from Jamaica and father from Scotland. Nightingale and Seacole both became famous for their work with the troops in Crimea, but for different areas of care. Seacole ran a hostel for soldiers to recuperate in, and she treated their ailments on the battlefield with herbal remedies she had learned from her doctress mother. Nightingale was a statistician and collected data as well as tending to the sick men in a field hospital, organising a team of nurses and lobbying for cleaner conditions, better food and safe water. None of this history is disputed (Nelson & Rafferty, 2010), and in different ways, in response to the suffering they witnessed in conflict, both shaped the role of nursing (Dumitrascu et al., 2020; McDonald, 2020). They serve as examples, not only of the impact that nurses working in emergencies can have and the wider advancements in practice that can result from this, but also some of the wider challenges faced by nurses in the modern era, such as subservience to physicians, racism and sexism.

Nightingale is remembered largely in the public consciousness as 'the lady with the lamp', but she was so much more. She was a formidable statistician and became the first female member of the Royal Society of Statisticians at a time when a female's place was most certainly held to be in the home (Nelson, 2010). The lamp that Nightingale carried illuminated her work as she provided bedside care to wounded soldiers in the darkness of military hospitals during the Crimean War. Whilst bedside care is a vital part of Nightingale's career, it should be viewed alongside the panoply of her other achievements, which are often forgotten.

The career and status of Seacole point toward another core issue of nursing workforce development and nurses' role in emergencies—that of formalised regulation. As a step toward standardised care, most health systems develop a system of maintaining a register of nurses, placing conditions on their practice and ensuring compliance with agreed norms of professionalism often framed as a code of professional conduct. Modern nursing concerns regarding the scope of practice and effective regulation are evidenced in the career of 19th-century Seacole. There is an ongoing historical debate surrounding her formal and informal qualifications, the work that she undertook and its relevance to nursing (Staring-Derks et al., 2015). This debate goes so far as to question if Seacole was a 'nurse' at all, with some writers describing her as a 'doctress' (Anionwu, 2012) and others as a nurse practitioner (Messmer & Parchment, 1998). Unfortunately, Seacole was lost to history for around 100 years—and this may have been because of her mixed-race heritage—until nurses from the Caribbean visited her grave in northwest London and lobbied for her recognition. In 2004, Mary Seacole was voted the Greatest Black Briton, and in 2016, her statue was finally unveiled in the grounds of St Thomas' Hospital on London's Southbank. The Mary Seacole Trust continues her legacy.

FROM CRISIS TO REGULATION

Efforts to standardise and regulate nursing in the early 20th century were led by Dame Sarah Swift, founder of the Royal College of Nursing and Ethel Gordon Fenwick, who was instrumental in developing the Nursing Registration Act of 1919 (Attenborough, 2021). These advancements pushed nursing toward the profession we recognise today. It is unlikely that these changes would have occurred at the same rate without the strides in nursing prompted by the progress made by wartime nurses in the 19th century, which were brought to the attention of policymakers and the public by Nightingale.

Health emergencies can place nurses at the very edge of their regulatory parameters and clinical competence, as they are confronted with a mix of overwhelming needs coupled with limited human and physical resources within a confused and fluctuating environment. Nursing practice in emergency response has evolved, but many of the current health system issues that nurses face have echoed the challenges faced by nurses in centuries past. For example, think of the challenges of the recent COVID pandemic when there was inadequate supply of personal protective equipment (PPE) in almost all countries. Nurses were reported using plastic bags as PPE (Lee et al., 2020), and there were accounts of the reuse of 'single use' equipment (Rowan & Laffey, 2021). As the largest group of frontline health workers, nurses in every emergency are most likely to be using their problem-solving skills and innovating their way out of the overwhelming challenges they face. (Dawson et al. 2017) suggest that although nurses are recruited and participate in health-focused humanitarian activities in low- to middle-income countries, there is limited research into the nature of care that nurses—rather than teams—provide in this context. Further targeted research is needed to enable greater understanding of nursing care in this context.

We would argue there is a golden thread that runs between changes in nursing practice regulation and nursing responses to disasters and health emergencies. Fletcher et al. (2022) also note the parallel progression of developments in nursing and nursing in emergencies, highlighting the multidimensional roles of a nurse that take on disaster response challenges. In other words, there is a tense feedback loop as chaotic environments, caused by natural or human-made disasters, place structured and standardised care under overwhelming pressure to which nursing responds in an ad hoc way, and in turn, the regulation seeks to address new realities that emerge from crises. Responding to global emergencies moulded the modern nurse, and to this day, nursing practice development and humanitarian response remain inextricably interwoven.

THINK BOX 4.2

The global pandemic demanded much of health workers around the world.

- Were there examples from your location where nursing regulation did not keep pace with the nursing responses?
- Have there been long-lasting changes in regulation as a result?

Examples may include nurse prescribing or nurses being the first point of contact in general practices or emergency rooms.

PREEXISTING HEALTH INFRASTRUCTURE

Before considering nurses' response to disaster and emergency, it is important to place these within the context of the affected health system, how effectively the country or region was managing 'business as usual' and how comprehensively it had prepared and planned for emergency response before its occurrence (Lantada et al., 2020).

The capacity of the existing system to deliver high-quality health care in 'normal times' is the most significant influencing factor in how that system will respond to emergencies. As described in other chapters, the global nursing workforce is not currently sufficient in terms of numbers to meet the goal of universal health coverage. There is also a significant maldistribution of the workforce, with 80% of nurses working in countries with only half the world's population (Fig. 4.1) (World Health Organization, 2020).

We know health worker maldistribution is a critical weakness at a global level, but the distribution of nurses and other health workers *within* a country is also important. Broadly, urban areas are more comprehensively served by health workers of all cadres in comparison to rural areas. In India, for example, approximately 66% of the population is found in rural areas but is served by only 33% of the nation's health workers (Karan et al., 2021).

Crises can act like a 'barium meal' on a health system, identifying the areas of weakness and concern and exacerbating existing health inequalities. When evaluating their health system, nurses should be aware of the existing health inequalities within their area, as any crisis is very likely to worsen these inequalities, with the most marginalised and vulnerable likely to feel the brunt of almost any crisis. Nurses need to advocate for the most marginalised, as in these contexts, the specific vulnerabilities of certain groups are not always appreciated. During the early stages of the coronavirus pandemic, UK Cabinet Office Minister Michael Gove suggested that the 'fact that both the prime minister and the health secretary have contracted the virus is a reminder that the virus does not discriminate' (Morgan, 2020). This was not borne out by evidence from the UK government's figures, and research eventually showed that those from the poorest areas of the

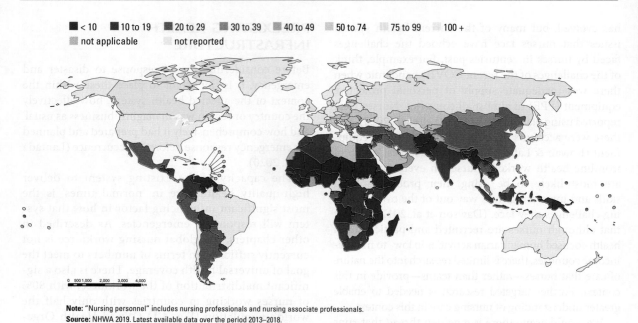

■ < 10   ■ 10 to 19   ■ 20 to 29   ■ 30 to 39   ■ 40 to 49   ■ 50 to 74   ■ 75 to 99   ■ 100 +
not applicable   not reported

Note: "Nursing personnel" includes nursing professionals and nursing associate professionals.
Source: NHWA 2019. Latest available data over the period 2013–2018.

Fig. 4.1 ■ Density of nursing personnel per population of 10,000 in 2018. From World Health Organization. (2020). *State of the world's nursing 2020.* https://www.who.int/publications/i/item/9789240003279.

United Kingdom were twice as likely to die as those in the richest areas (Office for National Statistics, 2020). There was also evidence that those classed as economically most disadvantaged were more likely than any other group to require critical care and a resulting higher adjusted 30-day mortality (Lone et al., 2021).

Alongside socioeconomic status, COVID-19 disproportionally affected black and ethnic minority individuals (Pathak et al., 2021). Race as a predictor of risk within a health emergency is far from a new concept, and the impact on black and ethnic minorities of coronavirus had been graphically predicted in the case of Hurricane Katrina in the United States in 2005. The hurricane caused widespread damage and huge loss of life, with those classified as Black 1.7 to 4 times more likely to die compared to Whites (Brunkard et al., 2005). It has been argued that the seeds of this appalling outcome were sown years before the crisis. Health services were not as responsive to those in predominately black areas, and the storm levees protecting predominately black neighbourhoods were in disrepair (Hartman et al., 2006). Further to this, evacuation plans were based on the use of private vehicles which those in poverty had less access to (White et al., 2007).

In both the cases of Katrina and coronavirus, the socioeconomic and racial inequalities that were present within the health system prior to the event were magnified and worsened by it. It is rarely, if ever, the case that risk of displacement, injury or death is evenly distributed across a population. The richest and most affluent are the most well insulated, and nurses and policymakers, when planning their health service response, should recognise that populations that were vulnerable before the crisis are likely to disproportionately suffer from its effects (Bambra et al., 2020). For nurses, the implications seem to be clear: it is critical that nurses have a good overview of the social determinants of health (SDH) (there is more in Chapter 1 about the SDH), as, even in emergency situations, this background will be vital to plan adequate care targeted to those who will be most affected. Nurses are also key in advocating for awareness of the impact of SDH on health risks and outcomes. The first step may be simply to include questions about social issues during routine health checks in a sensitive way. For example, including a simple question such as 'Do you ever have difficulty making ends meet at the end of the month?' may accurately identify patients living below the poverty line (Andermann, 2016).

THINK BOX 4.3

- Where could you find out about discrepancies in population health in your location?
- What statistics are available to you and health service managers?

RESPONDING TO EMERGENCIES

The response to a localised health emergency will differ greatly depending on the locally available information, resources and the ability of the country to bring in support from other areas and possibly coordinate additional supplies and human resources provided by the international community.

The widely accepted traditional approach to disaster management has four phases (Nojavan et al., 2018):

- Mitigation
- Preparedness
- Response
- Recovery

Recently, a fifth phase has been added before mitigation: Prevention (Veenema, 2018). Prevention refers to proactive planning that might include the forecasting of possible emergencies (for example, coastal flooding or extreme weather events) and ensuring there are proactive measures in place for communities as well as an opportunity for anticipatory planning. There is clearly overlap between prevention, mitigation and preparedness: earlier, we addressed the critical role that nurses might have in prevention with specialist and in-depth community knowledge. In the following sections, we explore each of the other areas in more depth.

MITIGATION

This stage includes assessing the ability of the local health system to respond to emergencies or disasters. This is notoriously difficult given the considerable uncertainty which exists in evaluating the various threats to a health system and their likelihood. Indeed, it is often said that disaster planners fall into the trap of preparing for the last disaster rather than for the next one.

Nurses working to plan for an emergency should therefore evaluate their workplace and regional and wider health systems' strengths and weaknesses as they assess their ability to respond effectively to emergencies and be able to contribute to neighbourhood, regional and national emergency preparedness plans. Such an assessment requires a level of macro-, meso- and microlevel planning that nurses can be uniquely placed to undertake, especially nurses who work in, and are familiar with, a community. As already mentioned, there will be predisposing factors that can make a section of the population particularly vulnerable, and here, nurses' knowledge of the SDH plus their knowledge of people in their communities can be critical information for planning responses. The vital importance of appraisal was demonstrated in the early stages of the COVID-19 pandemic, which highlighted the risks associated with presumptions of health system preparedness and workforce capacity in supposedly advanced health systems, including Western Europe and North America.

In October 2019, the Global Health Security Index (GHSI) rated the United States and the United Kingdom to be world leaders in outbreak planning and effective response. This assessment turned out to be overly optimistic and based on flawed projections of the nature of the likely spread of disease, underestimating the speed of transmission and the capacity of existing stockpiles of equipment (Patel & Sridhar, 2021). In the United Kingdom, for example, a retrospective analysis of pandemic stockpiles found that millions of items of equipment were 'potentially unusable' (Livingston et al., 2020).

The assumptions of readiness were to have tragic consequences, and despite the favourable assessments of high income, developed countries they were to suffer significant mortality and partial health system collapse in the early pandemic waves. In any context, the lesson that nurses should draw from this is that there is a pressing need to assess the mitigation for major incidents. This includes identifying and addressing weaknesses in the nursing workforce and the systems that are needed to support its effective functioning, such as equipment, medication and safe hospital environments (see the use of the World Health Organization [WHO] health system building blocks for an example).

PREPAREDNESS

The phrase 'history may not repeat itself, but it often rhymes' is often attributed to Mark Twain, and it can be a useful starting point when considering how to effectively prepare a health service for a crisis or emergency. This type of preparation requires nurses not to be fortune tellers with a focus on guessing the precise nature of events that may occur in the future but, rather, historians who examine crises in their own country and others to reflect on both the mistakes and missteps and also the successes and developments of the response to these events. Taking an approach of scientific curiosity toward previous crises and 'war gaming'* what the approach would be should such an incident happen within one's workplace can provide useful insight and provide nurses with indications of areas within their direct supervision that can be improved. The crucial next step is to undertake a comprehensive capability assessment.

When we consider preparedness, it can be challenging to consider the possible eventualities that may occur. It is certainly true that flexibility is a vital component of the planning process, as all emergencies are unique events with distinct challenges. However, there are core components of any major incident which can be predicted. This includes preparing for increases in capacity of the health facility, effective triage and the redeployment of staff into areas where they are unfamiliar.

It may be helpful to view preparedness through the prism of the WHO's six building blocks of health systems (World Health Organization, 2010):

- Service delivery
- Health workforce
- Health information
- Access to essentials
- Health financing
- Leadership and governance.

Through assessing each of these building blocks for current resilience and challenges, nurses can begin to gain a rounded picture of the strengths and weaknesses of their workplace and the health systems that surround them. This is not to argue that nurses must have

all the answers or, indeed, have managerial oversight over the various levers of power that would be required to make changes across all six building blocks. In truth, very few, if any, decision-makers within a health system would have the authority to directly influence all the building blocks. This does not negate the importance of a well-rounded assessment as a way nurses can prepare for an emergency within their context; awareness of potential pitfalls beforehand is hugely preferential to having to rapidly improvise when a crisis occurs. Forewarned is, after all, forearmed.

Preparedness can only be applied to resources that exist or can be obtained within an appropriately brief time frame. On this basis, the question of what size of event to prepare for is more a policy issue than a planning one. Hence, funding for preparedness for disasters is predominantly a consideration for regional and national governments, although private sector providers, including hospitals and other organisations, may have internal plans in place. There is fiscal tension here, as preparedness, particularly at a national level, can mean considerable upfront costs preparing for events that may never happen. A degree of wastage, even in a highly organised system, is an inevitable consequence of stockpiling, and a rate-limiting factor may be policymakers' and taxpayers' willingness to fund vast piles of equipment that may expire without ever being used. In resource-poor settings, where there are already very significant budgetary pressures on day-to-day health systems running, the stockpiling of equipment and preparation of staff are often impossible.

THINK BOX 4.4

If you were assessing your local (the region where you work) preparedness for a disaster—for example, another pandemic or an earthquake—where would you look for information? Under each of the WHO health system building blocks, list what information sources are available to you.

RESPONSE

As previously described throughout this book, nurses are the foundation of most modern health workforces and central to the emergency response of any country faced with natural or human-made disaster. In high-performing health systems, the emergency response

---

*War gaming describes analytic games that simulate aspects of warfare at the tactical, operational or strategic level. The phrase here is suggesting simulations that would do the same in health care to plan for disruptions.

will, in most cases, be largely through the country's existing health workforce, and in this context, an adaptable and well-developed nursing cadre is an essential component of a coherent and well-organised response. Alarmingly, a survey of 32,000 nurses by the American Nurses Association undertaken during the pandemic revealed that 87% of nurses were afraid to go to work. Nurses reported an urgent need for education on caring for COVID-19 patients, PPE usage, personal safety and COVID-19 testing (Forbes, 2020). All of this shows clearly that this nursing workforce was unprepared to respond to this crisis, and those findings have been mirrored all over the world (Downey et al., 2023; also see Chapter 5).

Within a well-funded and flexible system, nurses can be redeployed relatively quickly based on evolving needs. This approach is not new: throughout the 1919 influenza pandemic, nurses in many richer countries responded in this way (Wood, 2017). This approach was mirrored and advanced in the recent coronavirus pandemic which saw, for example, nurses from other clinical areas redeployed to intensive care wards and, in the United States, nurses deployed to states with the greatest needs. In low-resource settings, the emergency response often requires support from other nations, not only in the initial response but also in the rebuilding effort. Each step is a process with distinct challenges and appropriate actions. The United Nations (UN) classification is outlined in Table 4.1.

The underlying principle is that a low-resource setting with less health system resilience is likely to reach the limits of its capabilities more rapidly and more frequently compared to its more affluent counterparts.

BANGLADESH—A CASE STUDY

Bangladesh is known to be highly prone to natural disasters such as tropical cyclones and storm surges,

flooding, tornadoes, earthquakes and riverbank erosion. This means that to a certain extent, Bangladesh can understand which types of disasters are more likely to occur and prepare. Over time, Bangladesh has built a comprehensive disaster response system that has developed to help the country counter the damage from critical incidents. In 1988, flooding caused severe damage to crops, infrastructure and the economy. Just a few years later in 1991, a cyclone claimed the lives of over 138,000 people. These disasters prompted the change from responding to incidents to preparedness for incidents (Sabur, 2012).

Before the serious incidents of 1988 and 1991, Bangladesh had responded to disasters after each event with relief and rehabilitation efforts. The significant loss of life and damage to the economy and livelihood of so many prompted a shift in perception of disaster management, and the concept of total disaster management emerged. As already laid out in this chapter, Bangladesh began to consider all aspects of disaster management and used the four-stage theory (Sabur, 2012). Although they are named differently, the concepts remain the same.

1. Normal phase: No immediate threat from a known hazard. The opportunity to plan and prepare for possible hazards.
2. Alert and warning phase: During this phase, an official warning is placed, and precautionary measures are taken until either the disaster makes an impact or the period passes.
3. Disaster phase: During this phase, the disaster hits, plans are carried out and emergency management takes place.
4. Recovery phase: The period after the acute disaster where efforts are made to restore infrastructure and livelihoods. This can often be the longest period.

TABLE 4.1
United Nations Classification of Emergencies
Level 1: a localised emergency (often confined to a single region/area)
Level 2: an emergency that is at a larger scale but can still be dealt with within the capacity of the agencies, government and other actors who are present in-country.
Level 3: the largest type of emergency and requires an international response, with the need for capacity and resources to be 'surged' into the country to help with the response.

(UNICEF Level-3 and Level-2 Emergencies. Available from: https://www.corecommitments.unicef.org/level-3-and-level-2-emergencies.)

Implementation of this theory in Bangladesh has highlighted three key learning points for other communities.

Firstly, traditionally, disaster management followed a hierarchical chain of command structure, with instructions being given out from a central command. This was found to limit community engagement and reduce the effectiveness of relief. This learning led to community-based disaster management, where a bottom-up approach is taken alongside a more traditional top-down approach. Communities are encouraged to assess local risks to them and work to build strategies.

The second learning point is that of gender inclusion. Gender inclusion has been discussed for some time, and the work is ongoing. A recent policy analysis of gender-inclusive disaster management policy in Bangladesh found that access to the early warning system and discussion of gender was present in the legal frameworks, equal participation in decision-making was moderately addressed and gender-based violence was mildly addressed (Hasan et al., 2019). When providing care and participating in disaster relief, nurses must be aware of these issues, as nurses are well placed to advocate for adjustments or developments in programs of care that are available and include all who need support.

Thirdly, the coordination and collaboration of government and nongovernmental organisations (NGOs) in Bangladesh are important to note. Bangladesh has many NGOs working within the country, and without coordination, this may lead to repeated coverage of certain areas and missing others. To ensure coordination and good coverage, all disaster relief is coordinated by the government. This collaboration can mitigate some of the challenges highlighted earlier; for example, NGOs provide the majority of the resources for relief during the emergency phase, reducing the pressure placed on existing limited resources. Financial support is also provided, with some countries supporting with significant budgets (Saudi Arabia provided $100 million USD after the cyclone in 2008) (Sabur, 2012).

THINK BOX 4.5

- Would a 'community-based disaster management' approach be useful where you work?
- Could it be used for other health planning initiatives beside disasters?
- What differences in responses might you expect to see?

THE 'REAL POLITIC' OF INTERNATIONAL RESPONSE

The scale and effectiveness of international responses to events remain problematic, with slowly evolving, longer-term crises often receiving less comprehensive support when compared to emergencies that are more rapid in onset. Layered on top of this are societal, geopolitical, media and cultural forces which sway public opinion, policymakers and health care workers and thus influence the response. The classification of emergencies, particularly moving between the levels outlined in Table 4.1, is sometimes inconsistent. This is despite the death tolls and impact being similar or much worse in scale—and in some cases, the response fails to match the need.

The Boxing Day Tsunami of 2004 is estimated to have killed 230,000 people (Nugroho and Fahmi, 2021) and saw an unprecedented global response, with significant resources mobilised to Southeast Asia and East Africa very rapidly. This is almost identical to the number of females who die globally each year in pregnancy and childbirth (Kurjak et al., 2022) without the same public call to arms and action. It is argued that the invention of modern telecommunications, improved global televising of conflict and natural and human-made disasters in the later part of the 20th century changed the way that richer nations responded to global emergencies (Gebbie and Qureshi, 2006); this is undoubtedly true and will be explored in more detail in this chapter.

It is, however, a mistake to presume that the international response to comparably significant emergencies is broadly similar, as there is strong evidence to suggest the opposite remains the case.

THE RIGHT 'TYPE' OF EMERGENCY FOR AN INTERNATIONAL RESPONSE

Following a ponderous start, hundreds of international nurses and other health workers were deployed to West Africa to assist in containing the Ebola outbreak. The international response was huge, with many NGOs and governments from richer nations responding with supplies and technical expertise. This included many nurses from across the world. The United Kingdom alone deployed more than 150 health workers to support the response to the outbreak, part

CASE STUDY 4.2
Ebola 2014–2016 and the Yemen Civil War

With over 28,000 confirmed cases, the 2014–2016 West African Ebola virus disease epidemic is documented as the largest in history, surpassing all previous outbreaks combined (Cenciarelli et al., 2015). The rapid cross-border spread of the Zaire strain from rural Guinea to neighbouring Liberia and Sierra Leone was exacerbated by poor public health infrastructure and grossly inadequate surveillance. Shultz et al. (2016) condemn the prevalence of fear-related behaviours alongside inaccurate public health messaging for their role in expediting the spread of the virus, whilst the slow and poorly coordinated international response served to further exacerbate the situation (Moon et al., 2015).

of a huge international effort. The support from the United States, United Kingdom and Germany alone was estimated to cost $3.611 billion in the first year of the outbreak (Centers for Disease Control [CDC], 2019). International nurses played a significant role in the response to the Ebola outbreak, providing extra capacity within the systems and supporting clinical care across all three countries. Analysis of the response highlighted the initial hesitancy of the international community but also praised nurses, both local and international, amongst the wider international community (Coltart et al., 2017).

There is no doubt that the Ebola outbreak caused very significant mortality and morbidity, not only directly, where it is estimated that 11,000 people died, but also through the widespread impact on general health services, with females and children's health particularly adversely affected (Delamou et al., 2017). The impact of Ebola was significantly mitigated by the prompt international response and the role of health workers, including nurses, who, at considerable personal risk, undertook to deliver high-quality health care in very challenging circumstances. They were supported by the rapid development of pharmaceuticals, a multimillion-dollar logistical supply chain and a global public who lauded their efforts.

The crisis that emerged in parallel in Yemen did not attract the same response. In 2014, a civil war erupted

in Yemen between the country's official government and Houthi rebels. As the Ebola crisis was taking hold in West Africa, the situation in Yemen was becoming increasingly grim. Yemen's health system was historically weak, and half of its population lived in poverty (He et al., 2018). However, in the years leading up to the war, outcomes had begun to improve 'including increased life expectancy, reduced infant, under-5 child and maternal mortality' (Qirbi & Ismail, 2017). The effects of war caused a rapid regression in the progress that was being made and brought the health system to the brink of collapse. Evidence of this collapse was seen in significant outbreaks of diseases which are part of standard vaccination programmes across the world, including diphtheria (Dureab et al., 2019)l and diseases of poor water and sanitation, including a prolonged cholera outbreak (He et al., 2018).

By 2017, it was estimated that more than 24,382 children alone had died as either a direct or indirect result of the conflict (Jenkins et al., 2018), which is more than double the total number of adults and children killed as a result of Ebola in the West African outbreak. By 2021, the estimated civilian death toll in Yemen stood at 233,000, mostly from 'indirect causes' (OCHA, 2022).

The magnitude of the health catastrophe in Yemen dwarfed the response from the international community which, in turn, was very far removed from the response to Ebola. Few international nurses worked in the Yemen during the war, and Yemen's nurses were left to work in a system that was collapsing around them. In 2015, the UN estimated that international aid for Yemen was only 55% of what was required for an adequate response (Financial Tracking Service, 2016). In the same period, millions of dollars in arms sales from the United Kingdom and the United States were found to have escalated the conflict in Yemen and been responsible for significant civilian casualties (Feinstein & Choonara, 2020). The impact of the war on the Yemeni nursing workforce was disastrous. Between 2014 and 2015, the number of nurses and midwives per head of population in Yemen fell by a third (Downey et al., 2023), and whilst this has now recovered a little, there is evidence that nurses have suffered from a lack of rudimentary professional development, including in topics as fundamental as basic life support (Alkubati et al., 2022).

THINK BOX 4.6

Before you read the next section, reflect on the responses to these two disasters and the effects of the response on both the outcomes and the nursing workforces.

- Why do you think the responses were so different?

What these two crises, which began within months of each other, demonstrate is the asymmetric nature of international crisis response. Geography, media, race, perceived threat to one's own country and type of disaster all influence the global response to a crisis. However, regardless of international support, nursing care continues in almost all contexts. This is most often through the courageous work of the existing nurses and health workforce.

The impact of politics on the lives of those affected by the crisis is clear—Yemen is not a political priority and has not been funded or supported as such. We draw the comparison between Yemen and Ebola not in any way to denigrate the international response to the Ebola outbreak in West Africa but, rather, to hold it as an exemplar of what is possible when international actors work effectively. It is also clear that the international response to the crisis is not always based on need, even as crises develop and worsen over years.

It is vital for nurses, as a global community, to advocate for compatriots facing impossibly difficult challenges in many wars and disasters across the world, including forgotten or ignored crises and conflicts which rarely lead nightly news bulletins or feature highly in the wider public consciousness.

RECOVERY

Even in the event of a short-term localised emergency, it can take a significant period for health services to recover. The backlog in delayed care alongside the need for staff recovery, both physical and mental, can make recovery problematic. As the world emerges from the coronavirus, we see significant pressure on health services as staff deal both with fatigue and the effects of stress while health services grapple with unmet needs. In some cases, the response of the international community can worsen the situation. Perhaps the most obvious example of this was the Haiti earthquake in

2010 which killed 149,095 people, of which 6300 died in a potentially preventable cholera outbreak which was most likely brought to the country by those who had come to assist (Bayntun et al., 2012). It is almost inevitable that the delay and disruption in core health system functions can lead to a secondary wave of mortality and poor health outcomes. This is being seen now as the world emerges from COVID but was also seen during many previous crises, including Ebola's extraordinarily damaging effect on routine maternal and child health care due to health system collapse (Delamou et al., 2017).

Perhaps unsurprisingly, the inequalities that were identified before and during the crisis are also in evidence as the country and health system emerge from it. For example, research has demonstrated that just as race was predictive in identifying poor health outcomes before and during Hurricane Katrina, racial background may play a role in how likely a person is to recover from the event. A study of African American survivors of the hurricane found higher rates of unemployment and psychological distress compared to white survivors (Elliott & Pais, 2006). Nurses involved in supporting the recovery of a health system must be aware of the inequalities that existed before the event and mindful that the crisis is almost always going to have worsened these disparities in outcome. Recovery should focus, alongside a return to business as usual, on a system that reduces inequality as part of a broader health strategy so that when the next crisis occurs, the disproportionate impact is more effectively mitigated.

The recovery phase is often made more challenging by the effect of the crisis or event on health workers. Alongside the impact on patients, there is a significant impact on health workers who have worked during the crisis, either within their home country or abroad as part of an aid effort. Mental illness amongst health workers causes significant individual impact and health system stress. Evidence from the coronavirus pandemic challenges the assumption that it is only after the event that mental health conditions increase in health workers. Nearly half of a sample of newly qualified clinicians in Nepal were found to be displaying signs of anxiety, and a third were displaying signs of depression in the first 2 months of the global pandemic (Khanal et al., 2020).

Research conducted on those who returned from supporting the postwar crisis in South Sudan found there was a significant prevalence of mental health conditions, with nearly a quarter of aid workers displaying symptoms of posttraumatic stress disorder (Strohmeier et al., 2018). Nurses must develop support strategies for staff before the crisis and enact these quickly during the crisis to reduce the impact on individuals and the wider health system.

The recovery phase of the response can take many years and is fraught with challenges to individuals and the system they work in. However, it can also be, as was highlighted by Seacole and Nightingale, a time for reappraisal and redesign. The lessons learnt from a short- or long-term crisis can inform and improve service provision and redesign. The role of nurses to shape and develop services in this context is endless, and the positive lessons to emerge from a crisis must not be forgotten in the rush to return to how things were before.

LOOKING TO THE FUTURE

Do undergraduate nursing curricula prepare nurses for emergencies? Whether during a hurricane or an infectious disease outbreak, nurses can help build community resilience by understanding how disasters affect people's health and restrict access to resources like transportation, medical care, food, shelter and jobs. With the right training and support, nurses can play a role in everything from distributing vaccines equitably to ensuring evacuees in shelters receive the physical and mental health care they need to recover. Current evidence suggests that nurses are not prepared for this role in preservice education. For example, undergraduate teaching curricula in many developed nations barely mention tropical diseases (Flaherty et al., 2015) even though the ease of global travel makes their occurrence possible anywhere. Only those nurses in infectious diseases and specialist units acquire significant clinical expertise in conditions such as malaria, cholera or dengue haemorrhagic fever. Even this clinical exposure is set within the familiarity of a well-funded health system, unlike many low-resource health settings, so it does not prepare nurses to work in low-resource emergency settings. Preservice nursing curricula seldom teach students about health care emergency preparedness, though recent experience of a pandemic may (and should) prompt future changes.

THINK BOX 4.7

Looking back at your own education in nursing, do you feel you have been prepared to deal with emergencies? Maybe you were nursing during the global pandemic and experienced the need for additional skills and knowledge:
- If so, what would you have liked to know?
- If you were to rewrite the nursing curriculum to deal with emergencies, what might you include?

Even at a postgraduate level, most disaster nursing education programmes occur in countries where, overwhelming, disasters are exceptionally rare (Kalanlar, 2018). There is no association between the location of specialist disaster nursing courses, which are most commonly hosted in Europe and North America, and regions where such an event is most likely to occur, for example, sub-Saharan Africa and Southeast Asia (Loke et al., 2021). Disaster nursing as a discipline still requires significant support to develop and teach, and curricula and learning outcomes are currently not harmonised between courses, leading to a wide variety of graduate skills and expertise. Previous attempts to provide oversight, including the International Nursing Coalition for Mass Casualty Education, have ended when funding was not maintained. The result of this lack of coordination is that the nursing profession is not as represented as it should be at policy and strategic forums. This mirrors a much broader global picture of nurses, discussed earlier in this chapter, as critical first-line workers, the largest cadre of health workers, with little input into policy and strategic decision-making. In Chapter 8, there is more about nurses and power related to nursing being a predominantly female workforce.

The coronavirus pandemic has given the global nursing workforce a significant opportunity to enhance and develop its role and political clout within the global health community. Not for the first time in history, nurses have proved both their capabilities and capacity to adapt and deliver high-quality care in the most exceptionally challenging environments. Slowly, the world is waking up to nurses being far from an optional extra to health system functioning but, in fact, the driving force of every health system across the globe. As the nurses that pioneered care more than a century ago proved, the opportunities to innovate and succeed are possible if nurses seize them.

REFERENCES

Alkubati, S. A., McClean, C., Yu, R., Albagawi, B., Alsaqri, S. H., & Alsabri, M. (2022). Basic life support knowledge in a war-torn country: A survey of nurses in Yemen. *BMC Nursing, 21*(1), 1–7.

Andermann, A. CLEAR Collaboration. (2016). Taking action on the social determinants of health in clinical practice: a framework for health professionals. *CMAJ, 188*(17-18), E474–E483. doi:10.1503/cmaj.160177. Epub 2016 Aug 8. PMID: 27503870; PMCID: PMC5135524. 2016.

Anionwu, E. N. (2012). Mary Seacole: Nursing care in many lands. *British Journal of Health care Assistants, 6*(5), 244–248.

Attenborough, J. (2021). A century of professional regulation: What does it mean for nurses today? *Nursing Times, 117*(9), 18–21.

Bambra, C., Riordan, R., Ford, J., & Matthews, F. (2020). The COVID-19 pandemic and health inequalities. *Journal of Epidemiology and Community Health, 74*, 964–968. https://jech.bmj.com/content/74/11/964.

Bayntun, C., Rockenschaub, G., & Murray, V. (2012). Developing a health system approach to disaster management: A qualitative analysis of the core literature to complement the WHO Toolkit for assessing health-system capacity for crisis management. *PLoS Currents, 4*, e5028b6037259a. doi:10.1371/5028b6037259a. PMID: 23066520; PMCID: PMC3461970. Last accessed March 2024.

Bostridge, M. (2015). *Florence Nightingale: the woman and her legend*. Penguin Random House UK.

Brunkard, J., Namulanda, G., & Ratard, R. (2008). Hurricane Katrina deaths, Louisiana, 2005. *Disaster Medicine and Public Health Preparedness, 2*(4), 215–223. doi: 10.1097/DMP.0b013e31818aaf55. PMID: 18756175. Last accessed March 2024.

Cenciarelli, O., Pietropaoli, S., Malizia, A., Carestia, M., D'Amico, F., Sassolini, A., Di Giovanni, D., Rea, S., Gabbarini, V., Tamburrini, A., Palombi, L., Bellecci, C., & Gaudio, P. (2015). Ebola virus disease 2013-2014 outbreak in west Africa: an analysis of the epidemic spread and response. *International Journal of Microbiology, 2015*, 769121. doi: 10.1155/2015/769121. Last accessed March 2024.

Centers for Disease Control and Prevention, (CDC). (2019). Cost of the Ebola Epidemic | History | Ebola (Ebola Virus Disease) | CDC. Available from: https://www.cdc.gov/vhf/ebola/history/2014-2016-outbreak/cost-of-ebola.html [Accessed Jun 4, 2022].

Coltart, C. E., Lindsey, B., Ghinai, I., Johnson, A. M., & Heymann, D. L. (2017). The Ebola outbreak, 2013–2016: Old lessons for new epidemics. *Philosophical Transactions of the Royal Society B: Biological Sciences, 372*(1721), 20160297.

Dawson, S., Jackson, D., & Elliott, D. (2021). Understanding the motivation of nurses volunteering for non-disaster humanitarian service. *Collegian, 28*(6), 645–651.

Delamou, A., El Ayadi, A. M., Sidibe, S., Delvaux, T., Camara, B. S., Sandouno, S. D., Beavogui, A. H., Rutherford, G. W., Okumura, J., & Zhang, W. (2017). Effect of Ebola virus disease on maternal and child health services in guinea: A retrospective observational cohort study. *The Lancet Global Health, 5*(4), e448–e457.

Downey, E., Fokeladeh, H. S., & Catton, H. (2023). *What the COVID-19 pandemic has exposed: the findings of five global health workforce professions*. Geneva, Switzerland: World Health Organization. (Human Resources for Health Observer Series No. 28).

Dumitrascu, D. I., David, L., Dumitrascu, D. L., & Rogozea, L. (2020). Florence Nightingale bicentennial: 1820–2020. Her contributions to health care improvement. *Medicine and Pharmacy Reports, 93*(4), 428.

Dureab, F., Al-Sakkaf, M., Ismail, O., Kuunibe, N., Krisam, J., Müller, O., & Jahn, A. (2019). Diphtheria outbreak in Yemen: The impact of conflict on a fragile health system. *Conflict and Health, 13*(1), 1–7.

Elliott, J. R., & Pais, J. (2006). Race, class, and hurricane Katrina: Social differences in human responses to disaster. *Social Science Research, 35*(2), 295–321.

Feinstein, A., & Choonara, I. (2020). Arms sales and child health. *BMJ Paediatrics Open, 4*(1), 1–5. https://bmjpaedsopen.bmj.com/content/bmjpo/4/1/e000809.full.pdf. Last accessed March 2024.

Financial Tracking Service. (2016). Appeals and response plans 2015. Available from: https://fts.unocha.org/appeals/overview/2015. Last accessed March 2024.

Flaherty, G., Scott, A., Malak, M., Avalos, G., & O'Brien, T. (2015). Recognition of imported tropical infectious disease in returned travellers in a university hospital emergency department. *Emergency Medicine Open Journal, 1*(2), 39–45.

Forbes. (2020). 'Why Americas nurses were not prepared for the pandemic. Health Report. https://www.forbes.com/sites/coronavirusfrontlines/2020/06/04/why-americas-nurses-were-not-prepared-for-the-coronavirus-pandemic/?sh=729921c2164b. Last accessed November 2022.

Fletcher, K. A., Reddin, K., Tait, D. (2022). The history of disaster nursing: from Nightingale to nursing in the 21st century. *Journal of Research in Nursing, 27*(3), 257–272. doi:10.1177/17449871211058854.

Gebbie, K., & Qureshi, K. (2006). A historical challenge: Nurses and emergencies. *OJIN: The Online Journal of Issues in Nursing, 11*(3), 1–8.

Hartman, C. W., Squires, G., & Squires, G. D. (2006). *There is no such thing as a natural disaster: Race, class, and Hurricane Katrina*. Taylor & Francis. New York Routledge. https://doi.org/10.4324/9780203625460.

Hasan, M. R., Nasreen, M., & Chowdhury, M. A. (2019). Gender-inclusive disaster management policy in Bangladesh: A content analysis of national and international regulatory frameworks. *International Journal of Disaster Risk Reduction, 41*, 101324.

He, D., Wang, X., Gao, D., & Wang, J. (2018). Modeling the 2016–2017 Yemen cholera outbreak with the impact of limited medical resources. *Journal of Theoretical Biology, 451*, 80–85.

Helmstadter, C., & Godden, J. (2016). *Nursing Before Nightingale* (pp. 1815–1899). Routledge. https://doi.org/10.4324/9781315598628.

Jenkins, D., Marktanner, M., Merkel, A. D., & Sedik, D. (2018). Estimating child mortality attributable to war in Yemen. *International Journal of Development Issues, 17*(3), 372–383. https://doi.org/10.1108/IJDI-02-2018-0031.

Kalanlar, B. (2018). Effects of disaster nursing education on nursing students' knowledge and preparedness for disasters. *International Journal of Disaster Risk Reduction, 28*, 475–480.

Karan, A., Negandhi, H., Hussain, S., Zapata, T., Mairembam, D., De Graeve, H., Buchan, J., & Zodpey, S. (2021). Size, composition and distribution of health workforce in India: Why, and where to invest? *Human Resources for Health, 19*(1), 1–14.

Khanal, P., Devkota, N., Dahal, M., Paudel, K., & Joshi, D. (2020). Mental health impacts among health workers during COVID-19 in a low resource setting: A cross-sectional survey from Nepal. *Globalization and Health, 16*(1), 1–12.

Kurjak, A., Stanojević, M., & Dudenhausen, J. (2022). Why maternal mortality in the world remains tragedy in low-income countries and shame for high-income ones: Will sustainable development goals (SDG) help? *Journal of Perinatal Medicine, 51*(2), 170–181. https://doi.org/10.1515/jpm-2022-0061.

Lantada, N., Carreño, M. L., & Jaramillo, N. (2020). Disaster risk reduction: A decision-making support tool based on the morphological analysis. *International Journal of Disaster Risk Reduction, 42*, 101342.

Laurent, C. (2019). *Rituals & Myths in Nursing: A Social History*. Pen and Sword Yorkshire UK. www.pen-and-sword.co.uk.

Lee, E., Loh, W., Ang, I., & Tan, Y. (2020). Plastic bags as personal protective equipment during the COVID-19 pandemic: Between the devil and the deep blue sea. *Journal of Emergency Medicine, 58*(5), 821–823.

Livingston, E., Desai, A., & Berkwits, M. (2020). Sourcing personal protective equipment during the COVID-19 pandemic. *JAMA, 323*(19), 1912–1914.

Loke, A. Y., Guo, C., & Molassiotis, A. (2021). Development of disaster nursing education and training programs in the past 20 years (2000–2019): A systematic review. *Nurse Education Today, 99*, 104809.

Lone, N. I., McPeake, J., Stewart, N. I., Blayney, M. C., Seem, R. C., Donaldson, L., Glass, E., Haddow, C., Hall, R., Martin, C., Paton, M., Smith-Palmer, A., Kaye, C. T., & Puxty, K. (2021). Influence of socioeconomic deprivation on interventions and outcomes for patients admitted with COVID-19 to critical care units in Scotland: A national cohort study. *The Lancet Regional Health - Europe, 1*, 100005. https://doi.org/10.1016/j.lanepe.2020.100005.

Messmer, P. R., & Parchment, Y. (1998). Mary Grant Seacole: the first nurse practitioner. *Clinical excellence for nurse practitioners, 2*(1), 47–51. 1998.

Moon, S., Sridhar, D., Pate, M. A., Jha, A. K., Clinton, C., Delaunay, S., Edwin, V., Fallah, M., Fidler, D. P., & Garrett, L. (2015). Will Ebola change the game? ten essential reforms before the next pandemic. the report of the Harvard-LSHTM independent panel on the global response to Ebola. *The Lancet, 386*(10009), 2204–2221.

McDonald, L. (2020). Florence Nightingale: The making of a hospital reformer. *HERD: Health Environments Research & Design Journal, 13*(2), 25–31.

Morgan, M. (2020). Why meaning-making matters: The case of the UK government's COVID-19 response. *American Journal of Cultural Sociology, 8*(3), 270–323.

Nelson, S. (2010). The Nightingale Imperative. In S. Nelson, & A.-M. Rafferty (Eds.), *Notes on Nightingale*. Ithaca and London: Cornell University Press.

Nelson, S., & Rafferty, A.-M. (Eds.). (2010). *Notes on Nightingale*. Ithaca and London: Cornell University Press.

Nojavan, M., Salehi, E., & Omidvar, B. (2018). Conceptual change of disaster management models: A thematic analysis. *Jamba, 10*(1), 451. doi:10.4102/jamba.v10i1.451.

Nugroho, A., & Fahmi, M. (2021). *The 2004 Indian Ocean Earthquake and Tsunami: Resettlement and Demographic Challenges*. In *Climate Change, Disaster Risks, and Human Security* (pp. 317–331). Springer: Singapore. https://doi.org/10.1007/978-981-15-8852-5_15.

OCHA. (2022). Yemen | Global Humanitarian Overview. Available from: https://gho.unocha.org/yemen. [Accessed Aug 4, 2022].

Office for National Statistics. (2020). Deaths involving COVID-19 by local area and socioeconomic deprivation: deaths occurring between 1 March and 31 July 2020. Released 28 August 2020. https://www.ons.gov.uk/peoplepopulationandcommunity/birthsdeathsandmarriages/deaths/bulletins/deathsinvolvingcovid19bylocalareasanddeprivation/deathsoccurringbetween1marchand31july2020.

Patel, J., & Sridhar, D. (2021). Better pandemic preparedness, Finance & Development. www.meetings.imf.org.

Pathak, E. B., Menard, J. M., Garcia, R. B., & Salemi, J. L. (2021). Social class, race/ethnicity, and COVID-19 mortality among working age adults in the United States, medRxiv. https://www.medrxiv.org/content/10.1101/2021.11.23.21266759v1.full.

Qirbi, N., & Ismail, S. A. (2017). Health system functionality in a low-income country in the midst of conflict: The case of Yemen. *Health Policy and Planning, 32*(6), 911–922.

Rowan, N. J., & Laffey, J. G. (2021). Unlocking the surge in demand for personal and protective equipment (PPE) and improvised face coverings arising from coronavirus disease (COVID-19) pandemic–implications for efficacy, re-use and sustainable waste management. *Science of the Total Environment, 752*, 142259.

Sabur, A. A. (2012). Disaster management system in Bangladesh: An overview. *India Quarterly, 68*(1), 29–47.

Shultz, J. M., Cooper, J. L., Baingana, F., Oquendo, M. A., Espinel, Z., Althouse, B. M., Marcelin, L. H., Towers, S., Espinola, M., & McCoy, C. B. (2016). The role of fear-related behaviors in the 2013–2016 West Africa Ebola virus disease outbreak. *Current Psychiatry Reports, 18*(11), 1–14.

Staring-Derks, C., Staring, J., & Anionwu, E. N. (2015). Mary Seacole: Global nurse extraordinaire. *Journal of Advanced Nursing, 71*(3), 514–525.

Strohmeier, H., Scholte, W. F., & Ager, A. (2018). Factors associated with common mental health problems of humanitarian workers in South Sudan. *PLoS One, 13*(10), e0205333.

Veenema, T. G. (2018). *Disaster nursing and emergency preparedness for chemical, biological, and radiological terrorism and other hazards* (4th ed.). New York: Springer Publishing Company.

White, I. K., Philpot, T. S., Wylie, K., & McGowen, E. (2007). Feeling the pain of my people: Hurricane Katrina, racial inequality, and the psyche of black America. *Journal of Black Studies, 37*(4), 523–538.

Wood, P. J. (2017). Managing boundaries between professional and lay nursing following the influenza pandemic, 1918–1919: Insights for professional resilience today? *Journal of Clinical Nursing, 26*(5-6), 805–812.

World Health Organization. (2010). *Monitoring the building blocks of health systems: a handbook of indicators and their measurement strategies*. Geneva, Switzerland: World Health Organization.

World Health Organization. (2020). *State of the world's nursing 2020: Investing in education, jobs and leadership*. Geneva, Switzerland: WHO.

World Health Organization. (2022). World health organization's global health workforce statistics - Yemen. Available from: https://data.worldbank.org/indicator/SH.MED.NUMW.P3?locations=YE.

5

NURSING WORKFORCE ISSUES DURING COVID-19

GREG SHARPLIN ▪ IMOGEN RAMSEY ▪ MARION ECKERT

INTRODUCTION

In 2020, the International Year of the Nurse and Midwife, health care workers across the globe faced unprecedented challenges in managing the COVID-19 pandemic. COVID-19 is an infectious respiratory illness caused by the severe acute respiratory syndrome coronavirus 2 (SARS-CoV-2) virus, which was first identified in December 2019 in the city of Wuhan, Hubei Province, China. In the months that followed, COVID-19 spread to every inhabited continent. The World Health Organization (WHO) declared COVID-19 a global pandemic on 11 March 2020 (World Health Organization, 2020).

The COVID-19 virus mutated into numerous variants or strains and subvariants. By June 2022, WHO had identified five variants of concern, classified as such because they may either have higher transmissibility, cause more severe symptoms or respond less effectively to vaccines or treatments than previous strains (World Health Organization, 2022). Of these, the Omicron variant, which WHO declared a variant of concern on 26 November 2021, was the dominant strain circulating throughout much of the world in 2022 (World Health Organization, 2022). Early evidence suggested that the Omicron variant was associated with less severe disease, higher transmissibility, higher risk of reinfection and lower vaccine effectiveness compared to other variants (Araf et al., 2022). Its rapid spread in late 2021 caused record-breaking numbers of COVID-19 cases and strained health systems around the world.

The rapid spread of COVID-19 had the potential to overwhelm primary and acute health care services, and this was the case in many countries. Globally, daily new infections peaked in January 2022. By December 2022, approximately 645 million cases of COVID-19 had been reported globally, and an estimated 6.64 million people had died. A significant number of these deaths were health care workers who met evolving challenges on the front lines of the pandemic. In the pandemic's early stages, the world's health care workforces faced an unknown pathogen, and they had limited knowledge, personal protective equipment (PPE) and tools for diagnosis and treatment (Grinspun et al., 2022). The challenge to deliver health care services was compounded by the spread of COVID-19, particularly the highly infectious Omicron variant, among health care workers, which affected staffing levels. To create new COVID-19 services, health resources were continuously reshuffled and reallocated, which placed additional strain on existing services. Staff shortages increased the pressure on already overwhelmed health systems, prompting urgent action in many countries to try and secure more health care workers (Buchan et al., 2022). Throughout this global health crisis, nurses were the largest health care professional group providing frontline care (Paterson et al., 2020).

The impacts of the pandemic on the global health care workforce have extended far beyond dealing with immediate cases. Throughout the pandemic, health care workers have been confronted with risk to their personal safety as well as highly stressful working conditions. Health care workers, and nurses in particular, are at increased risk of COVID-19 infection because of increased contact time with people who are infected (Zheng et al., 2020). The pandemic also exposed nurses to increased patient loads, uncertainty around disease outcomes, workforce shortages and rapidly changing organisational policies and practices. A *Nursing Times* survey conducted in January 2021 in the United Kingdom showed that almost all nurses were working shifts that were short-staffed due to colleagues being too unwell or isolating (Ford, 2021). A European Federation of Nurses (EFN) Associations report identified major concerns about inconsistent and uncertain provision of PPE and COVID-19 testing for nurses (European Federation of Nurses Associations, 2020). In addition to these challenges, nurses have reported that other significant stressors have impacted their physical, mental and emotional well-being during the pandemic (Catania et al., 2021; Delgado et al., 2020; Maben & Bridges, 2020; Spoorthy et al., 2020). Long shifts, wearing PPE, community aggression and abuse, and concerns for the safety of loved ones and patients added to these difficulties. Awareness of these issues raised concern about increasing levels of burnout among nurses and the lack of psychological and social support available in many countries (European Federation of Nurses Associations, 2020).

RESEARCH INTO NURSING WORKFORCE CHALLENGES DURING COVID-19

To understand how the COVID-19 pandemic impacted nurses and midwives, the Rosemary Bryant AO Research Centre conducted climate surveys of the nursing and midwifery workforces in Australia, Canada and internationally. In 2020, we surveyed 11,902 Australian nurses, midwives and personal care workers in collaboration with state and territory branches of the Australian Nursing and Midwifery Federation. Although the Australian COVID-19 outbreak was relatively contained by global standards at this time, this was a year of unprecedented stress and concern for health care workers. In 2021, together with the Registered Nurses' Association of Ontario, we surveyed 5200 Canadian nurses. In the same year, in partnership with Nursing Now, we surveyed 1500 nurses and midwives from 125 countries, using English, French and Spanish (with participation highest in North America and Europe). The timing of our Canadian and international surveys coincided

with the downward trend of Europe's second wave of COVID-19, increasing case numbers across North America and other parts of the world, and more virulent strains of the virus emerging. At the time, ongoing global surges of COVID-19 meant that nurses and midwives had not had a reprieve from the first wave of the pandemic. Prior studies exploring the impact of the first wave of the pandemic on the health care workforce had focused largely on the availability of PPE and treatment regimens (Galanis et al., 2021; Morgantini et al., 2020; Zheng et al., 2021). As concerns shifted to staff shortages and workforce burnout, our 2021 surveys captured a global snapshot of factors influencing nurses' clinical practice, workforce environment and well-being during the pandemic as it entered its second year as a global crisis. This chapter provides a critical reflection on challenges faced by nursing workforces globally during the COVID-19 pandemic, based on our research findings and other literature. They are summarised into the following themes:

- Global and regional leadership
- Workplace safety
- Personal concerns related to COVID-19
- Workloads and staffing
- Well-being, burnout and access to support

GLOBAL AND REGIONAL LEADERSHIP

The nurses at the front line of the COVID-19 pandemic need and deserve strong leaders who will speak with courage and sound knowledge to ensure that their interests are front and centre at the decision-making table (Daly et al., 2020).

Leadership is key to strengthening the nursing workforce (Shalala et al., 2011). As respected collaborators across multidisciplinary teams, leaders can contribute to enhanced quality and safety structures within their organisations (Wymer et al., 2021). Leadership has been highlighted by nurses in the literature as a key factor in supporting quality care (Heinen et al., 2019). Authentic nurse leadership and a healthy work environment have been found to contribute positively to staff and patient outcomes in studies conducted before and during the pandemic (Raso et al., 2021). Authentic

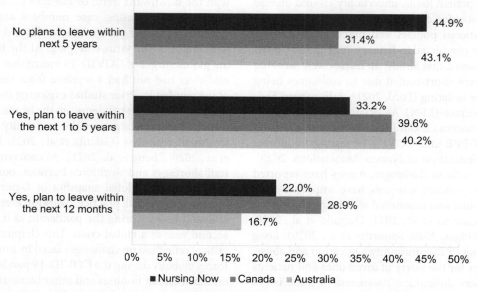

Fig. 5.1 ■ Nurses' and midwives' intentions to leave their current position across three surveys.

nursing leadership has also been linked to job satisfaction, turnover, work-related attitudes and behaviours, and staff empowerment (Wong & Walsh, 2020). However, although they make up more than half of the health workforce, nurses are the least represented health profession in leadership positions and decision-making (World Health Organization, 2020).

Effective nurse and midwife leadership is critical to addressing global and regional challenges for maintaining long-term nursing and midwifery workforce stability. The 'State of the World's Nursing 2020' report, coauthored by the WHO, the International Council of Nurses (ICN) and Nursing Now, recommended that nursing leadership is developed at regional, national and global levels to address the projected worldwide shortage of 7.8 million nurses by 2030 (World Health Organization, 2020). Addressing this projected resource shortage is particularly important in developing countries and environments where nurses and midwives play a critical role in community health care. The COVID-19 pandemic has exacerbated long-standing issues for the nursing workforce, and some authors have warned that nursing faces an impending leadership crisis (Daly et al., 2020). Over half of the respondents from the Nursing Now and Australian surveys, and more than two-thirds of the

respondents from the Canadian survey reported having plans to leave their job within the next 5 years (see Fig. 5.1). Of these, around 12%–17% intended to exit their profession to work in another field, and around one-quarter intended to retire. Nurses most likely to report intentions to exit the profession were those aged 40–49 years, around the mean age of nurse leaders in US hospitals (Westphal, 2012). In a study exploring the impacts of the pandemic on nursing leaders, one-quarter of participants reported poor emotional well-being, and their intent to leave the nursing profession increased by 123% in 6 months (American Organization for Nursing Leadership & Joslin Marketing, 2021). Turnover intentions in nurses have been found to be driven by several factors, including workload, work–life interference, burnout, engagement and leadership support (Labrague et al., 2020).

The COVID-19 pandemic disrupted existing systems and challenged nurse leaders to develop and implement novel policies while seeking to minimise transmission of COVID-19 to patients and staff. Nurse leaders have described various challenges during the pandemic, including the lack of a playbook, shortage of PPE and supplies, ever-changing information, changes in workplace culture and dynamics and the financial impact on staff (Joslin & Joslin, 2020). The American

Organization for Nursing Leadership conducted a longitudinal study of nurse leaders during COVID-19 and found that the greatest challenges they reported were communicating and implementing changing policies; surge staffing, training and reallocation; emotional well-being of staff; and access to PPE and other equipment (Joslin & Joslin, 2020). On average, respondents self-reported that they had handled challenges during the COVID-19 pandemic adequately (Joslin & Joslin, 2020). In the face of these challenges, nurse leaders played a key role in generating solutions to limit the spread of COVID-19, support health care workers and improve the pandemic response (Wymer et al., 2021). They implemented rapid changes across health systems in response to changing local and national policies, emerging data trends, scientific discoveries and surge capacity requirements (Wymer et al., 2021).

Perceptions of nursing leadership and policy during the COVID-19 pandemic varied. The Nursing Now international survey indicated a workforce perception of average nursing leadership present in the practice environment, along with insufficient staff and inappropriate skill mix to effectively deal with the health care burden of COVID-19. Participants reported moderate satisfaction with work, scheduling flexibility and collegial relationships and moderate dissatisfaction with extrinsic rewards and leadership and career opportunities. Participants identified that stronger leadership and policy would help mitigate personal risk in key areas of concern, including PPE practices, working within scope of practice and reported incidences of threats or abuse by members of the public. Collectively, these findings highlight that increasing the presence, authority and visibility of nurse leadership is critical for creating supportive work environments in which nurses and midwives can provide safe care. To achieve this, structural and policy changes are needed to empower and protect individuals at a system level (Schlak et al., 2022).

THINK BOX 5.1

- What leadership approaches and skills are required in a crisis like the COVID-19 pandemic?
- What strategies have been, or could be, put in place to support nurse leaders in managing a future health crisis?

WORKPLACE SAFETY

The value of nurses has never been clearer, not only to our health care systems but also to our global peace and security, nor could it be any clearer that not enough is being done to protect nurses and other health workers, tragically underscored by the more than 180,000 health worker deaths due to COVID-19. ICN Chief Executive, Howard Catton (International Council of Nurses, 2022).

Navigating the pandemic in the face of significant workplace risks to health and safety has been a major challenge for the nursing and midwifery workforces. The COVID-19 pandemic posed a direct threat to the health and safety of all frontline health care workers, who have an increased risk of contracting COVID-19 compared with the general community, even after allowing for other risk factors. The first reported infection rates among health care workers were for those in Wuhan, China, where 29% of all COVID-19 infections were among health care workers (Wang et al., 2020). Evidence suggested that staff working in inpatient care where PPE was reused or in nursing homes with inadequate PPE had the greatest risk (Nguyen et al., 2020). In a report by the European Centre for Disease Prevention and Control on occupational exposure, the majority of COVID-19 clusters and outbreaks were found in the health and social care sector (European Centre for Disease Prevention and Control, 2020). In a prospective cohort UK study of more than 120,000 employees, the risk of health care workers testing positive for COVID-19 was over seven times higher than for non-essential workers (Mutambudzi et al., 2021).

The emergence of highly transmissible COVID-19 strains increased the risk of COVID-19 infection for health care workers. However, the exact number of health care workers that have died from or contracted COVID-19 is unknown and underreported. The WHO Director-General's opening remarks at the World Health Assembly on 24 May 2021 estimated that at least 115,000 health and care workers had lost their lives due to the pandemic (World Health Organization, 2021a), and more recent estimates suggest this number may be closer to 180,000 (World Health Organization, 2021b). In the Nursing Now international survey, 70% of respondents had provided direct care to patients with confirmed COVID-19, and approximately 9% of respondents had themselves tested positive for COVID-19 in the past 4 weeks. Most of those who tested positive believed they had contracted COVID-19 through workplace exposure. Respondents were not specifically asked if they had tested positive since the pandemic began, so the proportion of those who have tested positive at any point since the start of the pandemic is likely higher. The results were similar to a study investigating COVID-19 infection in Spanish health care workers over a 2-month study period in which 11% had COVID-19 (Suárez-García et al., 2020). Suárez-García et al. (2020) reported that the profession with the highest proportion of confirmed infections in their study was nurse supervisors (37.5%).

Health care workers often put their own health and safety at risk when they provide care and treatment to patients. It is vital that governments and organisations therefore commit to providing a safe workplace environment in which they can practice by ensuring preparedness and implementing safe organisational policies (Berger, 2021). In the Nursing Now international survey, less than half of respondents reported that their respective organisations had a COVID-19 workplace plan or protocol in place when the pandemic was declared. However, at the time of the survey, almost all reported that their workplace had a plan in place. Although most staff reported that they had received infection prevention and control training, less than half were confident to practice safely because of this training. This supported findings from a longitudinal study by the American Organization for Nursing Leadership, which indicated concerns among nurse leaders about organisational preparedness well into the pandemic. Specifically, it found that nurse leaders' confidence in preparedness for a future surge, variant or pandemic declined by 34% in 1 year, from 87% in mid-2020 to 57% the following year (American Organization for Nursing Leadership & Joslin Marketing, 2021). Most participants rated their organisation's policies and procedures for staff screening for risk factors or symptoms of COVID-19, general cleaning and cleaning of isolation rooms as good to excellent. In contrast, more than half of the survey participants assigned ratings from fair to very poor for their organisation's policies and procedures regarding preventing staff abuse, accessing workplace psychological or mental health

support, debriefing, being able to deploy more staff if required and accessing alternative accommodation between shifts.

The risk of contracting COVID-19 within the workplace may be reduced by uptake of safe, effective vaccines among health care workers. A prospective multicentre study of 7445 health care workers in Greece found that vaccination significantly reduced morbidity, COVID-19, absenteeism and duration of absenteeism (Maltezou et al., 2021). In a case-control study of breakthrough COVID-19 infections, out of 1497 fully vaccinated health care workers who were tested for COVID-19 during the third and largest pandemic surge in Israel, only 39 breakthrough cases (18 of which were nurses) were detected (Bergwerk et al., 2021). Most breakthrough cases were mild or asymptomatic, with the suspected source of infection being an unvaccinated person (Bergwerk et al., 2021).

Challenges to the uptake of COVID-19 vaccines by the nursing workforce included initial issues with supply and availability and vaccine hesitancy. The issue of mandatory vaccination for health care workers divided many countries; some made it mandatory for all health care workers, and others mandated proof of vaccination for certain sectors such as aged care (Stokel-Walker, 2021). Most, but not all, of the nurses (77%) who participated in the Nursing Now survey reported that they were vaccinated. This was lower than the proportion of participants in the Canadian (94%) survey who were vaccinated. A systematic review found that, on average, 23% of more than 76,000 health care workers worldwide reported COVID-19 vaccination hesitancy (Biswas et al., 2021). Primary reasons for not being vaccinated were concerns about vaccine safety, efficacy and side effects (Biswas et al., 2021). Factors associated with the uptake of vaccines by health care workers in the literature were being involved in the care of patients with COVID-19 (Dror et al., 2020; Shekhar et al., 2021), male gender, older age, higher education, perceived risk of contracting COVID-19 and history of influenza vaccination (Biswas et al., 2021). Health care organisations have legal and ethical responsibilities to provide a safe health care environment for staff and patients (Biswas et al., 2021). Nurses have a duty of care to their patients, many of whom may be from vulnerable populations. As they are role models for engaging in preventative health behaviours, some have argued that nurses also have a moral imperative to promote vaccine acceptance (Biswas et al., 2021). The existing research suggests that additional education and policy-based interventions are required to encourage compliance with vaccination among health care workers to reduce risk to the workforce and the public (Biswas et al., 2021).

PROVISION OF PERSONAL PROTECTIVE EQUIPMENT

A significant contributor to the high rates of infection among health care workers early in the pandemic, and an ongoing concern for health care workers worldwide, has been the lack of sufficient and appropriate PPE (The Lancet, 2020). Requiring nurses to provide care to patients with insufficient personal protection risks their safety and well-being, their ability to work and provide care to the community and the safety of their loved ones (Morley et al., 2020). Workplaces have a duty of care to health care workers to provide them with adequate and appropriate PPE (Morley et al., 2020). It was an immense challenge for governments and workplaces to provide adequate and appropriate supplies of PPE for health care workers throughout the COVID-19 pandemic, and these shortages came under considerable public scrutiny (Key et al., 2020).

A lack of PPE was among top concerns for nurses in a survey conducted by the American Nurses Association (ANA) in May 2020 (American Nurses Association, 2020). Out of more than 32,000 responses, 74% of respondents were 'extremely concerned' about PPE (American Nurses Association, 2020). PPE items in shortest supply were full and partial face shields, N95 masks, goggles, reusable respirators, surgical masks, isolation gowns and sanitary wipes (American Nurses Association, 2020). A follow-up survey found that 79% of respondents were encouraged or required to reuse PPE, and 59% felt unsafe doing so. Further evidence indicates that a PPE shortage was a significant factor in nurses' mental health. A study of 695 Michigan nurses, conducted in May 2020, found that nurses who lacked access to adequate PPE (25%) were more likely to report symptoms of depression, anxiety and posttraumatic stress disorder (Arnetz et al.,

2020). More frequent exposure to COVID-19 and poorer availability of adequate PPE were both associated with worse mental health outcomes (Arnetz et al., 2020).

By 2022, initial issues of PPE supply and availability had improved, but concerns around PPE distribution and standards had emerged. The European Federation of Nurses reported that many countries had taken initiatives to ensure adequate supplies of PPE by ordering directly from China or repurposing some factories. However, some countries still have concerns about having adequate supplies to manage future surges (European Federation of Nurses Associations, 2020). In the Nursing Now international survey, most respondents reported having access to the right types of PPE, but over half of respondents reported that they had PPE concerns, and over a third reported not having breaks while working in full PPE. In our Australian, Canadian and international surveys, the proportion of participants who reported feeling confident in their PPE training, supported by their workplace regarding PPE concerns and requirements and adequately resourced to deliver high-quality PPE training ranged from around 30%–50% (see Fig. 5.2).

Since an association has been found between nurses' self-reported stress and increased duration of mask-wearing time (Hoedl et al., 2021), further consideration of policies and procedures regarding breaks while wearing PPE is needed. Ongoing issues around PPE distribution, standards, wearability and vigilance regarding respiratory fit testing have required attention as the transmissibility of emerging disease variants has increased. It is imperative that PPE concerns and requirements continue to be addressed by management to ensure the effective control of COVID-19 infections. Any harm to patients because of a lack of PPE is not the responsibility of individual health care workers but of systems and organisations (Morley et al., 2020).

THINK BOX 5.2

- Why might wearing PPE for longer durations be associated with stress? If you were a manager, how would you seek to address this?

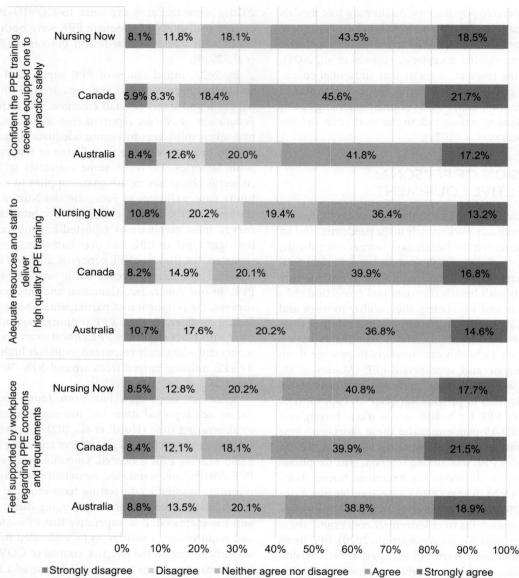

Fig. 5.2 ■ Personal protective equipment (PPE) organisational support and training across three surveys.

PERSONAL CONCERNS RELATED TO COVID-19

The emerging evidence suggests that there is a global phenomenon of mass trauma experienced by nurses working in the COVID-19 response. The phenomenon is complex and intertwined with various issues, including persistently high workloads, increased patient dependency and mortality, occupational burnout, inadequate PPE, the fear of spreading the virus to families and relatives, an increase in violence and discrimination against nurses, COVID-19 denial and the propagation of misinformation and a lack of social and mental health support. The *potential longer-term impacts of COVID-19, including posttraumatic stress disorder and long COVID, are currently unknown but are potentially extremely significant (International Council of Nurses, 2021).*

The physical and psychological strain on health care workers during a large-scale public health event such as COVID-19 is significant. In addition to workplace safety, nurses and midwives were concerned about keeping the people they live with and vulnerable family members safe during the COVID-19 pandemic. Out of more than 32,000 nurses who participated in the ANA COVID-19 survey, 64% were 'extremely concerned' about the safety of their family and friends. This ranked above personal safety, caring for COVID-19 patients and having adequate test kits and training. These findings were consistent with other studies documenting that the main concern of health care staff during the COVID-19 outbreak in China was fear of bringing the virus to their home and families (Liu et al., 2020). In the Nursing Now international survey, about a quarter of participants reported that they had chosen to self-isolate from their families. A moderate level of work–life conflict was reported by all respondents, and this was highest for respondents working in hospitals. Having worked through pandemic surges for over 18 months at the time of the survey, it is not surprising that so many nurses and midwives were experiencing work–family tension and challenges. Half of all nurses and midwives who participated were also concerned about their own psychological well-being, although less than a quarter had sought mental health well-being support.

The pandemic also contributed to heightened moral distress among nurses. Moral distress occurs when constraints prevent health care workers from acting in accordance with their core moral values to provide good patient care (Silverman et al., 2021). When a person has identified the ethically appropriate response to a situation but is unable to take that action, their moral integrity is challenged, which may cause them to experience physical and psychological distress (Silverman et al., 2021). Psychological manifestations of moral distress include negative feelings, decreased self-esteem, ambiguity, avoidance, frustration, anger, sadness, guilt and shame. Physical symptoms include loss of appetite, nausea, diarrhoea, migraines and heart palpitations

(Silverman et al., 2021). Nurses have reported a range of circumstances that prompted moral distress in relation to the COVID-19 pandemic. These included helplessness from the numbers and severity of COVID-19 patients, lack of knowledge and uncertainty regarding how to treat a new illness, fear of virus exposure leading to suboptimal care, policies to reduce transmission (e.g., visitation and PPE policies) preventing nurses from fulfilling their caring role, changes in practice models, intraprofessional tensions, practising under a crisis standard of care, increased workloads and dealing with medical resource scarcity due to the confines of allocation policies (Silverman et al., 2021). Emerging evidence suggests associations between moral distress and increased levels of burnout, staff turnover and poorer patient care.

Nurses and midwives received public acknowledgment for the sacrifices they made during the pandemic, but many also experienced discrimination and harassment at work and outside of work. Around 60%–70% of respondents in our Australian, Canadian and international surveys had experienced community support for their work. However, around one-third of participants in the Australian and international surveys and half of participants in the Canadian survey had experienced abuse or felt threatened at work (see Fig. 5.3), while up to a quarter had experienced stigmatisation or abuse outside of work.

During public health crises such as the COVID-19 pandemic, when work environments undergo rapid change, frontline health care workers are more vulnerable to workplace bullying (Somani et al., 2022). Organisational factors that may contribute to workplace bullying include rapid changes with inadequate guidelines, high staff turnover, increased workloads, inadequate resourcing and lack of training (Somani et al., 2022). Individual factors that may contribute to workplace bullying include discrimination, leadership style, increased stress and undue expectations (Somani et al., 2022). Rates of workplace bullying against nurses have increased since the pandemic and were as high as 71% in one international survey (Dye et al., 2020). Among members of the public, this behaviour is thought to be commonly driven by stigmatisation due to fear that frontline health care workers are sources of COVID-19 infection, as well as frustration in response to changed policies (e.g., regarding mask wearing or

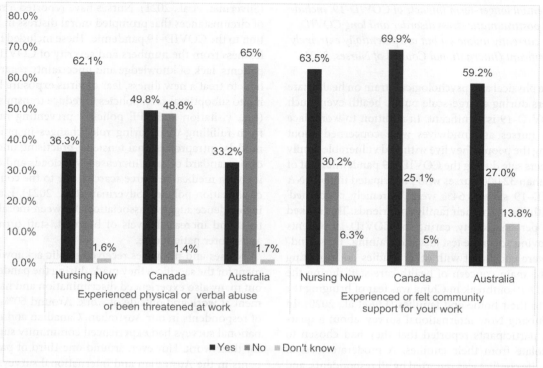

Fig. 5.3 ▪ Participants' experiences of community support and abuse across three surveys.

visitation rights). In a random sample study of 3551 members of the North American public, a high proportion of participants believed that health care workers should not be allowed to go out in public, should be allowed to have restrictions on their freedoms, should be isolated from the community and should be separated from their families (Taylor et al., 2020).

THINK BOX 5.3

Nurses are rated as the most trusted profession in the United States (see Chapter 10 for more on this).
- Why was the public so suspicious of nurses and other health workers during the pandemic?
- Why did the trust seem to be broken—and will it return?
- What's the evidence from your location?

WORKLOADS AND STAFFING

Any preexisting understaffing and resource limitations have been exposed and amplified by the

pandemic and have added to the stress and workload of the nurses who are at work. In addition, the pandemic has directly impacted nurses as people—they have suffered higher than average incidence of infection, illness and mortality whilst also carrying the pressures of trying to avoid infecting friends and families (Buchan et al., 2022).

The pandemic created additional demand for nurses, who provided patient care and conducted testing and vaccination. The increased demand for nurses was compounded by staff absenteeism due to COVID-19 exposure or infection as well as other workload and staffing issues, which varied across settings and contexts (Lopez et al., 2022). For example, it was critical in Italy and Spain, which were severely impacted by the first wave of the pandemic, to relocate and redefine the tasks of health care professionals (García & Calvo, 2021). In Spain, the nurse-to-patient ratio increased from 8.8 patients per nurse to 13, and working hours per shift increased to 12 hours (García & Calvo, 2021).

In the United Kingdom, ICU nurse-to-patient ratios increased from one patient per nurse to six or more, with the shortfall made up by staff without ICU experience (Maben & Bridges, 2020). Under increased demands for nursing staff, many countries fast-tracked final-year nursing students to join the nursing register early and encouraged retired colleagues back to practice (Jackson et al., 2020). Nurses and other health care workers were redeployed to new specialties or higher-acuity areas (Graichen, 2021). Collectively, these factors likely added to stress on existing staff, with additional implications for the well-being of new team members (Maben & Bridges, 2020).

Patients with COVID-19 require measures to limit spread of the virus, such as donning PPE, decontamination procedures and dedicated isolated areas, all of which increase nursing workload in terms of time, organisation and management (Lucchini et al., 2020b). Studies have found evidence of higher nursing workload for COVID-19 patients (Lucchini et al., 2020a; Reper et al., 2020) due to not only the severity of the illness but also the need to provide care in the absence of family. Nurses working in ICUs were expected to provide the usual high standard of care to high-complexity COVID-19 patients, many of whom were dependent on organ and system support. Moreover, they did so while managing PPE and decontamination requirements, the need for distanced communication between patient and relatives and increased incidence and severity of agitation due to the isolated environment (Lucchini et al., 2020b). Higher than usual workloads and associated staffing issues throughout the pandemic contributed to high levels of exhaustion, particularly for nurses and midwives who worked in settings providing direct clinical care. Systematic review findings indicate that nurse outcomes associated with staffing were burnout, fatigue, emotional exhaustion, depersonalisation and stress (Bae, 2021).

The Nursing Now international survey found that over two-thirds of respondents were moderately to extremely concerned about having adequate staffing levels (i.e., number of staff/ratios of staff to patients or clients). In addition, over half were moderately to extremely concerned about having the right skills mix (i.e., number/ratio of the right kinds of staff) in their workplace (*n* = 520, 57.6%) and about their ability to manage their workload. These were the three most

significant concerns highlighted by participants in the Nursing Now, Canadian and Australian surveys, with staffing levels the top concern. Approximately one-third of respondents from Nursing Now, one-quarter from Canada and fewer than one in five from Australia said they had been asked to work outside their usual scope of practice during the pandemic. Of these respondents, around half from Nursing Now and two-thirds from the Canadian and Australian surveys reported that they did not receive appropriate education and training to work outside their usual scope of practice (see Fig. 5.4). Approximately one in eight participants said they had been redeployed to a different hospital or speciality of work. Nealy half reported that their organisation had increased staff numbers to cope with extra demand, and a quarter reported recruiting student nurses or midwives to support the regular workforce to cope with demand. Importantly, survey respondents who were moderately to extremely concerned about their current workload, staff levels or skills mix reported higher levels of stress, symptoms of anxiety and depression, exhaustion and disengagement compared with those who were not as concerned.

THINK BOX 5.4

- What did you learn during the pandemic in your location (facility, region or country) about staffing levels?
- Has what you learned resulted in lasting change?
- Has the workforce recovered?

WORKFORCE WELL-BEING, BURNOUT AND ACCESS TO SUPPORT

The prepandemic shortage of nurses has been exacerbated by the cumulative and increasing negative impact of successive waves of the pandemic. Nurse burnout is linked to poorer quality of care, lower patient satisfaction and reduced productivity. Prepandemic causes of burnout, related to work environment and workload, have been magnified. Nurses have died; others are ill. Burnt-out nurses are leaving employment or taking absence. Those who remain at work report increasing levels of stress and an increasing propensity to consider leaving their job or profession. There is a huge concern that high

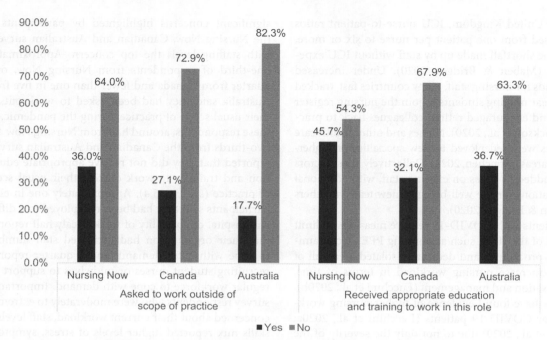

Fig. 5.4 ▪ Participants' scope of practice and training across three surveys.

levels of nurse burnout are reported in many of these studies and that the increased 'intention to leave', expressed in so many of the surveys, will become 'nurses who have left' (Buchan et al., 2022).

A meta-analysis found that mental health concerns, a lack of support at work, emotional exhaustion and increased work demands were among the leading cases of illness, absenteeism and workplace disabilities in nursing prior to the pandemic (Gohar et al., 2020). For nearly 3 years, nurses have felt the impacts of the pandemic constantly at work and home. The ongoing threat to their own health and safety, compounded by high workloads and staff shortages, has created a perfect storm of persistent work–life stress. It therefore comes as no surprise that the pandemic has significantly impacted nurses' well-being and contributed to burnout within the workforce. Recently named an 'occupational phenomenon' by the World Health Organization (2019), burnout is a persistent dysfunctional state resulting from a chronically stressful working environment. It is commonly thought to arise when an individual's job demands exceed the resources available to manage them (Jourdain & Chenevert, 2010).

Resources may be individual (e.g., competence), interpersonal (e.g., team support), or organisational (e.g., developmental opportunities) (Jourdain & Chenevert, 2010). Nursing and midwifery are highly skilled professions involving work that is inherently demanding and emotionally strenuous. This workforce is particularly vulnerable to work strain and burnout, which can negatively impact job performance, mental and physical well-being, and the quality of nursing care (Dall'Ora et al., 2020).

Burnout is commonly measured in terms of three key indicators (Maslach & Jackson, 1984):

- Emotional exhaustion (i.e., feeling overextended and drained by work)
- Depersonalisation (i.e., feelings of detachment, cynicism or a loss of empathy)
- A reduced sense of personal accomplishment (i.e., feeling incompetent or dissatisfied with one's performance at work)

Emotional exhaustion closely resembles stress and is often considered the primary element of burnout. However, workers who are burnt out are not just exhausted—they have often lost a sense of meaning and psychological connection to their work (Leiter & Maslach, 2016). A lack of empathy, which is crucial to clinical competence, means that nurses and midwives may be present in their jobs but not engaging with their patients (Wilkinson et al., 2017), while a lack of accomplishment signals that nurses and midwives feel unable to provide patient care to their satisfaction. All three indicators are independent precursors to job dissatisfaction, turnover and poor quality of care (Poghosyan et al., 2010; Van Bogaert et al., 2013; Van Bogaert et al., 2014).

The frontline caring role of nurses and midwives leaves them particularly susceptible to burnout because they are frequently exposed to trauma, make critical decisions under time pressure and experience difficult and emotionally demanding interactions with clients (Montgomery et al., 2015). This may be compounded by an excessive workload, a lack of autonomy and systemic issues such as working irregular hours, high administrative burden and understaffing (Woo et al., 2020). Burnout can affect individuals physically and mentally in a range of ways. Symptoms may include decreased concentration and memory, fatigue, anxiety, sleep problems, headaches, reduced immune function, interpersonal conflict, moodiness, irritability, withdrawal, a loss of purpose, disillusionment, and feeling underappreciated and/or overworked (Portnoy, 2011; Woo et al., 2020). Any one of these factors can detrimentally affect a nurse or midwife's capacity to provide optimal patient care (Hall et al., 2016; McHugh et al., 2011). Nurse absenteeism and turnover due to burnout also come with significant financial costs (Halter et al., 2017).

In studies of the Australian nursing and midwifery workforce conducted in 2017 and 2019, participants showed signs of burnout even before the COVID-19 pandemic. These surveys found concerningly high levels of emotional exhaustion and a high proportion of staff intending to leave their positions or the profession entirely. Research into the well-being of Australian nurses and midwives has identified that intensifying workloads, unsatisfactory working conditions and other workplace issues within the control of management and policymakers were contributing to burnout long before the COVID-19 pandemic (George, 2017; Holland et al., 2013; Holland et al., 2018). Most respondents in our Australian, Canadian and international

surveys reported working in fast-paced and cognitively and emotionally demanding conditions during the pandemic (see Fig. 5.5), with those working in aged care reporting the highest levels of workplace, emotional and cognitive demand. Across all workplace settings, respondents who worked in hospitals rated their satisfaction with work scheduling, flexibility and extrinsic rewards the lowest.

In a recent umbrella review examining emotional exhaustion and burnout in health care workers during the COVID-19 pandemic, prevalence rates of burnout (about one-third of health care workers) were found to be comparable with earlier SARS and MERS outbreaks (Magnavita et al., 2021). Similarly, a meta-analysis that pooled results from 16 studies examining nurses' burnout during the COVID-19 pandemic, involving nearly 19,000 participants in total, found indicators of burnout present in up to 34% of nurses (Galanis et al., 2021). Our Australian, Canadian and international surveys found high rates of workforce exhaustion and disengagement (see Fig. 5.6), which were comparable to findings from studies conducted in Singapore (Tan et al., 2020), Italy (Bellanti et al., 2021) and Sweden (Peterson et al., 2008).

Despite the high prevalence of mental health problems reported by health care workers during the pandemic, research suggests that access to mental health support could be improved (Greenberg et al., 2020). In the Nursing Now international survey, around 60% of respondents rated access to workplace psychological or mental health support as fair to very poor, and less than 25% had sought well-being support. This was similar to a large study of Australian health care workers, where 26% reported that they had accessed formal support during the pandemic, despite a much higher proportion reporting that they had experienced anxiety (62%), burnout (58%) or depression (28%) (Smallwood et al., 2021). Many countries have dedicated teams to provide mental health support for health care workers, including China, Italy, Spain, the United Kingdom and the United States (Moreno et al., 2020). Evidence-based psychological support for nurses and nurse leaders during the COVID-19 pandemic is critical and should include strategies and interventions aimed at the individual, team and managers and leaders in organisations (Hofmeyer & Taylor, 2021; Maben & Bridges, 2020). Support needs to be carefully planned and executed

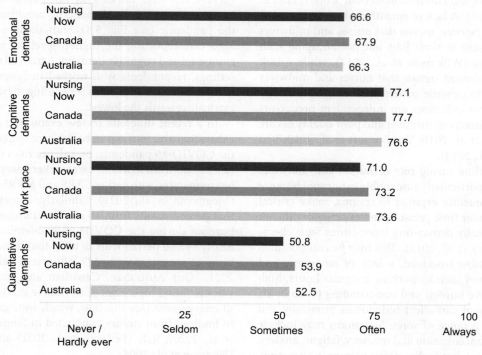

Fig. 5.5 ■ Participants' work demands and pace across three surveys.

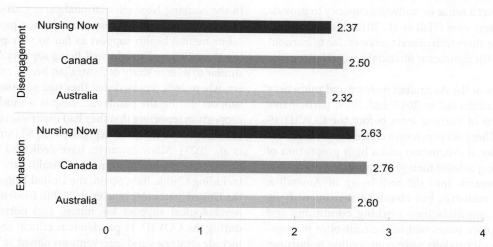

Fig. 5.6 ■ Participant's burnout subscale scores for exhaustion and disengagement across three surveys.

so that interventions do no harm, are tailored to individual need and provide effective services (Maben & Bridges, 2020; Moreno et al., 2020).

THINK BOX 5.5

This chapter provides evidence about the effects of the pandemic on nurses personally and professionally.
- If you think about lessons learned, where do you think health policymakers should be investing in health systems for the future?

REFERENCES

American Nurses Association. (2020). Initial COVID-19 Survey results, May 2020. The American Nurses Association & American Nurses Foundation's Pulse on the Nation's Nurses, COVID-19 Survey Series [Online]. Available: https://www.nursingworld.org/practice-policy/work-environment/health-safety/disaster-preparedness/coronavirus/what-you-need-to-know/covid-19-survey-results/ [Accessed 25 Aug 2021].

American Organization for Nursing Leadership & Joslin Marketing. (2021). AONL COVID-19 Longitudinal Study August 2021 Report: Nurse Leaders' Top Challenges, Emotional Health, and Areas of Needed Support, July 2020 to August 2021.

Araf, Y., Akter, F., Tang, Y. D., Fatemi, R., Parvez, M. S. A., Zheng, C., & Hossain, M. G. (2022). Omicron variant of SARS-CoV-2: genomics, transmissibility, and responses to current COVID-19 vaccines. Journal of Medical Virology, 94, 1825–1832.

Arnetz, J. E., Goetz, C. M., Sudan, S., Arble, E., Janisse, J., & Arnetz, B. B. (2020). Personal Protective Equipment and Mental Health Symptoms Among Nurses During the COVID-19 Pandemic. Journal of Occupational and Environmental Medicine, 62, 892–897.

Bae, S.-H. (2021). Intensive care nurse staffing and nurse outcomes: A systematic review. Nursing in Critical Care, 26, 457–466.

Bellanti, F., Lo Buglio, A., Capuano, E., Dobrakowski, M., Kasperczyk, A., Kasperczyk, S., Ventriglio, A., & Vendemiale, G. (2021). Factors Related to Nurses' Burnout during the First Wave of Coronavirus Disease-19 in a University Hospital in Italy. International Journal of Environmental Research and Public Health, 8(10), 1–14.

Berger, D. (2021). Up the line to death: Covid-19 has revealed a mortal betrayal of the world's healthcare workers. BMJ Opinion [Online]. https://blogs.bmj.com/bmj/2021/01/29/up-the-line-to-death-covid-19-has-revealed-a-mortal-betrayal-of-the-worlds-healthcare-workers/. [Accessed 29 Jan 2021].

Bergwerk, M., Gonen, T., Lustig, Y., Amit, S., Lipsitch, M., Cohen, C., Mandelboim, M., Gal Levin, E., Rubin, C., Indenbaum, V., Tal, I., Zavitan, M., Zuckerman, N., Bar-Chaim, A., Kreiss, Y., & Regev-Yochay, G. (2021). Covid-19 Breakthrough Infections in Vaccinated Health Care Workers. New England Journal of Medicine, 385, 1474–1484.

Biswas, N., Mustapha, T., Khubchandani, J., & Price, J. H. 2021. The Nature and Extent of COVID-19 Vaccination Hesitancy in Healthcare Workers. Journal of Community Health, 46, 1244–1251.

Buchan, J., Catton, H., & Shaffer, F. (2022). Sustain and Retain in 2022 and Beyond. International Council of Nurses, 71, 1–71.

Catania, G., Zanini, M., Hayter, M., Timmins, F., Dasso, N., Ottonello, G., Aleo, G., Sasso, L., & Bagnasco, A. (2021). Lessons from Italian front-line nurses' experiences during the COVID-19 pandemic: A qualitative descriptive study. Journal of Nursing Management, 29, 404–411.

Dall'Ora, C., Ball, J., Reinius, M., & Griffiths, P. (2020). Burnout in nursing: a theoretical review. Human Resources for Health, 18, 41.

Daly, J., Jackson, D., Anders, R., & Davidson, P. M. (2020). Who speaks for nursing? COVID-19 highlighting gaps in leadership. Journal of Clinical Nursing, 29, 2751–2752.

Delgado, D., Wyss Quintana, F., Perez, G., Sosa Liprandi, A., Ponte-Negretti, C., Mendoza, I., & Baranchuk, A. (2020). Personal safety during the COVID-19 pandemic: Realities and perspectives of healthcare workers in Latin America. International Journal of Environmental Research and Public Health, 17, 2798.

Dror, A. A., Eisenbach, N., Taiber, S., Morozov, N. G., Mizrachi, M., Zigron, A., Srouji, S., & Sela, E. (2020). Vaccine hesitancy: the next challenge in the fight against COVID-19. European Journal of Epidemiology, 35, 775–779.

Dye, T. D., Alcantara, L., Siddiqi, S., Barbosu, M., Sharma, S., Panko, T., & Pressman, E. (2020). Risk of COVID-19-related bullying, harassment and stigma among healthcare workers: an analytical cross-sectional global study. BMJ Open, 10, e046620.

European Centre for Disease Prevention and Control. (2020). COVID-19 clusters and outbreaks in occupational settings in the EU/EEA and the UK. https://www.ecdc.europa.eu/sites/default/files/documents/COVID-19-in-occupational-settings.pdf.

European Federation of Nurses Associations. (2020). COVID-19 impact on nurses and nursing: a perspective of crisis management at national level. Brussels, Belgium: The European Federation of Nurses Associations (EFN).

Ford, M. (2021). Nursing Times survey reveals extent of Covid-19 workforce pressures [Online]. Nursing Times Available: https://www.nursingtimes.net/news/workforce/nursing-times-survey-reveals-extent-of-covid-19-workforce-pressures-03-02-2021/. [Accessed 5 August 2021].

Galanis, P., Vraka, I., Fragkou, D., Bilali, A., & Kaitelidou, D. (2021). Nurses' burnout and associated risk factors during the COVID-19 pandemic: A systematic review and meta-analysis. Journal of Advanced Nursing, 77, 3286–3302.

García, G. M., & Calvo, J. C. A. (2021). The threat of COVID-19 and its influence on nursing staff burnout. Journal of Advanced Nursing, 77, 832–844.

George, T. (2017). A workforce in crisis: Has anything changed? Australian Midwifery News, 17, 24.

Gohar, B., Lariviere, M., Nowrouzi-Kia, B. (2020). Sickness absence in healthcare workers during the COVID-19 pandemic. Occupational Medicine, 70, 338–342.

Graichen, H. (2021). What is the difference between the first and the second/third wave of Covid-19?—German perspective. Journal of Orthopaedics, 24, A1–A3.

Greenberg, N., Docherty, M., Gnanapragasam, S., & Wessely, S. (2020). Managing mental health challenges faced by healthcare workers during covid-19 pandemic. BMJ, 368, m1211.

Grinspun, D., Perry, L., Abu-Qamar, M. E. Z., Stannard, D., & Porritt, K. (2022). Nursing crisis: Challenges and opportunities for our profession after COVID-19. *International Journal of Nursing Practice, 28*, e13075.

Hall, L. H., Johnson, J., Watt, I., Tsipa, A., & O'connor, D. B. (2016). Healthcare staff wellbeing, burnout, and patient safety: a systematic review. *PloS One, 11*, e0159015.

Halter, M., Boiko, O., Pelone, F., Beighton, C., Harris, R., Gale, J., Gourlay, S., & Drennan, V. (2017). The determinants and consequences of adult nursing staff turnover: a systematic review of systematic reviews. *BMC Health Services Research, 17*, 824.

Heinen, M., Van Oostveen, C., Peters, J., Vermeulen, H., & Huis, A. (2019). An integrative review of leadership competencies and attributes in advanced nursing practice. *Journal of Advanced Nursing, 75*, 2378–2392.

Hoedl, M., Eglseer, D., & Bauer, S. (2021). Associations between personal protective equipment and nursing staff stress during the COVID-19 pandemic. *Journal of Nursing Management, 29*, 2374–2382.

Hofmeyer, A., & Taylor, R. (2021). Strategies and resources for nurse leaders to use to lead with empathy and prudence so they understand and address sources of anxiety among nurses practising in the era of COVID-19. *Journal of Clinical Nursing, 30*, 298–305.

Holland, P. J., Allen, B. C., & Cooper, B. K. (2013). Reducing burnout in Australian nurses: The role of employee direct voice and managerial responsiveness. *The International Journal of Human Resource Management, 24*, 3146–3162.

Holland, P. J., Tham, T. L., & Gill, F. J. (2018). What nurses and midwives want: Findings from the national survey on workplace climate and well-being. *International Journal of Nursing Practice, 24*, e12630.

International Council of Nurses. (2021). *Mass trauma experienced by the global nursing workforce.* Geneva: Switzerland.

International Council of Nurses. (2022). "The greatest threat to global health is the workforce shortage" - International Council of Nurses International Nurses Day demands action on investment in nursing, protection and safety of nurses [Online]. Available: https://www.icn.ch/news/greatest-threat-global-health-workforce-shortage-international-council-nurses-international [Accessed 5 Aug 2022].

Jackson, D., Bradbury-Jones, C., Baptiste, D., Gelling, L., Morin, K., Neville, S., & Smith, G. D. (2020). Life in the pandemic: Some reflections on nursing in the context of COVID-19. *Journal of Clinical Nursing, 29*, 2041–2043.

Joslin, D., & Joslin, H. (2020). Nursing Leadership COVID-19 Insight Survey: Key Concerns, Primary Challenges, and Expectations for the Future. *Nurse Leader, 18*, 527–531.

Jourdain, G., & Chenevert, D. (2010). Job demands-resources, burnout and intention to leave the nursing profession: a questionnaire survey. *International Journal of Nursing Studies, 47*, 709–722.

Key, T., Mathai, N. J., Venkatesan, A. S., Farnell, D., & Mohanty, K. (2020). Personal protective equipment during the COVID-19 crisis: A snapshot and recommendations from the frontline of a university teaching hospital. *Bone & Joint Open, 1*, 131–136.

Labrague, L. J., De Los Santos, J. A. A., Falguera, C. C., Nwafor, C. E., Galabay, J. R., Rosales, R. A., & Firmo, C. N. (2020). Predictors of nurses' turnover intention at one and five years' time. *International Nursing Review, 67*, 191–198.

Leiter, M. P., & Maslach, C. (2016). Latent burnout profiles: A new approach to understanding the burnout experience. *Burnout Research, 3*, 89–100.

Liu, Q., Luo, D., Haase, J. E., Guo, Q., Wang, X. Q., Liu, S., Xia, L., Liu, Z., Yang, J., & Yang, B. X. (2020). The experiences of healthcare providers during the COVID-19 crisis in China: a qualitative study. *The Lancet Global Health, 8*, e790–e798.

Lopez, V., Anderson, J., West, S., & Cleary, M. (2022). Does the COVID-19 Pandemic Further Impact Nursing Shortages? *Issues in Mental Health Nursing, 43*, 293–295.

Lucchini, A., Giani, M., Elli, S., Villa, S., Rona, R., & Foti, G. (2020a). Nursing Activities Score is increased in COVID-19 patients. *Intensive and Critical Care Nursing, 59*, 102876.

Lucchini, A., Iozzo, P., & Bambi, S. (2020b). Nursing workload in the COVID-19 era. *Intensive and Critical Care Nursing, 61*, 102929.

Maben, J., & Bridges, J. (2020). Covid-19: Supporting nurses' psychological and mental health. *Journal of Clinical Nursing, 29*, 2742–2750.

Magnavita, N., Chirico, F., Garbarino, S., Bragazzi, N. L., Santacroce, E., & Zaffina, S. (2021). SARS/MERS/SARS-CoV-2 Outbreaks and Burnout Syndrome among Healthcare Workers. An Umbrella Systematic Review. *International Journal of Environmental Research and Public Health, 18*, 4361.

Maltezou, H. C., Panagopoulos, P., Sourri, F., Giannouchos, T. V., Raftopoulos, V., Gamaletsou, M. N., Karapanou, A., Koukou, D. M., Koutsidou, A., Peskelidou, E., Papanastasiou, K., Souliotis, K., Lourida, A., Sipsas, N. V., & Hatzigeorgiou, D. (2021). COVID-19 vaccination significantly reduces morbidity and absenteeism among healthcare personnel: A prospective multicenter study. *Vaccine, 39*, 7021–7027.

Maslach, C., & Jackson, S. E. (1984). Burnout in organizational settings. *Applied Social Psychology Annual, 5*, 133–153.

McHugh, M. D., Kutney-Lee, A., Cimiotti, J. P., Sloane, D. M., & Aiken, L. H. (2011). Nurses' widespread job dissatisfaction, burnout, and frustration with health benefits signal problems for patient care. *Health Affairs, 30*, 202–210.

Montgomery, A., Spânu, F., Băban, A., & Panagopoulou, E. (2015). Job demands, burnout, and engagement among nurses: A multi-level analysis of ORCAB data investigating the moderating effect of teamwork. *Burnout Research, 2*, 71–79.

Moreno, C., Wykes, T., Galderisi, S., Nordentoft, M., Crossley, N., Jones, N., Cannon, M., Correll, C. U., Byrne, L., Carr, S., Chen, E. Y. H., Gorwood, P., Johnson, S., Kärkkäinen, H., Krystal, J. H., Lee, J., Lieberman, J., López-Jaramillo, C., Männikkö, M., Phillips, M. R., Uchida, H., Vieta, E., Vita, A., & Arango, C. (2020). How mental health care should change as a consequence of the COVID-19 pandemic. *The Lancet Psychiatry, 7*, 813–824.

Morgantini, L. A., Naha, U., Wang, H., Francavilla, S., Acar, Ö., Flores, J. M., Crivellaro, S., Moreira, D., Abern, M., & Eklund, M. (2020). Factors contributing to healthcare professional burnout during the COVID-19 pandemic: a rapid turnaround global survey. *PloS one, 15*, e0238217.

Morley, G., Grady, C., Mccarthy, J., & Ulrich, C. M. (2020). Covid-19: Ethical challenges for nurses. *Hastings Center Report, 50*, 35–39.

Mutambudzi, M., Niedwiedz, C., Macdonald, E. B., Leyland, A., Mair, F., Anderson, J., Celis-Morales, C., Cleland, J., Forbes, J., & Gill, J. (2021). Occupation and risk of severe COVID-19: prospective cohort study of 120 075 UK Biobank participants. *Occupational and Environmental Medicine, 78*, 307–314.

Nguyen, L. H., Drew, D. A., Graham, M. S., Joshi, A. D., Guo, C.-G., Ma, W., Mehta, R. S., Warner, E. T., Sikavi, D. R., Lo, C.-H., Kwon, S., Song, M., Mucci, L. A., Stampfer, M. J., Willett, W. C., Eliassen, A. H., Hart, J. E., Chavarro, J. E., Rich-Edwards, J. W., Davies, R., Capdevila, J., Lee, K. A., Lochlainn, M. N., Varsavsky, T., Sudre, C. H., Cardoso, M. J., Wolf, J., Spector, T. D., Ourselin, S., Steves, C. J., Chan, A. T., Albert, C. M., Andreotti, G., Bala, B., Balasubramanian, B. A., Beane-Freeman, L. E., Brownstein, J. S., Bruinsma, F. J., Coresh, J., Costa, R., Cowan, A. N., Deka, A., Deming-Halverson, S. L., Elena Martinez, M., Ernst, M. E., Figueiredo, J. C., Fortuna, P., Franks, P. W., Freeman, L. B., Gardner, C. D., Ghobrial, I. M., Haiman, C. A., Hall, J. E., Kang, J. H., Kirpach, B., Koenen, K. C., Kubzansky, L. D., Lacey, J. J. V., Le Marchand, L., Lin, X., Lutsey, P., Marinac, C. R., Martinez, M. E., Milne, R. L., Murray, A. M., Nash, D., Palmer, J. R., Patel, A. V., Pierce, E., Robertson, M. M., Rosenberg, L., Sandler, D. P., Schurman, S. H., Sewalk, K., Sharma, S. V., Sidey-Gibbons, C. J., Slevin, L., Smoller, J. W., Steves, C. J., Tiirikainen, M. I., Weiss, S. T., Wilkens, L. R., & Zhang, F (2020). Risk of COVID-19 among front-line health-care workers and the general community: a prospective cohort study. *The Lancet Public Health, 5*, e475–e483.

Paterson, C., Gobel, B., Gosselin, T., Haylock, P. J., Papadopoulou, C., Slusser, K., Rodriguez, A., & Pituskin, E. (2020). Oncology nursing during a pandemic: critical reflections in the context of COVID-19. *Seminars in Oncology Nursing*, 151028 Elsevier.

Peterson, U., Demerouti, E., Bergström, G., Samuelsson, M., Åsberg, M., & Nygren, Å. (2008). Burnout and physical and mental health among Swedish healthcare workers. *Journal of Advanced Nursing, 62*, 84–95.

Poghosyan, L., Clarke, S. P., Finlayson, M., & Aiken, L. H. (2010). Nurse burnout and quality of care: Cross-national investigation in six countries. *Research in Nursing & Health, 33*, 288–298.

Portnoy, D. (2011). Burnout and compassion fatigue: watch for the signs. *Health Progress (Saint Louis, Mo.), 92*, 46.

Raso, R., Fitzpatrick, J. J., Masick, K., Giordano-Mulligan, M., & Sweeney, C. D. (2021). Perceptions of Authentic Nurse Leadership and Work Environment and the Pandemic Impact for Nurse Leaders and Clinical Nurses. *JONA: The Journal of Nursing Administration, 51*, 257–263.

Reper, P., Bombart, M. A., Leonard, I., Payen, B., Darquennes, O., & Labrique, S. (2020). Nursing Activities Score is increased in COVID-19 patients. *Intensive and Critical Care Nursing, 60*, 102891.

Schlak, A. E., Rosa, W. E., Rushton, C. H., Poghosyan, L., Root, M. C., & Mchugh, M. D. (2022). An expanded institutional- and national-level blueprint to address nurse burnout and moral suffering amid the evolving pandemic. *Nursing Management, 53*, 16–27.

Shalala, D., Bolton, L., Bleich, M., Brennan, T., Campbell, R., & Devlin, L. (2011). *The future of nursing: Leading change, advancing health*. Washington DC: The National Academy Press doi, 10, 12956.

Shekhar, R., Sheikh, A. B., Upadhyay, S., Singh, M., Kottewar, S., Mir, H., Barrett, E., & Pal, S. (2021). COVID-19 Vaccine Acceptance among Health Care Workers in the United States. *Vaccines (Basel), 9*(2), 119.

Silverman, H. J., Kheirbek, R. E., Moscou-Jackson, G., & Day, J. (2021). Moral distress in nurses caring for patients with Covid-19. *Nursing Ethics, 28*, 1137–1164.

Smallwood, N., Karimi, L., Pascoe, A., Bismark, M., Putland, M., Johnson, D., Dharmage, S. C., Barson, E., Atkin, N., Long, C., Ng, I., Holland, A., Munro, J., Thevarajan, I., Moore, C., Mcgillion, A., & Willis, K. (2021). Coping strategies adopted by Australian frontline health workers to address psychological distress during the COVID-19 pandemic. *General Hospital Psychiatry, 72*, 124–130.

Somani, R., Muntaner, C., Smith, P., Hillan, E. M., & Velonis, A. J. (2022). Increased workplace bullying against nurses during COVID-19: A health and safety issue. *Journal of Nursing Education and Practice, 12*, 47.

Spoorthy, M. S., Pratapa, S. K., & Mahant, S. (2020). Mental health problems faced by healthcare workers due to the COVID-19 pandemic—A review. *Asian Journal of Psychiatry, 51*, 102119.

Stokel-Walker, C. (2021). Covid-19: The countries that have mandatory vaccination for health workers. *BMJ, 373*, n1645. doi: https://doi.org/10.1136/bmj.n1645.

Suárez-García, I., Martínez De Aramayona López, M. J., Sáez Vicente, A., & Lobo Abascal, P. (2020). SARS-CoV-2 infection among healthcare workers in a hospital in Madrid, Spain. *Journal of Hospital Infection, 106*, 357–363.

Tan, B. Y. Q., Kanneganti, A., Lim, L. J. H., Tan, M., Chua, Y. X., Tan, L., Sia, C. H., Denning, M., Goh, E. T., Purkayastha, S., Kinross, J., Sim, K., Chan, Y. H., & Ooi, S. B. S. (2020). Burnout and Associated Factors Among Health Care Workers in Singapore During the COVID-19 Pandemic. *Journal of the American Medical Directors Association, 21*, 1751–1758. e5.

Taylor, S., Landry, C. A., Rachor, G. S., Paluszek, M. M., & Asmundson, G. J. G. (2020). Fear and avoidance of healthcare workers: An important, under-recognized form of stigmatization during the COVID-19 pandemic. *Journal of Anxiety Disorders, 75*, 102289.

The Lancet. (2020). COVID-19: Protecting health-care workers. *Lancet, 395*, 922.

Van Bogaert, P., Kowalski, C., Weeks, S. M., & Clarke, S. P. (2013). The relationship between nurse practice environment, nurse work characteristics, burnout and job outcome and quality of nursing care: a cross-sectional survey. *International Journal of Nursing Studies, 50*, 1667–1677.

Van Bogaert, P., Timmermans, O., Weeks, S. M., Van Heusden, D., Wouters, K., & Franck, E. (2014). Nursing unit teams matter: Impact of unit-level nurse practice environment, nurse work characteristics, and burnout on nurse reported job outcomes, and quality of care, and patient adverse events—A cross-sectional survey. *International Journal of Nursing Studies, 51*, 1123–1134.

Wang, D., Hu, B., Hu, C., Zhu, F., Liu, X., Zhang, J., Wang, B., Xiang, H., Cheng, Z., & Xiong, Y. (2020). Clinical characteristics of 138 hospitalized patients with 2019 novel coronavirus–infected pneumonia in Wuhan, China. *JAMA, 323*, 1061–1069.

Westphal, J. A. (2012). Characteristics of nurse leaders in hospitals in the USA from 1992 to 2008. *Journal of Nursing Management, 20*, 928–937.

Wilkinson, H., Whittington, R., Perry, L., & Eames, C. (2017). Examining the relationship between burnout and empathy in healthcare professionals: A systematic review. *Burnout Research, 6*, 18–29.

Wong, C. A., & Walsh, E. J. (2020). Reflections on a decade of authentic leadership research in health care. *Journal of Nursing Management, 28*, 1–3.

Woo, T., Ho, R., Tang, A., & Tam, W. (2020). Global prevalence of burnout symptoms among nurses: A systematic review and meta-analysis. *Journal of Psychiatric Research, 123*, 9–20.

World Health Organization. (2019). *Burn-out an "occupational phenomenon": International Classification of Diseases.* Geneva, Switzerland: World Health Organization.

World Health Organization. (2020). *WHO Director-General's opening remarks at the media briefing on COVID-19 - 11 March 2020 [Online].* WHO. Available:. https://www.who.int/dg/speeches/detail/who-director-general-s-opening-remarks-at-the-media-briefing-on-covid-19-11-march-2020. [Accessed 10 Jul 2020].

World Health Organization. (2021a). Director-General's opening remarks at the World Health Assembly - 24 May 2021.

World Health Organization. (2021). *The impact of COVID-19 on health and care workers: a closer look at deaths.* Geneva, Switzerland: World Health Organization.

World Health Organization. (2022). Tracking SARS-CoV-2 variants [Online]. Available: https://www.who.int/activities/tracking-SARS-CoV-2-variants [Accessed 5 Aug 2022].

Wymer, J. A., Stucky, C. H., & De Jong, M. J. (2021). Nursing Leadership and COVID-19: Defining the Shadows and Leading Ahead of the Data. *Nurse Leader, 19*, 483–488.

Zheng, L., Wang, X., Zhou, C., Liu, Q., Li, S., Sun, Q., Wang, M., Zhou, Q., & Wang, W. (2020). Analysis of the infection status of healthcare workers in Wuhan during the COVID-19 outbreak: A cross-sectional study. *Clinical Infectious Diseases, 71*, 2109–2113.

Zheng, R., Zhou, Y., Fu, Y., Xiang, Q., Cheng, F., Chen, H., Xu, H., Wu, X., Feng, M., & Ye, L. (2021). Prevalence and associated factors of depression and anxiety among nurses during the outbreak of COVID-19 in China: A cross-sectional study. *International Journal of Nursing Studies, 114*, 103809.

Section 2

GLOBAL ROLE AND IDENTITY OF NURSES TODAY

SECTION OUTLINE

6

DECOLONISING GLOBAL NURSING: CONCEPTS, BARRIERS AND STRATEGIES

RADHA ADHIKARI ■ PAM SMITH

INTRODUCTION

Recent decades have witnessed a significant increase in literature, policy debates, changes in academic curricula, seminars, conferences, webinars and civil rights movements focusing on 'decolonising' higher education, global health and international development and exploring possible strategies to move forward with more fair, just and inclusive policy and practices. However, globally, professional nursing has yet to join the mainstream debate and actively engage in decolonising activities. This chapter offers a perspective on why the nursing profession needs to join the debate and actively engage in decolonising nursing education, research and practice.

WHY DO WE NEED TO DECOLONISE NURSING?

Long-standing structural inequality across the world, in tandem with colonial mindsets, continues to prevail today, manifesting in social exclusion, exploitation, discrimination and the marginalisation of minority and less powerful people and communities, who find themselves facing numerous barriers in accessing key social and organisational positions and true recognition of their contribution to organisations, societies and politics, nationally and internationally. This is especially true for minority nurses in accessing jobs, progressing in their careers and attaining decision-making roles in nursing and the wider health care sector. The concept of 'decolonisation' has emerged from this context of structural inequality and widespread social injustice and become much debated, in many

arenas, including that of global health (Chaudhuri et al., 2021; Jacubec & Bourque Bearskin, 2020; Shahjahan et al., 2022). However, given the limited critical discussion of, and research and academic engagement on, the concept of decolonising within nursing, this chapter engages with relevant literature on decolonising higher education and global health, as these disciplines are close to professional nursing.

THINK BOX 6.1

What does the term 'decolonising nursing' mean to you?
- In order to find out, you might decide to search the literature on 'decolonising nursing'.
Which key words would you use?
- We used the following: 'decolonisation', 'nursing', 'global health' and 'higher education.'
- Our results gave us many references to decolonisation, global health and higher education in non-nursing disciplines but few references specific to nursing.
- These results are surprising given nurses make up over 50% of the global health care workforce.
- It looks as if there is not much written specifically about nursing and decolonisation.
Why do you think this might be the case?

In order to help you explore 'decolonising nursing' further to answer these and other questions, the chapter is divided into three parts. Each part addresses key aspects of the debate. Part one explores the historical and colonial context of nursing globally, part two examines the various barriers to decolonisation of global nursing and global health, and part three illustrates some approaches and practical strategies to decolonise nursing and global health.

PART ONE: CONTEXT

Contradiction and Tension Within Global Nursing

There is an apparent contradiction and tension within global nursing in relation to decolonising professional education and practice, as nursing is a colonial product and discipline. Throughout the professional history of nursing globally, it has had a strong connection with nurse and health worker migration, discussed in detail in Chapter 9: 'Unravelling the Complexities of Global Nurse Migration'. It took the form of early establishers (nurses and health care workers) from Europe and North America moving to various countries and continents to set up nursing education and the current practice of international recruitment from low-income countries, including former colonies of rich nations (Choy, 2003; Stilwell et al., 2004).

With nursing widely perceived as females' work, its professional values and practices are firmly set for universal use within unequal intra- and interprofessional structures and hierarchies. Yet at the same time, nursing workforces are some of the most diverse professional groups in the world. The Nursing Now Challenge (n.d.) website testifies to this, with its leadership programme aiming to champion 100,000 nurses and midwives in 150 countries.

Therefore, given this diversity, it is important to unpack the professionalisation of nursing within the context of historical colonisation and the gendered division of labour and critically examine the impact it has had until now.

Further, with a specific focus on nursing education, research and practice, relevant concepts and practices of internationalisation, globalisation, modernisation of nursing and professional competencies are some of the main global drivers that are being explored in this chapter. It is important to engage with these areas, as they raise critical ethical questions and debates around barriers to decolonising professional nursing and global health across the world, and they help us to understand relationships between the internationalization of nursing and professional competencies with decolonisation in an age of globalisation and international migration.

These global drivers play central roles within nursing today and shape the future of the profession.

While a clear concept and practical roadmap to the decolonisation of global health, higher education and global nursing has yet to be found and implemented, the arguments for it are compelling. Scholars and activists, working on decolonising higher education and global health, argue that decolonising is urgently needed to address existing power imbalances between affluent and low-income countries, as well as within societies, to address inequalities within the profession and health care systems (Chaudhuri et al., 2021; Hirsch, 2021; Kulesa & Brantau, 2021).

Clearly, the concept of decolonising global nursing and global health indicates a need to acknowledge and value social diversity, and to decentre power or dismantle the 'old boys club', and remove the practice of discrimination and social exclusion that is based on socioeconomic class, race, ethnicity and gender, among others. Therefore, decolonising any professional discipline, or any field of study, is a complex political and economic concept and process. Trying to address existing power imbalances, both intra- and interprofessionally, particularly in relation to medical domination, can destabilise the current social order and organisational structure and/or pose a threat to those who hold power.

The 'doctor–nurse game', first described in 1967 and revisited in 1990 and 2008, is a classic illustration of these power imbalances reflected in the traditional male–female relationships in medicine and nursing which shape professional practice today (Reeves, 2008; Stein 1967; Stein et al., 1990).

Colonisation, Origin and Meaning of Nursing

In order to clarify the concept of decolonising, it is useful to discuss what colonising means. As the Cambridge Dictionary (n.d.) states, it is 'filling a particular place or taking control of a particular area of activity'. In simple terms, it is about those in power, be it economic, political, religious or professional, having domination or control over minority or less powerful groups. Colonising has been widely experienced globally, at various levels and in various forms, for many centuries and for many generations in human history, and of course, it still occurs today.

Stemming from history and widely perceived as the Euro-American political and economic powers dominating most parts of Africa, Asia and South America, colonising is not only about the influence of British, European and North American colonial or imperial expansion and their control over less powerful countries, communities and peoples. It also includes any group of people with power systematically suppressing less powerful and minority groups in their community, or professional colleagues at work, over a period of time, thus shaping social and professional concepts and values. These can be transmitted through educational curricula or simply by everyday social interactions, by workforce recruitment and employment practices, and also by social policy and/or political practices. Colonisation can also happen unconsciously, so it can be invisible. As such, decolonising is perforce a complex process, requiring a great amount of political commitment, reflection and sensitivity.

Written historical accounts suggest today's nursing originates from the familial practice of looking after or caring for the sick, children and young people, both in a society and across the world. Versluysen observes that over the centuries, 'women have always been the main healers in English (sic) society. They have delivered babies, rendered first aid, prescribed and dispensed remedies for the sick, infirm and dying, both as a neighbourly service and as paid work' (Versluysen, 1981, p. 175). Similar practices existed in most societies across the world.

THINK BOX 6.2

Can you imagine what caring practices were like in the past, before modern nursing education/training was established?

To start you thinking, consider:
- Caring as females' 'natural' work
- Supporting a female during labour
- Treating fever before the discovery of antibiotics

Perhaps this caring practice was known differently in different societies, but the term 'nursing' currently used globally is itself a colonial term which was universalised by Euro-American colonisers. During the Dutch colonial period in Indonesia (1816–1942), female servants, or 'helpers' known as 'babus' and 'Mantri

nurses', worked as nurses in the newly established hospitals. This legacy continues to have a negative impact on nursing's image today (Juanamasta et al., 2021). India provides another example of the negative effects of colonialism on the professional development of nursing. During the British colonial period (1906–48), local nurses were stigmatised as low-status 'menials' who were subject to poor pay and working conditions (Healey, 2010). It is ironic that Florence Nightingale, famous for her role in reforming the Indian Public Health System (1859), paid little attention to the development of Indian nursing, limiting her recommendations to the care of British soldiers by British nurses. Indeed, Fitzgerald (2006) suggests there was a 'growing self-perception of nurses as agents of Empire'. Therefore, exploring the historical context and understanding the local terms and practices of care and caring (before the present form of 'nursing' was introduced in a society and countries) is a massive global project, which is why we have given you some examples to get you thinking, although a wider discussion is beyond the scope of this chapter.

According to the International Council of Nurses (ICN, n.d.), in the modern day:

> *Nursing encompasses autonomous and collaborative care of individuals of all ages, families, groups and communities, sick or well and in all settings. Nursing includes the promotion of health, prevention of illness, and the care of ill, disabled and dying people. Advocacy, promotion of a safe environment, research, participation in shaping health policy and in patient and health systems management, and education are also key nursing roles.*

THINK BOX 6.3

Explore the history of care and caring in your community and/or in your country. Can you think of examples how history has influenced present-day nursing, both positively and negatively?

In order to prepare for these key roles, it is common in most countries that nurses undertake a period of university-level education, resulting in a professional licence to practise nursing and provide care.

THINK BOX 6.4

At this point, we suggest you look at Chapter 7, 'The Same but Different—Nursing Roles in the World for the Next Century', where Barbara Stilwell and Sally Kendall encourage you to explore nursing roles in your country.

Global Nursing, a Colonial Legacy: The Role of Christian Missionaries and Foreign Aid Workers in the Establishment of Nursing Education and Health Care

As discussed, nursing, as a professional discipline in the vast majority of countries, was introduced by the colonial rulers (Adhikari, 2019; Carter, 2019; Choy, 2003; Horwitz, 2011; Juanamasta et al., 2021; Msila, 2017; Nair & Healey, 2006). For example, nursing education in India was set up (after 1800) by the British, in Indonesia (in 1799) by the Dutch rulers first, then supported by British and later by North Americans, and in South Africa by Anglican sisters in 1877 (Horwitz, 2011; Juanamasta et al., 2021; Nair, 2018). Therefore, nursing's professional education, values, principles and practices are firmly shaped by Euro-American sociocultural, religious and political values. As such, professional nursing has been a colonial product.

After the Second World War, a significant proportion of nursing education and health systems globally have been further shaped by international development assistance, which again has a colonial root, influenced by colonial values (Adhikari, 2019; Banda, 2023; Choy, 2003; Juanamasta et al., 2021; Nair & Healey, 2006). Christian missionaries and foreign aid workers from Europe and North America went to low-income countries or to their former colonies to establish health care systems, including nursing education. Horwitz (2011), in her examination of the professionalisation and development of nursing in South Africa, suggests that, as nursing education was set up by Christian missionary nurses, it has therefore been completely influenced by Western Christian values. This remains the case in Malawi and many other African countries (Grigulis, 2011; Msila, 2017).

Nursing in India and in wider Asian contexts such as in the Philippines and Indonesia, was also set up with external support (Carter, 2019; Choy, 2003; Nair & Healey, 2006). Established at different periods of colonial expansion and during post–World War II international development and influenced primarily by Western sociocultural, political and religious values, nursing education has resulted in becoming a global professional discipline today.

CASE STUDY 6.1

Nursing Education and Practice in Nepal

The history of nursing education in Asia is similar. Nepal is an example of this. Regularly represented as an 'exotic Himalayan country', it was never formally ruled or officially colonised by a Western, or any other, imperial power. Therefore the country has no direct or official colonial links. Nevertheless, the profession has been significantly influenced by Western ideas of modernity, development and Christian sociocultural values. European and North American missionary nurses and development workers established professional nursing in Nepal. Its nursing curriculum and, indeed, its medical curriculum, have always been based on Euro-American education systems and health care values and principles. Nepali nurses and health care professionals have learned those principles and professional values throughout their education and professional practice which continues until February 2024 (Adhikari, 2019). As such, their concept of nursing has emerged to be, and remains to be, based on colonial values; nothing has changed until recently. Nepal's nursing curriculum has followed the principles and practices of the textbooks produced in the English language by Western scholars and practitioners, such as British and American nurses.

Further, current-day practices of international nurse recruitment, internationalisation of the profession and professional competency continue to sustain colonial practice to exploit the nursing workforce. Therefore any debates on the decolonisation of professional nursing demand closer and critical analysis. We now consider some of the key drivers that sustain colonial practice and exploitation of the global nursing workforce that are central to the decolonisation debate.

THINK BOX 6.5

- International recruitment, social and professional diversity and the inclusion debate
- Global economy knowledge and political power: centre and periphery

Read and consider how each driver:

1. Shapes global nursing education and professional practice today
2. Is central to the decolonisation debate

International Recruitment, Social and Professional Diversity and the Inclusion Debate

Social diversity increases with population mobility. People have moved across the globe throughout human history looking for such opportunities as land to settle, work or business, and education. However, global mobility has intensified in the past four to five decades. As a result, our world has become an incredibly diverse place in terms of race, religion, culture, language, social class, social and political values, gender, ability and access to resources. Nursing is integral to all societies and is a global profession. It is currently also one of the most diverse professions in the world. Unfortunately, stemming from colonial hierarchy, discriminatory practices, exclusion and marginalisation are widely experienced by minority groups of professional nurses across the world.

Currently, migrant nurses comprise a significant proportion of most countries' nursing workforces (Adhikari & Plotnikova, 2023; Kingma, 2006; Stilwell et al., 2004). Given the current global nursing shortage and the prevalence of international recruitment, the diversity of the nursing workforces and also that of the service recipients are expected to expand across the world. With this increased diversity of health care workers and health service recipients, the need for, and the value of, inclusive workplace culture at all levels has been recognised (Kingma, 2006; Smith et al., 2006; Winkelmann-Gleed, 2006). In response to this, initiatives in diversity management and culturally sensitive care provisions as an approach to manage social diversity have been recognised and are being adopted in the wider global context (Coronado et al., 2020; World Health Organization, 2020). However, meaningful implementation of any policy in practice has been an ongoing challenge in the United Kingdom, the United States and many other countries (Adhikari, et al., 2023; Iheduru-Anderson, 2021; Kline, 2014).

Global Economy, Knowledge and Political Power: Centre and Periphery

Scholars (such as Thomas and Wilkin, 2004; Tickner, 2013) assert that global political and economic power is centred in the rich countries of Europe and North America, also commonly categorised as the Global North, which disadvantages people (and politics) in low-income countries in the Global South: Asia, Africa and South America. Scientific evidence and knowledge are produced and controlled in the Global North and diffused or distributed to the periphery in the Global South. Powerful institutions (that hold political and economic power and knowledge), situated in the Global North, control so-called 'scientific inventions', run global economies and produce knowledge for wider global use. This has created a mindset, both colonial and stereotypical, that scientific facts and theories, invented by powerful institutions located in the Global North, have more credibility. Traditional local knowledge and practices in countries in the Global South are not valued in the same way. This has created not only the North–South divide but also a system that determines what is scientific, gold standard and more credible and what is not. Unfortunately, nursing globally is plagued by the same mindset.

Scholars working in higher education and global health sectors in the United Kingdom, North America and in countries in Africa and Asia have recognised the prevailing mindset and begun to challenge this, through the promotion of 'decolonising' ideas and approaches, to address long-standing social injustice and improve race relations (Banda, 2023; Batty, 2020; Moncrieffe et al., 2019). Universities, higher education institutions (HEIs) and global health institutions, as major sources of global knowledge and teaching pedagogy, have begun working towards promoting inclusivity within this sector. The introduction of race relations, gender equality, social diversity and inclusion in curricula forms part of the plan to decolonise higher education in the United Kingdom in addition to changing approaches and methods in teaching and learning (Batty, 2020; Moncrieffe et al., 2019). By the same token, governmental and nongovernmental organisations are exploring and implementing strategies to improve equality, diversity and inclusion (EDI) agendas in order to manage workplace diversity.

However, with advances in communication technology and improvements in global connectivity and mobility, higher education, including nursing education, has increasingly become international and global and therefore very diverse. Professionalisation of nursing has been part of a wider and global colonial project. As highlighted earlier, global health has been completely colonised, and decolonising debates have been initiated and are currently in progress. Here, we present an example of how global health industries associated with colonial institutions in the Global North have systematically supressed local capacity to produce medicines in Africa.

CASE STUDY 6.2

How the Global North Suppresses Local Capacity to Produce Medicines in the Global South

By providing evidence from a research study, Banda persuasively argues that the African pharmaceutical industry has been systematically supressed by powerful Northern pharmaceutical institutions that have extractive objectives. As a result, African capacity to use local engineering and technology to produce medicines has been completely undermined and underdeveloped, and the sector has become fully dependent on external supplies. Without any appropriate intervention, powerful institutions based in the Global North will continue to dominate the production of medical supplies. Banda concludes decolonisation to reactivate and strengthen African industry is urgently needed (Banda, 2023).

THINK BOX 6.6

Banda's (2023) research demonstrates the importance of understanding the impact of persistent colonial extractive institutions on the African pharmaceutical industry. The main objective of these institutions is to exploit and profit from, rather than develop, local industry (capacity). Consider how this situation might affect the delivery of nursing and global health care.

We have clarified the concept of colonisation by providing examples of colonisation of nursing and global health with case studies of nursing education in Nepal, colonisation of the pharmaceutical industry in Africa and historical accounts of the early establishment of nursing in India, Indonesia and South Africa. We have illustrated how nursing within the field of global health has been a colonial product and decolonising is urgently needed to make it a fair, just and inclusive profession. Part two explores existing barriers to decolonisation and global health in the contemporary world.

PART TWO: EXISTING BARRIERS TO THE DECOLONISATION OF NURSING

A critical question emerges here: is the current process and practice of internationalisation and globalisation complementary or contradictory to the process of decolonising higher education and professional nursing?

This is a complex question which we examine in some detail in the following sections and demonstrate how barriers to decolonisation are created and sustained.

Internationalisation of Nursing: (Un)Equal Opportunities and Power Relations

While the 'internationalisation' and 'globalisation' of nursing have been discussed and debated in recent decades, 'decolonising global nursing' is a very new concept. Internationalisation is understood as the process whereby the value and practices of a country are maintained and retained alongside their interactions with other countries (Allen & Ogilvie, 2004). The internationalisation of nursing begins with introducing this concept into nursing curricula, research and professional practice. Again, in practice, the process of internationalisation appears to be that powerful institutions in the Global North impart their practices and values in less powerful countries. The HEIs, including nursing, achieve this by actively collaborating with nursing education and research institutions in the Global South.

The internationalisation of professional nursing appears to have moved forward with three dominant concepts and practices. These are:

1. Developing curricula on cultural awareness and including the meaning and value of cultural competencies in nursing education. This is to be

achieved by the introduction of diverse sociocultural practices in the teaching curriculum and developing international exchange programmes (Law & Muir, 2005).

2. Creating international standards by harmonising and standardising nursing curricula within the global context.

3. Promoting international student exchange, international partnerships and learning and exchanging knowledge and practices. The justification for, and discussion of, internationalisation focuses on learning from diverse groups of people and offering culturally sensitive and respectful nursing care to all.

Within the context of internationalisation of nursing education, research and practice, let's examine existing barriers to decolonising.

Example 1 Sustaining Colonial Practice

Globalisation and Internationalisation of Nursing Education Curricula

There is economic interest in the internationalisation of HEIs, which is perhaps not openly admitted by institutions. Most of the HEIs in the United Kingdom and other economically rich countries (Europe, North America, Australia and New Zealand) and, indeed, globally, have ambitious international outlooks. They actively forge partnerships with international education and research institutions and engage in the recruitment of students and academic faculties from international sources. Many of the HEIs are proactive in their promotion of attractive educational and career prospects for students and graduates. Their recruitment adverts are designed to attract fee-paying international students and talented academic faculty members. Further, many UK HEIs, for example, have successfully established satellite campuses in Asia: in Hong Kong, Singapore, Malaysia, China and the Persian Gulf countries. Working in collaboration with their international partners, HEIs continue to expand and strengthen their internationalisation agenda. Quite clearly, they are not only diversifying their economic opportunities but also becoming more diverse in their institutional capacity and workforce composition. Higher education in nursing is an important aspect of the overall internationalisation process. However, an area demanding critical understanding is to establish if the relationships between these partner organisations are equal and to determine whether they are colonial, dominant or 'extractive' in nature. Economists use the term 'extractive'

to analyse the process by which the Global North exploits any local resource in the Global South without building in renewal or replenishment plans (for example, Case Study 6.2; Banda, 2023).

Further, the trend in student mobility internationally through international exchange programmes particularly favours nursing and health care students from the Global North. This is because more of them are able to afford to travel, which gives them opportunities to learn cultural diversity within the wider global context. This, in turn, serves to better prepare them to provide culturally sensitive care to their diverse clients. It also leads to their becoming global leaders in this field in the future. They are placed in the position to have the knowledge and expertise to speak for and represent those who do not have access to the same knowledge and travel opportunities or are unable to speak for themselves, often minority groups and people from the Global South. However, corresponding opportunities are not available for those students receiving their nursing and other professional education in facilities in low-income countries or the Global South. Unfortunately, the structures of many immigration and border control policies and sociocultural and political order in the countries of the Global North are all designed to discourage immigration and thus retain colonial values and practices.

We live in a time-compressed and interconnected world. Our messages are transmitted instantly across the globe. In fact, global, economic and political processes shape the very core of the current global order in politics, health, education, economy, infrastructure, development and every other sector. Colonial mindsets are prevalent everywhere, and all aspects of our everyday life, local values and practices have gradually been eroded and reshaped and become influenced by global forces over a period of time. Appadurai (1996) terms this process as the 'globalisation', or 'homogenisation', of sociocultural values and ideas.

Example 2 Sustaining Colonial Practice

Evidence-Based Practice in Nursing: Whose Evidence Counts?

Ideas of evidence-based practice have become important in all areas. Health care institutions and professional practitioners are educated to provide evidence-based health care. Nursing has been driven increasingly as an evidence-based practice. Evidence considered relevant and best suited in one country, or in one part of the world, may not be the case elsewhere. However, due to colonial thinking or rigid mindsets, evidence and standards created in affluent and powerful institutions in the Global North are considered to be applicable to, and acceptable by, nurses working in all sociocultural contexts globally without any question. Practitioners in the Global South are rarely in a position to challenge these precepts and standards or promote their local practices to wider, global-level use.

As indicated earlier, institutions in the Global North are in politically and economically privileged positions to create gold-standard evidence, and countries in the South are to use the evidence generated by, and decided upon, in the Global North. Evidence generated and created by the health care systems, institutions and professional bodies in the Global South are not considered 'gold standard' and therefore are not considered as evidence by powerful nations. There is a mindset that anything and everything created by scholars in the Global North is better. As the standards are decided and supported by evidence, there is no space for alternative arguments and alternative evidence in current global health systems. Similarly, a significant proportion of publications are produced by authors based in affluent countries, even though the studies are conducted in low-income countries in partnership with professionals there (Kokutse, 2022).

For example, with regards to nursing professional ethics, the core guiding principles of the profession, globally, are based on the ICN's values, whose sociocultural, political and religious origins are Euro-American. As Wagoro & Duma (2018, p. 159) point out: 'Most of the literature that nurses in Africa refer to when confronted with ethical challenges is from high-income countries. Examples from such literature often do not resonate with the African sociocultural and religious contexts'.

We do have different sociocultural, political and professional contexts; therefore, our ethics and professional standards should be shaped according to local sociocultural values and ethics. Nurses and health care professionals across the world need to understand, acknowledge and embrace this truth. We need to expand our views and value others' ideas. Local evidence is perhaps more relevant to a particular context and should be considered for local use, but it is critical to have global consent on this.

Example 3 Sustaining Colonial Practice

Creating Professional Hierarchy and Rigid Competency

Further, as global health care systems become increasingly advanced, complex, and interconnected and workforces have become more diverse, so, too, have stricter professional regulations and competency frameworks

been developed and implemented. Colonial values and practices, in tandem with the creation of rigid professional regulations and competencies required for professional licences, favour majority health care professionals who are educated in the Global North which disadvantages, and marginalises those from minority backgrounds. Due to those rigid regulations, migrant nurses (and health care professionals) do not get the jobs that they are qualified to do, and their career progression is often delayed (Adhikari et al., 2023). This serves to further create and sustain the concept of professional class and therefore perpetuates structural inequalities and institutional racism.

The health care sector globally strives towards achieving and maintaining superior standards of service and standards in all key areas: professional education, regulation and practice and overall health system governance. Various measurement tools are created and used to monitor and maintain service standards. In this context, the ideas of excellence in any professional education and practice create a hierarchy of low- and high-income countries, which has not been adequately and critically examined in current literature.

Throughout the professional history of nursing in the United Kingdom, it is widely perceived that nursing education institutions and associated hospitals have certain images, and education quality and service standards are determined accordingly. This happens in most countries globally, for example, in Nepal, India and the United Kingdom. In Nepal, nurses educated in government-run or government-supported nursing colleges and teaching hospitals are deemed to be better qualified than nurses educated in the private sector (Adhikari, 2019). Similarly, in India, those nurses educated in government-run nursing colleges are considered better educated than those educated in private colleges (Tsujita & Oda, 2023). Further, it is regularly heard that nurses educated in London's larger teaching hospitals, for example, St Thomas' Hospital or King's College London, or at the University of Edinburgh, are perceived to have achieved higher professional standards than those educated/ trained in smaller hospitals and recently established colleges. In a similar fashion, nurses educated in the United Kingdom are credited with higher professional prestige than nurses educated in Nepal, India and the Philippines. As a result, they continue to be accorded this higher status and occupy privileged positions. Research evidence generated by these institutions is also considered more credible than that from smaller institutions. This mindset continues to sustain professional hierarchies and needs to be critically examined and challenged if nursing is to be decolonised.

Professional class and racial hierarchy have existed throughout the history of nursing in the United Kingdom and globally. Migrant nurses educated outside the United Kingdom, particularly in low-income countries in Asia and Africa, are seen as less skilled than those educated in the United Kingdom (Smith & Mackintosh, 2007). Parry (2002, p. 67) states: 'Any analysis of current migration cannot ignore this historical context' and the 'continuing presence of empire'. This is evident in the following quotation from a British African Caribbean nurse manager who describes a 'pecking order in the NHS (National Health System, United Kingdom) to get positions'. This 'pecking order', or 'hierarchy', appeared to be based on the nurse's race and country of origin, which is, if not Britain, then a former British colony.

CASE STUDY 6.3

Colonised Professional Nursing Hierarchies

People say that there is a pecking order in the NHS to get positions. So, it's White first, White British first, then White Australian, White South African. When you run out of all of that and you have only got Black left after all the Whites, it's Asians. After the Asians, you come down to Black, and if you have to differentiate, it's Black Caribbean then Black African...It's a pecking order

(SMITH ET AL., 2006, P. 61).

In order to decolonise professional nursing, there is a need to closely examine the structural issues and challenges in nursing education and workforce management practices.

Currently, such professional regulatory bodies as the Nursing and Midwifery Council (NMC) in the United Kingdom, the ICN (at a global level), the Indian Nursing Council, the Japanese Nursing Council and the Nursing Council of Nepal are responsible for creating professional competency standards at national and international levels. However, prevailing social and structural inequalities need to be acknowledged to avoid focusing solely on creating professional competency standards (Collier-Sewell et al., 2023). These standards and competency frameworks give little practical consideration of its impact on diverse and minority workforces

and current 'decolonising' and professional inclusion agendas.

The 'State of the World's Nursing' report (World Health Organization, 2020, p. 32) emphasises the importance of 'regulation which serves to protect the public through setting and enforcing education and practice standards'. 'Harmonisation' of educational standards is described as one approach to ensure local relevance and consistency within distinct global communities exemplified by the countries of the Caribbean Community of Education and the European Union (World Health Organization, 2020, p. 33, Box 4.9). However, this perspective comes with the caveat that these standards may have been originally influenced by colonial values and practices.

Unfortunately, these hierarchies continue to maintain prevailing structural inequalities, such as availability of, and access to, resources to run and regulate nursing education and practice. They continue to marginalise the views and values of the minority workforce and serve to maintain colonial order and practice. This form of discrimination is experienced every day but rarely reflected upon. Such practices need to be challenged.

Promoting and Maintaining Colonial Ideas and Mindsets

There is a prevailing idea that people in low- and middle-income countries lack modern Western-style biomedical health care services because the governments in those countries lack adequate resources to equip a health care system that is fit to provide optimal quality of care and service. These standards are measured using tools and criteria based on colonial values and practices. The current process of Objective Structured Clinical Examination (OSCE) undertaken by the UK NMC to assess overseas nurses to practise is a case in point (Foster, 2018). This process hugely undervalues overseas nurse skill and professional competency. Foster, a chief nurse at Oxford University Hospitals, United Kingdom, comments that candidates were advised to use an outdated manual developed in the United Kingdom, which did not accurately assess their clinical expertise and skills. These examinations are expensive, and failure rates are high (Foster, 2018).

CASE STUDY 6.4
Objective Structured Clinical Examination, UK Nursing and Midwifery Council

Foster (2018) states:

When my Trust went on a recruitment trip to India, last October I met with one of the first successful NMC registered nurses and discussed the OSCE process. This highly competent critical care cardiothoracic nurse had made two attempts at the OSCE before he passed. I was also told that we had had four further OSCE first attempt failures that week.

Colonial ideas have resulted in nurses and health care professionals in low-income countries being seen as lacking high standards of professional education and support, proper professional development opportunities and, finally, the resources needed to provide quality health care. This notion was amplified during the COVID-19 pandemic. The Western media regularly highlighted a risk of COVID-19 killing more people in poor countries than in affluent countries in the Global North, believing that people and health care systems in poorer countries lacked personal protective equipment, adequate personal hygiene and other essential health care supplies. However, as Oleribe and colleagues (2021) argue, this was not necessarily the case in sub-Saharan Africa at the start of the pandemic when factors such as favourable climate, younger populations and protective immunity against a range of infectious diseases resulted in a low prevalence of COVID-19 deaths. It is imperative therefore that the Global North is cautious in judging the Global South as a single entity without understanding the factors that come into play in specific countries and situations.

Therefore any effort towards decolonising professional disciplines is not possible without having an in-depth understanding of the local health care practices, colonial history and processes and how they have impacted and continue to impact the structure of society. Learning about, understanding and reflecting on colonial hierarchy and mindset and the colonial legacy are positive steps forward.

Example 4 Sustaining Colonial Practice
A Gendered Profession and Medical Domination

Globally, nursing and care have been seen as females' work. Almost 90% of nurses (and care workers) are female. Historically, medicine has been male dominated, with nurses viewed as doctors' assistants. There is a professional hierarchy within health care systems, with doctors generally accorded more professional authority and granted key decision-making positions within the organisation. Exploring deeper, in most sociocultural contexts, nursing was set up to assist doctors to provide care in institutional settings. In many instances, nursing schools were (and still are) located within medical schools (Horwitz, 2011; Juanamasta et al., 2011). Until now, nurses have been widely perceived as doctors' assistants.

However, new gender dynamics are emerging in medicine, too. In recent years, more females are joining medicine. It is likely that in the coming years, medicine will also be a female-dominated profession. However, professional and class hierarchies are likely to be sustained. Gender issues, combined with class and inter- and intra-profession hierarchy, need to be examined and addressed as a matter of urgency.

Even though nursing within the modern health care system has been revolutionised in the past decades to become an autonomous profession, much of its scope of practice and policy decisions are still controlled by medical professionals. This was made very clear during the COVID-19 pandemic response. While frontline nurses and health care professionals, a vast majority of whom were female, received praise globally for their selfless work, nurse leaders' voices were missing from the media, in policy decisions and in the boardrooms (Anders, 2020).

THINK BOX 6.7
Read Chapter 8: 'Gender, Nursing and Global Health: Why Does Gender Matter?'. Identify resonances with our discussion of gender as a factor in sustaining colonial practice.

PART THREE: APPROACHES AND STRATEGIES
Roadmap and Approaches to Decolonisation

Scholars propose and engage with various approaches to 'decolonise' global health, higher education and international development practices. Some suggest a complete systemic overhaul (Chaudhuri et al., 2021), and others propose a somewhat 'softer' approach through promoting EDI in organisations in a wide range of sectors, including health, higher education, international development and many others (Batty, 2020; Moncrieffe et al., 2019). EDI is considered to be one of the main organisational principles in the United Kingdom and, increasingly, in the wider world.

As our discussion of the literature demonstrates, the idea of decolonising is interpreted differently by different professionals, depending on their sociocultural and political backgrounds. It is therefore the case that any plan to decolonise the system has no clear and coherent universal approach.

Generally, in practice, professionals from the colonial side of the argument have perhaps considered decolonising to mean social inclusion, while, on the other hand, professionals from colonised backgrounds see the process as needing to undo all colonial structures and practices (Hellowell & Schwerdtle, 2021; Shahjahan et al., 2022). Scholars propound a complete systemic overhaul, with authority ceded to the colonised group; this is an interpretation of Frantz Fanon's ideas of total transformation, so it is a direct attack on White or Euro-American supremacy and power (Chaudhuri et al., 2021; Hirsch, 2021).

CASE STUDY 6.5
Frantz Fanon (1925–61)

Fanon was an African-Caribbean physician, psychiatrist, political thinker and activist from Martinique, a colony (now department) of France. He received his medical training in Lyon, France, and drew on phenomenology and psychoanalysis in his writings and practice. Fanon's most influential works include *Black Skin, White Masks* (1952) and *The Wretched of the Earth* (1961) in which he describes the 'black lived experience' and the dehumanising effects of colonisation on individuals and communities. Fanon inspired and influenced early decolonisation and liberation movements, particularly in Algeria and sub-Saharan Africa (Macey, 2000). The Wikipedia entry for Frantz Fanon reports that in his practice as a psychiatrist, Fanon used 'sociotherapy' as a way to connect with patients' cultural backgrounds and trained nurses and junior doctors in this approach. A recent book (Gibson, 2021) reflects on Fanon's visionary legacy and his contribution to decolonialise thought and struggles against racism, exploitation and injustice. The ongoing relevance of his (Fanon's) work is

embodied in the 'Black Lives Matter' movement, founded by African-American women activists in response to the murders of African-Americans Trayvon Martin, (Florida, 2013), Michael Brown (Ferguson, Missouri 2014) and others. The movement gained global traction and following George Floyd's murder by police in Minneapolis (2020) further ignited worldwide protests at state-sanctioned racist violence against Black citizens (Wikipedia).

Fanon's ideas of total transformation are so important to our understanding of the need for a systemic overhaul to cede authority from the coloniser to the colonised group. This observation is in line with Gibson (2021, p. 300), who notes: 'Fanon's new humanism is a politics of becoming, based on the fundamental transformation of paralysed black and colonized subjects into new human beings through liberation struggle'.

Similarly, Shahjahan et al. (2022, p. 83) described decolonising higher education in terms of 'decentring', destabilising, resisting, challenging, eliminating, divesting and 'dismantling' the monocultural perspective and practices.

On the other hand, when contextualising EDI in the UK's HEIs and professional nursing context, this is understood as having been mainly about being inclusive by inviting and welcoming professionals from minority and ethnic backgrounds into an organisation. However, quite often, this has been a tokenistic gesture, without valuing diverse opinions, offering adequate support to minority groups and sufficiently preparing organisations to accept diverse values and opinions.

As Shahjahan et al. (2022, p. 74) suggest, the curriculum and chosen style of pedagogy are deeply implicated in grounding, validating and/or marginalising or monopolising systems of knowledge production. For example, in Nepal, the pedagogy and the curriculum in nursing are both deeply grounded in and influenced by Western knowledge, but it would be impossible even to imagine this happening the other way around—that is, Nepali sociocultural values influencing British nursing education. Surely, it is important to realise and value the knowledge that is generated in other sociocultural contexts. In our view, a meaningful decolonisation would be to actively create space to learn, realise and embrace other values and approaches to learning and practice.

Decolonising medical curricula has been about designing and teaching cultural diversities, cultural competencies and cultural humility to medical students (Nazar et al., 2015). However, the professional nursing education system has still to actively engage in this discussion in order to have any meaningful impact on everyday practice in the United Kingdom, North America and globally.

Main Approaches and Practical Efforts to Decolonisation of Global Health and Higher Education Institutions

Scholars have highlighted two main approaches to decolonising the global sociopolitical order, which includes international development, education, health system governance and more. Proposed ideas, strategies and practices run in a continuum, from softer approaches of developing and implementing EDI to more radical systemic overhaul.

The softer approach suggests tackling the prevailing power imbalance by creating space for alternatives and valuing and recognising diversity. One example of this soft approach is teaching about decolonising in all education systems and through introducing equality, diversity and inclusivity policies into organisations (Hellowell & Schwerdtle, 2021).

Conversely, the other group of scholars highlights the need for a systemic overhaul (Chaudhuri et al., 2021). Both approaches constitute a threat to those who hold epistemic power or, indeed, any authority, organisation, government or individual who holds power to make major decisions which can significantly impact other people's lives. Those scholars, who propose a complete systemic overhaul, state that it is vital to recognise and challenge colonial arrogance and respect diverse care practices and that the current teaching pedagogy and practice hierarchy need to be completely restructured. They challenge the construction and maintenance of white supremacy and colonial hierarchy.

However, in recent years, there have been some efforts to decolonise professional nursing. We now present some examples of decolonising nursing education and practice in various settings to illustrate contemporary discussion, practical and policy efforts that have taken place to address oppressive and colonial nursing practice. The materials are available in the reference list in a PDF as resources for you to use.

CASE STUDY 6.6

Examples of Changes in Nursing Curriculum: Teaching and Practising Decolonising Nursing

- Decolonising and Anti-Oppressive Nursing Practice: Awareness, Allyship and Action', from Canada (Jacubec and Bourque Bearskin, 2020)

This example of educational materials suggests teaching and learning about diversity and discrimination, and understanding race relations is the first step to decolonising nursing. Case studies are presented which describe decolonising activities in the Canadian health care system. These include developing cultural competency, cultural awareness and culturally safe service through respect, trust and collaboration. Ways/approaches to learning about cultural humility and respectful care are illustrated to prepare nurses to become allies to racialised and diverse groups of people. Finally, this teaching resource suggests some questions to encourage professional nurses to think critically.

- Decolonisation of Nursing Education' (Zappas et al., 2021).

This short article highlights why nursing education needs decolonising and the role of the nursing faculty to prepare culturally sensitive nurses. Linking up with the structural context of marginalisation, this paper engages with DEI debates and the role of nurses in promoting racial and cultural humility and designing nursing curricula accordingly.

- 'Decolonising Nursing Education: Why Africanisation Matters' (Msila, 2017).

This example is based on a book chapter which illustrates how nursing in South Africa has been a colonial product and traditional knowledge of health and illness and caring practices, systematically erased by the South African colonial system and Africa at large. Now is the time to address racial, cultural, class and gender (paternalistic) divisions in nursing which need to be included in nursing education curricula.

In summary, there is a key argument to be made. Professional nursing, within the global health care sector, has been completely colonised, internationalised and globalised, and as such, the value of social and professional diversity is subsumed by universal standards and scope of practice models.

THINK BOX 6.8

This argument raises a critical issue regarding decolonising the profession, which is whether it is even possible for there to be a meaningful implementation of inclusive policies.

- Do we accept a softer approach to decolonisation to make nursing more inclusive and welcoming to diverse groups of people?
- How do we put these ideas into practice?
- How do we create a clear roadmap towards reforming professional nursing and making nursing more inclusive, attractive and a fair and just profession for a diverse group of people?

These questions merit in-depth exploration. Now is the time for those professionals who occupy privileged positions, which allow them to create and decide standards and evidence in nursing, to actively source diverse kinds of evidence that emerge from diverse populations. Ideas created out of their comfort zones are needed alongside the need to recognise evidence produced in a wider global context. In order for us to achieve this:

- It is vital to keep our minds open to understand and welcome ideas and evidence emerging from other parts of the world.
- Strategies are required to change the composition of research councils, funding bodies and ethics committees, so they are not dominated by members from the Global North. Membership should not be about an individual's nationality but their social values and viewpoints.

We present a case study of reflections on Chilean nursing, which sheds a light on global nursing.

CASE STUDY 6.7

Reflections on Chilean Nursing Shed a Light on Global Nursing

Dr Lissette Aviles, a nursing lecturer from Chile, draws on her experiences of educational developments and governance to reflect on decolonisation.

Lissette's reflections shed a light on:

- Hidden histories to understand resistance to Euro-American models of nursing education.
- The role of early medical domination in establishing university-based nursing education.
- Influence of politics, governance and trade unions to create a progressive clinical and public health nursing model.
- Nursing's value reflected in better salaries, high percentage of male nurses, and staff attraction and retention.
- Chilean nursing challenges the hegemony of the Global North and offers a positive example of global nursing.

Modern Chilean nursing training was initially influenced by the Euro-American model of in-hospital training. Yet despite this influence, the first university-based nursing school, the first in Latin America, was established in 1906. The school delivered a 3-year programme (University of Chile, n.d.) that was successfully replicated across the country. By 1920, the national census reported 1619 nurses, of whom 39% were male (Nunez et al., 2019). This is quite striking for a traditionally female-dominated profession. In 1927, a public health nursing degree was created to respond to local needs, followed in 1929 by a 4-year programme that combined both clinical and public health approaches. What is also striking is that in the English language literature, only four nursing schools, in Brazil, Argentina and Uruguay, followed the British-American model (Sand, 1924), which suggests resistance to the dominant colonising model at that time.

It is interesting to note that this groundbreaking and progressive approach to nursing education took place in nursing schools initially managed by physicians who arguably facilitated their development but at the expense of a legacy of patriarchy and male dominance. The political events during the 1970s, when a deadly dictatorship overthrew democracy, also undoubtedly affected nursing, eliminating unions, decreasing professional autonomy, closing some schools and barring males from nursing (Osses-Paredes et al., 2010). However, there is a lack of rigorous evidence which documents the impact of these seismic events.

Despite the challenges, Chilean nursing education progressed in the 1980s. Five-year programmes became the standard for all bachelor's degrees (including nursing) in Chile followed by postgraduate qualifications, including master's degrees. By 1995, Chilean nursing education comprised a bachelor's degree in nursing and the generalist registered nurse qualification. This led to the inclusion of nursing in the Health Act in 1996, which defined and established nursing's role and scope. This legislation led to recognition within health care institutions and the development of nursing care directives at the hospital level, gaining professional autonomy and social recognition. This progressive governance of the health care system and policies boosted nursing in Chile, positively affecting status and salaries. Since the 2000s, salary increases across public and private sectors attracted more applicants, including males, because nursing was seen as a scientific and well-paid profession rather than a vocational one. In 2016, males accounted for approximately 10%–20% of nurses, while my own experience suggests current nursing programmes train between 30%–40% of male nursing students.

To date, postgraduate qualifications are common among Chilean nurses, including diplomas, master's and PhD programmes. Recent studies report between 25%–42% of Chilean nurses had postgraduate education on top of their 5-year bachelor's degrees (Simonetti et al., 2020). Nowadays, Chilean nurses have achieved political and leadership roles in Parliament, hospital directorates and policy development, nationally and internationally. Yet arguably, because the Global North dominates the hegemony of evidence and knowledge, little is known about the progressive nature of nursing in Latin America. This knowledge could be used as an example to shed a light on the development of strategies and practices in the Global South that challenge the status quo, with the potential to decolonise nursing globally.

CONCLUSION

This chapter has presented the complex debate in relation to decolonising nursing within global health and higher education and also within the context of the internationalisation of professional nursing education and practice. The picture we have so far is a hazy one, and clearly, the concept of decolonisation faces significant challenges. Firstly, there is an apparent lack of meaningful professional engagement to explore professional perspectives, academic discussion and literature on the topic. Therefore the importance of exploring any possible practical approach to decolonising the profession cannot be clearly understood.

However, a wider discussion on decolonising higher education and global health suggests that there are no universal guidelines or approaches to decolonise any discipline and practice (Shahjahan et al., 2022). The available literature on the topic and institutional efforts to decolonise higher education in the United Kingdom have translated the concept into being primarily about improving social inclusion and race relations. This concept is applicable to nursing, too, as nurses are a highly diverse group. There is a huge diversity in nursing workforces in most countries: within Black, Asian and minority ethnic nurses in the United Kingdom, Black/African-American nurses in the United States and minority nurses globally (Adhikari et al., 2023; Iheduru-Anderson, 2021).

The current professional regulations, guidelines and rigid professional competencies treat nurses as a homogeneous group, which is a major barrier to decolonising nursing. It is critical to understand nursing workforce diversity, and there is a further need to address intersections within the diverse groups. The colonial construction of professional hierarchy and a homogenised professional image adds further complexity to the social diversity and emerging 'decolonising' debate. Professional practitioners and policymakers should improve their understanding of professional diversity and actively explore and embrace minority views, which have not been adequately valued in current professional educational practice. This should be taken into consideration when designing and implementing nursing curricula and practice guidelines. Inclusion should not just mean a representation of diverse and minority people in a workplace and in a team or to take a position to homogenise their ideas, values and practices, but diverse views and opinion should be valued and respected, and policy should have meaningful implementation and be monitored for effectiveness.

Another point this chapter raises is that the Euro-American value systems of education and health services have colonised the ideas of health and nursing across the world. Should there be a movement which starts from where colonial values and ideas have dominated local values and education systems? Should this movement be a global movement, and should the decolonising process be local with a global outlook? The literature on decolonising public health expresses a major concern that the voice from 'below' (i.e., from the Global South) is missing, which directs us to explore ways to hear the voices of those who have been colonised. Indeed, this leads us to question if it is actually possible to critically and genuinely discuss this issue and decolonise global health and nursing by scholars, whose values are shaped by education that is provided by institutions based in Global North?

Discussion in this chapter highlights the need to explore the concept in greater depth and for a movement to look at the impact of colonisation on the development of the profession at close range within our community in everyday practice. We argue, however, that it should go much further, beyond the United Kingdom and beyond the higher education sector. We need to expand our exploration and examine how nursing values and practices have been shaped globally by colonial influences across all societies. Furthermore, our professional values, principles and practices are not static but the result of a dynamic process, which should change over time.

And finally, decolonising nursing education and practice can improve nursing's professional image and create fair and just employment and a professional discipline that is able to attract more candidates, which is in the interest of the profession and society as a whole. It is vital therefore to expand our understanding of diversity and inclusion and create equal opportunities and a safe space for everyone. It is time to think differently.

REFERENCES

Adhikari, R., & Plotnikova, E. (2023). *Nurse Migration in Asia: Emerging Patterns and Policy Responses (Edit)*. Routledge, UK.

Adhikari, R., Corcoran, J., Smith, P., Rodgers, S., Suleiman, R., & Barber, K. (2023). It's ok to be different: Supporting black and minority ethnic nurses and midwives in their professional development in the UK. *Nurse Education in Practice, 66*. Available at: https://www.sciencedirect.com/science/article/pii/S1471595322002220 (Accessed: 8 December 2022).

Adhikari, R. (2019). *Migrant health professionals and the global labour market: the dreams and traps of Nepali nurses*. London: Routledge.

Allen, M., & Ogilvie, L. (2004). Internationalisations of higher education: Potentials and pitfalls for nursing education. *International Council of Nurses, International Nursing Review, 51*, 73–80. Available at: file:///Users/research1/Downloads/International%20Nursing%20Review%20-%202004%20-%20Allen%20-%20Internationalization%20of%20higher%20education%20%20potentials%20and%20pitfalls%20for%20nursing.pdf. (Accessed: 2 May 2023).

Anders, R. L. (2020). Engaging nurses in health policy in the era of Covid-19, Nursing Forum: An independent Voice for Nursing, available at: https://www.ncbi.nlm.nih.gov/pmc/articles/PMC7675349/pdf/NUF-56-89.pdf. (Accessed: 24 April 2023).

Appadurai, A. (1996). *Modernity at Large: Cultural Dimensions of Globalisation*. Minneapolis, MN: University of Minnesota Press.

Banda, G. (2023). Political Economy of the African Pharmacological Sector's "industrial underdevelopment" lock in: The importance of understanding the impact of persistent colonial extractive Institutions. *Frontiers in Research Metrics and Analytics.* open access. 10.3389/frma.2023.1020588, available at: https://www.ncbi.nlm.nih.gov/pmc/articles/PMC9947535/ (Accessed: 31 May 2023).

Batty, D. (2020) Only a fifth of universities, say they are 'decolonising' curriculum, Guardian, June 11. Available at: https://www.theguardian.com/us-news/2020/jun/11/only-fifth-of-uk-universities-have-said-they-will-decolonise-curriculum. (Accessed: 24 November 2022).

Carter, M. T. (2019). *Being a Nurse the Indian Way: An exploration of the lived experiences of Indian nurses, who came to the United Kingdom (UK) for higher education studies and work, a thesis submitted to degree of Doctor of Philosophy*. Brunel University.

Chaudhuri, M. M., Mkimba, L., Raveendran, Y., & Smith, R. D. (2021). Decolonising global Health: Beyond reformative roadmaps and towards decolonial thought. *BMJ Global Health, 6*, e006371. doi:10.1136/bmjgh-2021-006371.

Choy, C. (2003). *Empire of Care: Nursing and Migration in Filipino American History*. Duke University Press. Durham, USA.

Collier-Sewell, F., Atherton, I., Mahony, C., Kyle, R. G., Hughes, E., & Lasater, K. (2023). Competencies and standard in nurse education: Irresolvable tension. *Nurse Education Today, 125*, 105782. Available at: https://www.sciencedirect.com/science/article/pii/S026069172300076X?via%3Dihub , (Accessed: 2 June 2022).

Coronado, F., Beck, A. J., Shah, G., Young, J. A., Sellers, K., & Leider, J. P. (2020). Understanding the dynamics of diversity in the public health workforce. *Journal of Public Health Management Practice, 26*(4), 389–392. doi:10.1097/PHH.0000000000001075.

Fitzgerald, R (2006). "Making and Moulding the Nursing of the Indian Empire": Recasting Nurses in Colonial India". In Rhetoric and Reality: Gender and the Colonial Experience in South Asia, Edited by: Lambert-Hurley, S. & Powell, A. New Delhi: Oxford University Press.

Foster, S. (2018). Are the tests for overseas nurses fair? *British Journal of Nursing, 27*(9), 525.

Gibson, N. C. (2021). Fanon Today: Reason and Revolt of the Wretched of the Earth. *Zend Graphics Ltd.* Daraja Press, Quebec Canada.

Grigulis, A. (2011). *The lives of Malawian nurses: the stories behind the statistics.* Unpublished Ph.D. Thesis. London: University College.

Healey, M. (2010). 'Regarded, paid and housed as menials' Nursing in colonial India 1900–1948, South Asian. *History and Culture, 2*(1), 55–75. Available: https://doi.org/10.1080/19472498.2011.531609. (Accessed: 30 May 2023).

Hellowell, M., & Schwerdtle, P. N. (2021). Powerful ideas? Decolonisation and the future of global health. *BMJ Global Health, 7,* e006924. doi:10.1136/bmjgh-2021-006924.

Hirsch, L. A. (2021). The art of medicine: Is it possible to decolonise global health institutions? Perspective. *Lancet, 397.* Available at: https://www.thelancet.com/journals/lancet/article/PIIS0140-6736(20)32763-X/fulltext (Accessed: 10 May 2023).

Horwitz, S. (2011). The Nurse in the University: the History of University Education for South African Nurses a case study if the Witwatersrand. *Nursing Research in Practice, 2011.* doi:10.1155/2011/813270 Article ID 813270, 9 pages.

Iheduru-Anderson, K. C. (2021). The White/Black hierarchy institutionalizes White supremacy in nursing and nursing leadership in the United States. *Journal of Professional Nursing, 37,* 411–421. Available at: https://reader.elsevier.com/reader/sd/pii/S8755722320301113?token=B20507262B4AEBA79EE30D24A3-418E32F3828F5D7489532C53F15F1A52E53B7C2F7CA94FBC5EEE5EBADE1B4199B10A08&originRegion=eu-west-1&originCreation=20230325114600. (Accessed: 24 March 2023).

International Council of Nurses (n.d.), Nursing Definitions, available at: https://www.icn.ch/nursing-policy/nursing-definitions (Accessed: 14 May 2023).

Juanamasta, G., Iblasi, A. S., Aungsuroch, Y., & Yunibhand, J. (2021). Nursing Development in Indonesia: Colonialism, after Independence and Nursing Act. *Open Nursing, 7,* 1–10.

Jacubec, S.L. and Bourque Bearskin Lisa, R. (2020). Decolonising and anti-oppressive nursing practice: Awareness, allyship, and action, chapter 14. Available at: 9780323683364 Ch. 14 Decolonizing and Anti-Oppressive Nursing Practice.pdf (Accessed: 26 April 2023).

Kingma, M. (2006). *Nurses on the move: migration and global health care economy.* ILR press an imprint of Cornell University Press Ithaca and London.

Kline, R. (2014). *The "snowy white peaks" of the NHS: a survey of discrimination in governance and leadership and the potential impact on patient care in.* London and England: Available from Middlesex University's Research Repository. London, England.

Kokutse, F. (2022). In *Lead Authors from low income countries on the decrease.* University World News. Available at: https://www.universityworldnews.com/post.php?story=20220628095022532. (Accessed: 27 June 2023).

Kulesa, J., & Brantuo, N. A. (2021). Barriers to decolonising educational Partnership in global health. *BMJ Global Health, 6,* e006964. doi:10.1136/bmjgh-2021-006964.

Law, K., & Muir, N. (2005). The internationalisation of the nursing curriculum. *Nurse Education in Practice, 6,* 149–155.

Macey, D. (2000). *Frantz Fanon: A biography.* New York: Picador.

Moncrieffe, M., Asare, Y., Dunford, R., & Youssef, H. (2019). *Decolonising the Curriculum, Teaching and Learning About Race Equality.* University of Brighton. Available at: https://cris.brighton.ac.uk/ws/portalfiles/portal/6443632/Decolonising_the_curriculum_MONCRIEFFE_32_pages_4th_July.pdf (Accessed: 24 November 2022).

Msila, V. (2017). Decolonising nursing education: Why Africanisation matters. 2017. In Gumbo, M. T., & Msila, V. (Eds.), *African Voices on Indigenisation of the Curriculum: Insights from Practice.* available at: AFRICAN_VOICES_ON_INDIGENISATION_OF_THE.pdf (Accessed: 29 May 2023).

Nair, S. & Healey, M. (2006). A profession on the margins: Status issues in Indian nursing. Available at: https://archive.nyu.edu/bitstream/2451/34246/2/profession_on_the_margins.pdf. (Accessed: 17 April 2023).

Nazar, M., Kendall, K., Day, L., & Nazar, H. (2015). Decolonising medical curricula through diversity education: Lessons from students. *Medical Teacher, 37,* 385–393.

Nunez, E., Macias, L., Navarro, R., & DeSouza, S. (2019). Historia de la enfermeria chilena: una revision de fuentes. *Ciencia y Enfermeria, 25*(8).

Oleribe, O. O, Suliman, A. A. A., Taylor-Robinson, S. D., & Corrah, T. (2021). Possible reasons why sub-saharan Africa experienced a less severe COVID-19 pandemic in 2020. *Journal of Multidisciplinary Healthcare, 14,* 3267–3271. https://www.ncbi.nlm.nih.gov/pmc/articles/PMC8630399/. (Accessed: 2 July 2023).

Osses-Paredes, C., et al. (2010). Hombres en la enfermería profesional. *Enfermería Global.* Available: http://scielo.isciii.es/scielo.php?script=sci_arttext&pid=S1695-61412010000100016&lng=es&tlng=es . (Accessed: 14 June 2023).

Parry, B. (2002). "Directions and dead ends in postcolonial studies". In Goldberg, D. T., & Quayson, A. (Eds.), *Relocating Postcolonialism* (pp. 66–81). Oxford, UK: Blackwell.

Reeves, S. (2008). The doctor-nurse game in the age of interprofessional care: A view from. *Canada Nursing Inquiry, 15*(1), 1–2.

Sand, R. (1924). Notes on nursing schools in Latin America. *The American Journal of Nursing, 24*(8), 637–639.

Shahjahan, R. A., Estera, A. L., Suria, K. K, & Edwards, K. T. (2022). Decolonising curriculum and pedagogy: A comparative review across disciplines and global higher education contexts. *Review of Educational Research, 92,* 73–113.

Simonetti, M., Soto, P., Galiano, A., Ceron, M. C., Lake, E., & Aike, L. (2020). Hospital work environment, nurse staffing and missed care in Chile: A cross-sectional observational study. *Journal of Clinical Nursing, 31,* 2518–2529.

Smith, P., Allan, H., Henry, L. W., Larsen, J. A, & Mackintosh, M. M. (2006). *Researching Equal Opportunities for Internationally Recruited Nurses and Other Healthcare Workforce: Valuing and Recognising the Talents of a Diverse Healthcare Workforce.* University of Surrey Research Report. Guildford Surrey, England.

Smith, P., & Mackintosh, M. (2007). Profession, market and class: Nurse migration and the remaking of division and disadvantage. *Journal of Clinical Nursing, 16*(12), 2213–2220.

Stein, L. I. (1967). The doctor-nurse game. *Archives of General Psychiatry, 16,* 699–703.

Stein, L. I., Watts, D. T., & Howell, M. D. (1990). Sounding board: The doctor-nurse game revisited. *New England Journal of Medicine, 322*(8), 546–549.

Stilwell, B., Diallo, K., Zurn, P., Vujicic, M., Adams, O., & Dal Poz, M. (2004). Migration of health-care workers from developing countries: strategic approaches to its management. *Bulletin of the World Health Organization, 82*(8), 595–600.

The Cambridge Dictionary (online, no date), Colonize| English meaning, available at: https://dictionary.cambridge.org/dictionary/english/colonize, (Accessed: 30 November 2022).

The Nursing Now Challenge (n.d.) website: https://www.nursingnow.org/ (Accessed: 26 May 2023).

Thomas, C., & Wilkin, P. (2004). Still waiting after all these years: 'The third world' on the periphery of international relations. *The British Journal of Politics and International Relations, 6*, 241–258.

Tickner, A. B. (2013). Core, periphery and (neo)imperialist international relations. *European Journal of International Relations, 19*(3), 627–646.

Tsujita, Y., & Oda, H. (2023). Nursing education, employment and international migration: The case of India in Adhikari, & Plotnikova (Eds.), *Nurse Migration in Asia: Emerging Patterns and Policy Responses*. Routledge. Banbury, England.

University of Chile (n.d.) Historia de escuela de enfermeria. Available: https://medicina.uchile.cl/pregrado/resenas-escuelas/escuela-de-enfermeria. (Accessed: 8 June 2023).

Versluysen, C. M. (1981). Old Wives' Tales? Women Healers in English History. (1981). In Davies, C. (Ed.), *Rewriting Nursing History*. London: Croom Helm.

Wagoro, M. C. A., & Duma, S. E. (2018). Ethics in Nursing – An African Perspective. In: Nortjé, N., De Jongh, J. C., Hoffmann, W. (eds) *African Perspectives on Ethics for Healthcare Professionals. Advancing Global Bioethics*, vol 13. Springer, Cham. https://doi.org/10.1007/978-3-319-93230-9_12.

Wikipedia: Black Lives Matter. https://en.wikipedia.org/wiki/Black_Lives_Matter. (Accessed: 26 February 2024).

Wikipedia: Frantz Fanon. https://en.wikipedia.org/wiki/Frantz_Fanon (Accessed: 31 June 2023).

Winkelmann-Gleed, A. (2006). *Migrant Nurses: Motivation Integration and Contribution*. Radcliffe Publishing Oxford.

World Health Organization. (2020). *State of the world's nursing 2020*. Geneva, Switzerland.

Zappas, M., Walton–Moss, B., Sanchez, J., & Hildebrand, J. A (2021). The decolonisation of nursing education. *The Journal for Nurse Practitioners, 7*(2021), 225–229. Decolonisation of Nurse Education.pdf (Accessed: May 31 2023).

7

THE SAME BUT DIFFERENT— NURSING ROLES IN THE WORLD FOR THE NEXT CENTURY

BARBARA STILWELL ■ SALLY KENDALL

Nurses are found in every health system in the world, at every stage of health care—prevention, diagnosis, treatment, rehabilitation, end-of-life care—and in all places where health care is needed—schools, prisons, community facilities, hospitals and homes. Were it not for nurses, global health systems would collapse (Lancet, 2020). Given their crucial role in providing health care everywhere, it is surprising that nurses do not have a higher profile and status globally, and indeed, in some places, the work of nurses remains almost invisible (All-Party Parliamentary Group on Global Health, 2017). In this chapter, Sally Kendall offers a personal contribution that highlights the role of nurses as a constant in our lives no matter where we live, and in a world of uncertainty and chaos, the ever-present nursing role offers hope. Thinking back over the years of the pandemic, it is not difficult to see the resonance of this, as nurses have sought to find ways to offer physical, emotional and mental comfort to the critically ill, the dying and their relatives, often in the most challenging situations.

THINK BOX 7.1

If you have not yet viewed the series of films made by the BBC for International Council of Nurses (ICN) called *Caring with Courage*, it will be worth doing so now—you can choose a selection of them. You can find them here: https://www.icn.ch/what-we-do/projects/caring-courage.

As you watch them, think about what nurses are doing in different settings around the world.

- What makes them 'nurses'—what are the skills, knowledge and values that link nursing globally?
- Does nursing offer hope?
- Why do you think the series is called *Caring with Courage*?

In this chapter, we will explore nurses' roles worldwide and consider the interplay between the profession's development and the ways that global health has evolved. If you have not yet read Chapter 4 on nursing in emergencies, it would be helpful to read that chapter before this one. This chapter will explore how global health is defined and the potential of the nursing role to be pivotal to global health in the coming decades.

GLOBAL HEALTH

Global health is discussed in the first chapter of this book by Rosa and Mason and in Chapter 2 as it applies to globalisation. Here, the subject is once more raised to apply global health to nursing. A more developmental and historical lens is used to see ways in which the development of thinking in global health has influenced nursing. Rosa and Mason make important points about the Sustainable Development Goals (SDGs) and about planetary health, as do Lewis et al. in Chapter 2. The aim is for you, the readers, to be stimulated by all of these different perspectives about new ways to consider and advocate for the place of nursing practice in today's health landscape.

The term 'global health' is one that is commonly used but not necessarily with a common understanding of what it means. Recent discussion (Malqvist & Powell, 2022) has been useful in raising the issues inherent in using the term 'global health'. A common understanding is key if we are to agree on goals for global health, the approaches we should take, the skills that are needed and the ways that we should use resources (Koplan et al., 2009). The term 'global health' grew out of a blending of public health and international health, which started to happen in the 1940s. There is a fascinating early paper by Dunham (1945, p. 89) which, rather touchingly, begins:

Cooperation in protecting the health of an international public is requisite in a world that has outgrown isolationism. Not only the control of disease, but also improved social and economic relationships can result when people on different sides of the street or different sides of the world work together for health, the most valuable possession of man-'the greatest commodity in the world'.

Dunham was writing about the initial cooperation in the Americas which led to the formation of the Inter-American Cooperative Public Health programme, which later became the Pan-American Health Organization. His account tells the story of how international cooperation began late in the 19th century because of the cross-border spread of infectious diseases. But he goes on to say that the program allows for 'the pooling of our knowledge of public health measures and for the better utilization in all the American Republics of all the public health resources and knowledge available to us' (p. 91). In 1948, the World Health Organization (WHO) was established and essentially grew out of these early initiatives in international public health for the control of diseases.

In recent decades, the concept of global health has gained more attention with, for example, the establishment of the Global Fund for HIV/AIDS, TB and Malaria (The Global Fund, n.d.), founded in 2002; the Global Vaccine Initiative, GAVI (GAVI, n.d.), founded in 2000 and, more lately, the Global Health Workforce Alliance (World Health Organization, n.d.), founded in 2006 and now known as the Health Workforce Network. All of these entities have focused on knowledge sharing, some have channelled funds to specialist programmes in low-resource settings, and indeed, that is one accepted function of global health initiatives. Koplan et al. (2009) suggest that global health refers to the scope of health problems, not only infectious diseases, so this includes issues such as tobacco control, obesity, nutrition and migrant health. But of course, global health does still include those health issues that concern many countries, such as outbreaks—COVID-19 being the latest—and those issues that are relevant

to many countries, such as war (think of the global effects of the war in Ukraine in 2022), climate change, population movement and disease eradication (Koplan et al., 2019; Malqvist & Powell, 2022).

Most recently, there has been important discussion about the nature of partnerships between institutions in high-income countries (HICs) and low- and middle-income countries, which have been the structure of global collaboration for decades. Within the past few years, however, there has been a critical reevaluation of these partnerships and the power balance inherent in them. The consensus is that there is a need for a reexamination of the assumptions and practices underpinning global health partnerships (Finkel et al., 2022). The call to change the structures within which global health currently operates lies behind the global debates on decolonising global health, including nursing.

THINK BOX 7.2

Take a moment to reflect on what you have just read. What do you think about the definitions of global health? How might the way that global health is defined and operationalised affect a nursing role?

This might be a good moment to read Chapter 6 on decolonising nursing and also Chapter 3 on globalisation and its relevance to nursing.

Globalisation is the increasing interconnections between people, economies and societies, and it links inextricably with global health (see Chapter 3 for an in-depth discussion). It is interesting to see from early historical accounts of public and international health that even 150 years ago, there was a concern for illness travelling over borders (Dunham, 1945). Today, travel to another continent takes a matter of hours and facilitates our global connectedness, so we are interdependent in trade, even for daily food supplies. For example, the impact of the war in Ukraine has been felt globally as oil supplies are interrupted, transport and utility prices rise, and food cannot be delivered. The nutritional status of one country may be affected by war in another far away. There is a mutuality between nations that is at the heart of our global health efforts.

The reevaluation of global health has led those of us working in international health to recognise that in HICs, we do not necessarily have the best approaches for low- and middle-income countries. There has been a shift to real partnership in the last decade, with donors more likely to fund programmes implemented by a national programme than by a third-party international nongovernmental organisation acting as an intermediary. Instead of the international partner bringing the expertise from an HIC, there is a pooling of ideas with two-way learning. Malqvist and Powell (2022) argue for inclusion of planetary health in any discussion of global health, and indeed, it is included in this book as Chapter 2. Planetary health links with issues of sustainability, which have become key for human development in terms of environment as well as economics and society more generally.

THINK BOX 7.3

- Have you come across global nursing research?
- What would be a good global nursing research question?

Global partnership models lead to the global sharing of ideas, solutions, research and innovation and to the notion of global thinking but local action, where solutions can be adapted to local needs.

THINKING GLOBALLY, ACTING LOCALLY

The notion of 'thinking globally, acting locally' was first adopted by environmentalists to highlight that all of us should be making environmentally conscious decisions that might have a global impact on everyday life (Mikulska, n.d.). As thinking around global health has evolved, the benefits of mutual learning between countries have been discerned and used. In the Nursing Now campaign and especially through the pandemic, a feature of international webinars was the sharing of learning from different settings (Holloway et al., 2021). These webinars were an example of global thinking in nursing, which is now easy to share because of our global connectedness through technology. Social media offers a way of sharing information quickly and widely, though this raises the issue of false information, too. Finding ways to review information is critical if it is not in peer-reviewed journals, but this process is also facilitated by fast internet searches.

Thinking globally brings opportunities to conduct global health research and to be able to exchange research findings and experiences worldwide. Big data offer us a huge opportunity to explore not only diseases, their management and control but can also offer important insights into how behaviour can be modified to be healthier. Acting locally takes advantage of the scale of internet activity and the smaller handheld devices that allow individuals—even in more remote areas—to access global ideas and evidence. Read also Rosa and Mason in Chapter 1 on thinking locally and acting globally.

Considerations of global health are changing quickly, and as nurses, we have to consider where we are and want to be in this changing landscape. Other chapters in this book have discussed the SDGs, the social determinants of health and what the nursing contribution is to address them. Could nurses be more proactive in working for global health and addressing structural inequities? How would our role change? In the next section, the changing roles of nurses in global health will be explored.

THE CHANGING ROLES OF NURSES IN GLOBAL HEALTH CARE

The history of nursing at the WHO reveals an early interest in training for nurses in poorly resourced countries, but the model at that time, and until the 1960s, was a 'one-size-fits-all' approach in which ideas and approaches developed in well-resourced countries were simply imposed in lower-resourced countries (World Health Organization, 2017). The International Council of Nurses (ICN), founded in 1899, was the world's first and widest reaching international organisation for health professionals, and it worked closely with WHO in its early years to contribute to WHO's policies and activities related to nursing. There is more about ICN's role in Chapter 3 on power and governance in nursing. The first decade of WHO's work saw a nursing expert committee meet four times and give advice to the director-general, but nursing was essentially subsumed under 'auxiliary personnel', and nurses, midwives and other personnel were required because 'the physician by himself cannot cope fully with the health needs of his community' (World Health Organization, 2017, p. 6)

The second meeting of the Expert Committee on Nursing, in October 1951, posed four questions (World Health Organization, 2017):

1. What are the health needs of people and the methods of meeting them?
2. How can nursing help to meet these needs?
3. What principles are involved in planning a programme designed to prepare nursing personnel?
4. How can nursing make its maximum contribution?

In responding to these questions, examples were cited of the work being done by nurses even then: public health nursing in North Borneo, school health in the Amazon Valley, health visitors working with the malaria programme in India and nurses treating tuberculosis in India. All of these examples are described in the report (World Health Organization, 1951, p. 6), and what is fascinating about them is the ways in which nurses have innovated to provide missing pieces of care in their situations. In Chapter 11 in this book, which describes lessons learned from the Nursing Now campaign, there is much on the ways that nurses use innovations to provide care in changing situations: over more than 70 years, nurses continue to show their willingness to meet needs in new ways. This is a thread that runs through nursing, and Wootton and Davidson (2024, this book) discuss the way that nursing practice has been shaped over decades by nurses responding to emergencies.

Nursing and its potential contribution to health care provision came into a much sharper focus when primary health care (PHC) became a worldwide campaign in the 1970s. PHC was defined as 'essential health care based on practical, scientifically sound and socially acceptable methods, and technology made universally accessible to individuals and families in the community through their full participation and at a cost that the community and the country can afford to maintain at every state of their development in the spirits of self-reliance and self-determination' (Alma-Ata, 1978). In developing the PHC movement, the WHO was responding to findings from multi-country studies on the deployment and adequacy of the health workforce. What was found was a serious shortage of health personnel, especially nurses, and in all cases, inadequate training (World Health Organization, 2017).

The PHC approach was, in effect, a redesign of the health workforce. A mix of skills was needed, and there was a recognition that many minor problems encountered in communities could be managed by nurses, and sickness prevention and health promotion would improve community health. This new approach, which ensured better health for millions of people worldwide, relied on the nursing profession and required close collaboration within health care teams. It also highlighted the social determinants of health (though not called that at the time) and encouraged collaboration across sectors such as education and housing. Crucially, the active participation of communities was to be encouraged; they should not be passive recipients of care designed by someone else. In many places, these changing attitudes also led to a redefinition of the roles of doctors and nurses, with a break away from the traditional medical models. Change came gradually, implemented by the many nurses who were in the front line of PHC (World Health Organization, 2017). Later in this chapter, Dr Sally Kendall will discuss the importance of community nursing and the way that it has evolved; community nursing is one example of frontline PHC nursing.

By the 1970s, when PHC emerged, nurses were already developing advanced nursing roles in communities in rural areas of the United States as nurse practitioners, and this trend has continued ever since. Nurse practitioner roles are now common in many places, and in remote areas, nurses can safely provide the only community care available. The nurse practitioner role was based on a person-centred, holistic approach to care with the addition of diagnostic, treatment and management responsibilities previously limited to physicians. In the mid-1970s, Canada and Jamaica followed the United States's development, aiming to improve access to PHC for vulnerable populations in rural, remote and underserved communities. In the 1980s in Botswana, as the country responded to health care reform and population needs of the country spiralled, a family nurse practitioner role was launched. This was followed by the introduction of the nurse practitioner in the United Kingdom in the late 1980s, and the role has grown steadily worldwide.

Lately, the ICN has published guidelines on advanced practice nursing because many opportunities in advanced practice for nurses are emerging globally to meet new and unmet health care needs (International Council for Nurses [ICN], 2020). Both the nurse practitioner role and the clinical nurse specialist role are considered examples of advanced nursing practice roles. Since its beginnings, the focus of the NP has evolved to include general patient populations across the lifespan in PHC as well as to meet the complex needs of acute and critically ill patients. Nurse practitioners are expanding care in many settings—with ageing populations, for example, and for those having end-of-life care. The ICN report notes that the need for nurse practitioners often develops out of population health care needs (International Council for Nurses [ICN], 2020).

THINK BOX 7.4

Imagine you have to design a health workforce to meet population needs in the country where you live.
- What would it look like?
- Would there be more nurses than doctors?
- Would there be advanced nursing practice?
- In what settings?
- What information would you need in order to design the workforce?

The workforce challenges that the WHO identified in the 1970s continue. Nursing shortages remain critical in many countries, driven by international migration which, in turn, is driven by the failure of some governments to provide safe and decent working conditions for their health workforce. (Chapter 9 in this book discusses nurse migration in depth). The quality of training for nurses varies considerably from place to place, as does nursing regulation (World Health Organization, 2020).

In 1954, the WHO Expert Committee on Nursing noted the inadequate status of nursing and/or females and the insufficiency of financial support for nursing services. Nurses 'have been excluded from policy-making bodies…authority has been withheld, and the nurse has not been able, or has not been permitted, to assume the full responsibility of an administrator'. Sadly, this remains the case today; see Chapter 8, in this book, by Newman and Stilwell, for a deeper discussion of the factors that contribute to this. The Nursing Now campaign was formed to improve investment in nursing and is discussed in Chapter 11.

Although global nursing has come a long way in its development, it has not yet reached its full potential. In the next section, the role of nurses today will be explored together with some ideas about how it might—and perhaps should—change in the coming decades.

NURSING TODAY

The 'State of the World's Nursing' (SOWN) report (World Health Organization, 2020) revealed that, globally, there are now 144 distinct titles for nurses, ranging from 10 different titles in the Southeast Asia Region to over 30 in the European and American Regions. This is certainly an issue that concerns health workforce data collection, as counting nurses in the workforce becomes difficult if based on title alone. But it also highlights the challenges of defining and regulating nursing roles and assigning each of them a suitable title. The ICN films referred to at the beginning of this chapter show nurses working in many roles and in many places. Nurses provide health care in every setting—homes, schools and clinics, hospitals, prisons, mobile clinics and pharmacies. Nurses constitute the majority of the health workforce, and they work in every aspect of health care, so people are far more likely to encounter a nurse than any other health worker.

Looking at the history of nursing in the world, it

THINK BOX 7.5
- How is 'nurse' defined in your country?
- Who can use the title?
- Do you think the public understands the different roles that nurses have?

is clear that these many titles could well have derived from the many roles that nurses have, some of which develop from population need and some of which may not be properly regulated (World Health Organization, 2020). In the SOWN report in 2020, recommendations included ensuring that advanced nursing practice could be implemented to its full potential to meet population needs. While this is essential, it is also salutatory that 70 years after the first Expert Committee on Nursing, this recommendation is still necessary.

WHAT NURSES DO IN THE WORLD

The SOWN report (World Health Organization, 2020) described global roles and responsibilities of nurses contributing to SDG 3—that is, promoting good health and well-being for all. SOWN also points out that the nursing role is vital with respect to the WHO's mission 'to promote health, keep the world safe and serve the vulnerable'. The SOWN chapter on nursing roles then goes on to give a synthesis of evidence about nursing roles in global health systems in the 21st century. If you have not read this, then it is certainly worth doing so.

In summary, SOWN found that nurses work wherever health care is available, ranging from providing health information through hospital-based clinical care to care in the home. The ICN films reflect this variety of roles, too. They are likely called *Caring with Courage* because nurses often step up to take on missing pieces of care, even in situations where their safety may be compromised or where they face severe challenges in providing care.

Nursing is an extraordinary profession. Looking at global nursing roles—the ICN films are a great example (International Council for Nurses [ICN], 2022)— it is clear that nursing constantly adapts itself to the context and changing needs of health care and consequent changing demands of health systems. As health care has become more costly, sophisticated and highly technical, nurses have taken on tasks and treatments that were previously the business of medicine—such as managing chronic conditions, running PHC facilities and administering intravenous chemotherapy therapy. Distinguishing between medical diagnoses and nursing diagnoses has been a preoccupation of nurses as their roles have expanded and advanced practice has become commonplace. The roles are seldom without overlap, and there may be a lack of clarity, which may explain why nursing is often seen by the public as an assistant role—they perceive that the job of the nurse is to help the physician (Girvin et al., 2016). A fairly recent international systematic review of public perceptions of nursing found role incongruity among the public; they trusted nurses but did not necessarily respect them and did not understand their work (Girvin, 2016). Rather, the trust seemed to stem from the respect held for the traditional stereotypes of selfless, hardworking females. Nursing is a gendered occupation, with 90% of nurses worldwide being female. In Chapter 8, this is discussed extensively by Newman and Stilwell, who point out that the effects on the nursing profession of the place and self-esteem of females

in society are something that nurses in most countries have in common (World Health Organization, 2020). There are, in many places, outdated societal stereotypes about nurses and nursing that will affect who chooses nursing as a profession and how effective nurses are as leaders.

THINK BOX 7.6

- In your country, are most nurses female?
- Is nursing viewed as a profession for females?
- Why do you think people hold this view?
- What might make them change their view?

It is difficult to find a profession that reinvents itself quite as much as nursing. Yet changes in nursing have tended to happen in an ad hoc way without really having an impact on long-term health system design or formal recognition in legislative frameworks. Research shows (Dawson et al., 2015) that successful expansion of roles requires policy support, training and reward— and yet nurses are often invisible to policymakers (All-Party Parliamentary Group on Global Health, 2017). Is this invisibility to policymakers because nurses find it difficult to explain the value of what they do? Jones and Adynski in Chapter 3, Newman and Stilwell in Chapter 8 and Stilwell in Chapter 11 discuss the rather uneasy relationship of nurses to power and how the Nursing Now campaign offered an opportunity for nurses to be linked globally, share their experiences and lobby their politicians for greater investment in nursing. Global connectedness, mainly on social media, created a social movement which did have power because nursing became visible. Of course, the Nursing Now campaign ran during a pandemic, and the effects and aftershocks of the pandemic cannot be discounted in affecting the profile of nurses. Nevertheless, global connectedness offers nursing another way to draw the attention of policymakers to its value and its place in global health.

There is a new global health landscape emerging. We already know that people are living for longer, often with diseases that require long-term care, and maybe for many years. Those who forecast the future of health care predict a huge growth in virtual care stimulated by the COVID-19 pandemic, when consultations of all kinds had to go online. In February 2021, the use of telehealth in medicine was 38 times higher than prepandemic levels (Bestsennyy et al., 2022). In Chapters 11 and 12 in this book, some possible future scenarios are discussed in relation to where nurses see their future role. One of these scenarios is that care will be anywhere and not confined to health facilities (Khayat, 2019). New technologies make care at home—or indeed, anywhere—possible for more people. Remote patient-monitoring devices, for example, allow providers to monitor patient progress remotely and receive alerts if there are changes. Just-in-time decision-making is, of course, possible, aided by smaller and smaller handheld devices that connect to the internet. Symptoms, including photos, can be sent to a remote provider to assess. The future is most certainly different from the past.

THINK BOX 7.7

- Where do you see yourself as a nurse in future health care scenarios?
- What do you think is likely to be nursing's chief contribution to health care in 50 years' time?

There are amazing opportunities to improve economic prosperity in the future by implementing and using interventions that already exist. Using existing interventions, a 40% reduction in the global disease burden is possible, resulting in a USD $12 trillion boost to the global economy, and the economic return could be USD $2 to USD $4 for each USD $1 invested in better health. A 65-year-old might be as active as a 55-year-old (McKinsey Global Institute, 2020). Addressing the social determinants of health by creating cleaner and safer environments, supporting healthier behaviours and improving access to evidence-based treatments will lead us to this brighter future. For nurses everywhere, the key message is that this future can only be realised with investment in nursing and in the health workforce more generally.

Digital and technological transformations will take us far in expanding care, but we already have the knowledge of interventions that can work to result in a healthier population. Many of these are not the critical care interventions that tend to get the financial investment but are related to a way of life, planetary health and environment, and changing lifestyles. This book deals with global health, and it is no accident that there are chapters on all of these subjects, beginning with

the SDGs. Nurses work with people at every stage of life from birth to death and are already well placed as a trusted profession to lead the way in making better evidence-based care and health-related education available to all, no matter where they live. What is now needed is the investment in nursing that ensures that there are enough nurses in the places they need to be to make this vision a reality (International Council for Nurses [ICN], 2022; World Health Organization, 2021).

FINDING THE COMMON THEMES

Is there such a role as a global nurse? In looking at the history of nursing in the world and at the current proliferation of titles and scopes of practice, it is easy to see that nursing develops in response to where it is being practised and the needs of the people that nurses work with (Stilwell, 2020). But there are commonalities across nursing that are important because it is in these that the unique contribution that nurses can make to health can be found.

The Global Advisory Panel on the Future of Nursing was established by Sigma Theta Tau International to create a vision for the future of nursing and midwifery that will advance global health (Wilson et al., 2016). The panel defined global nursing as 'the use of evidence-based nursing processes to promote sustainable planetary health and equity for all people. Global nursing considers social determinants of health, includes individual and population-level care, research, education, leadership, advocacy and policy initiatives. Global nurses engage in ethical practice and demonstrate respect for human dignity, human rights and cultural diversity. Global nurses engage in a spirit of deliberation and reflection in interdependent partnership with communities and other healthcare providers' (Wilson et al., 2016, p. 9). (The definition is also in Chapter 1 of this book, related to SDGs.) This definition was based on themes in global nursing that were identified through an extensive literature review (Wilson et al., 2016, p. 6). Significant examples of these themes that relate to this book and especially to this chapter are:

- **Interdependence**
  This refers to the need to see people in their own context. It also addresses the requirement for systems thinking in nursing, which has always been used, though seldom named as such. Chapter 1

on the SDGs focuses on the need to consider the social determinants of health and essentially health as a 'big picture' that includes the environment, climate, social surroundings such as housing and community contacts, education and family. These are the systems in which people function, and overlaid on them is the health system in which the nurse is working—and that is another set of complex systems that will include referral pathways, care opportunities and funding mechanisms for health care. For nurses in any context, this points to the complexity of care. In a global context, the complexity is even deeper.

■ **Collaboration**
In a global nursing context, this refers to the role of nurses forging global partnerships. In Chapter 11 in this book, there is reference to the role of bridging between nurses and policymakers for nursing to become more influential. This is a critical role for global nurse leaders.

■ **Glocal**
This refers to nursing being able to take global ideas and evidence and adapt them to the local context—as well as taking what is local knowledge and use it globally. For example, the impact of natural disasters is felt most locally, and the lessons learned from the implementation and results of interventions after disasters can be of great global value.

■ **Advocacy**
Chapter 10 in this book discusses advocacy at length. In the context it is used here, it describes what nurses do as mediators between clients and the health system and also between client care and global evidence. One example might be the use of antibiotics. Evidence shows that they are overused, and this will lead to resistance to their effects. In practice, do nurses note their overuse? How do nurses help clients expecting antibiotics when they are perhaps not indicated? What is the nurse's role here as an advocate for their client?

■ **Caring**
Caring is a skilled part of nursing, central to its practice, and it refers to the ways that the nurse promotes an environment for healing within a relationship that allows full participation of the client and their family (Stilwell, 2020).

■ **Cultural competence**
With the ever-growing movement of people between countries, the practice of cultural competence has become ever more important in health care. It refers to the ability to be able to address social determinants of health with cultural humility and respect for diversity. Chapter 6 looks at decolonising nursing and why this is important.

■ **Sustainable**
This theme has emerged as a major theme in a concept analysis of the relevance of globalisation to nurses (Wilson, 2016; World Health Organization, 2021; also Chapters 1 and 2 in this book). It is not only the sustainability of the planet and ecosystem that is important but also of the nursing profession.

THINK BOX 7.8

Can you provide an example of each of the earlier themes from your own nursing practice?

THRIVING FOR ALL

Beyond the themes identified (Wilson et al., 2016), there is a growing preoccupation with thriving beyond recovery from illness and what this means for nursing (Crisp, 2020). Thriving is even more than being healthy; it is about flourishing as an individual, a member of a family and a community. We often use the word 'thriving' in relation to children, usually relating to physical development, but it can also mean that they are not reaching their potential in other ways, too.

This applies to all of us. In our daily lives, we want to be able to function fully and contribute as members of society. For nurses to have 'thrive' as a goal of care may mean stepping outside of what might be considered nursing boundaries—or perhaps extending them might be a better description.

Helping people to thrive means understanding the social determinants of their health—what helps them and what does not. This is always apparent in community nursing when nurses visit people in their homes and can see first hand if there is damp on the walls, if the home is warm and if there are health hazards in or around it. But nurses can and do go further by forming community groups or working among people who may not be in touch with the health system at all. Crisp (2020) tells the story of a nurse in London, United Kingdom, who works with parents and young people affected by drug-related crime. This nurse is originally from Zimbabwe and brings her experience from there to help in her work in London. She works in the neighbourhoods, seeking to understand the complex situations of gang boundaries and the impact on young people, as well as their relationships with school and with their cultural identities (Crisp, 2020, pp. 48–49). This is hugely complex work and mostly takes place outside of any health institution or place where nurses usually would provide care.

Thriving may be an unseen or unacknowledged goal of nursing care, but it underpins much of what nurses study. In the next section, a case study by Professor Sally Kendall brings greater clarity to why nursing is a therapy for an uncertain world.

THINK BOX 7.9

- Do you help people to thrive in your nursing practice?
- Are there ways you could improve this practice?

CASE STUDIES ON COMMUNITY NURSING

In a world where global change has had such a massive impact on the health, economics, resources and disasters across our regions and populations, it can seem as though chaos and uncertainty are the dominant constructs of our societies. Chaos and uncertainty leave us feeling as though life is unpredictable and out of our control, our governments don't do enough and we can't do enough for ourselves to stop pandemics, climate change, war and terrorism. Global organisations such as the WHO provide some structure and policy direction for countries through the SDGs, but even that can seem overwhelming and distant from individuals and communities, such as the people of Pakistan who, right now in 2022, suffer unimaginably from the effects of flooding that will continue for years ahead. In such times, it is important to remember what is constant in our lives. What can sustain life and hope when chaos predominates? In this chapter, I want to propose that nurses and nursing are global constants and that no matter what names we use and what educational provision or regulatory bodies are in place, nurses have

a place in the world that can and does make a difference to health, life and hope of our populations. Other authors have discussed specific aspects of global nursing; my interest and contribution are how community nursing and community nursing research can be constant and sustaining.

In my work as an academic nurse and health visitor, I have always endeavoured to stay close to practice; what happens in the everyday lives of individuals, families, communities, my students and the wider population nationally and internationally is important. For community nursing to be sustaining and for research to be meaningful, this is essential. The nurse in the community has both the privilege and the ability to hear, understand and respond to the needs of the community, and this is key to the global constancy that community nurses can offer, which is most effective when nurses can both make good use and generate evidence that supports and underpins practice. In 2006, Bryar and Kendall presented the debate and global challenge that community nursing faced in developing the evidence for practice and raising the quality of community nursing through a series of research studies conducted at that time. In the decades that have followed, there have been changes in how community health and nursing research are regarded internationally; as Mathieson et al. (2019)'s review reveals, there is a range of high-quality evidence of community nursing research available, but the greatest challenge is to find organisational and sustainable ways to implement it into everyday health care. Most recently in the United Kingdom, a priority-setting exercise conducted by the James Lind Alliance in collaboration with the public and the profession has nominated 20 priorities for community nursing research. The top priority is this research question:

How can community nurse teams better meet the complex needs of patients with multiple health conditions?

This illustrates, I believe, a global need that community nurses worldwide are addressing through their research which is best illustrated by some selected case studies drawn from my work as part of the International Collaboration for Community Health Nursing Research.

THINK BOX 7.10

- What do you know about what community nurses do?
- Is it a recognised speciality in your country?

CASE STUDY 7.1

ANNE SKOGLUND, NORWAY

Anne is a nurse in Norway who has a particular interest in the mental health and well-being of young people, in particular, those currently studying at university. This is a specific population that may be regarded as elite and privileged but where, nonetheless, there is a worrying increase in mental health problems and rising suicide rates. Anne's work is to support the student population in Norway and use her research to promote their mental health and well-being (Box 7.1).

CASE STUDY 7.2

ELLEN NKUMBULE, MALAWI

Ellen is a registered nurse in Malawi, currently working in Kamuzu College and undertaking research with people in the community with chronic conditions. In her recent research with people with insulin-dependent diabetes, she demonstrates the importance of uncovering the challenges that people face when they confront the complexity of a chronic condition such as diabetes alongside their daily lives in a challenging rural community, where it is estimated that 71% of Malawi people live in extreme poverty (Box 7.2).

CASE STUDY 7.3

BRENDA POKU, GHANA

Brenda is a registered nurse in Ghana with experience in neonatal care, currently working as an academic in the United Kingdom. She undertook her PhD in the United Kingdom with a focus on the experience of SCD amongst adolescents in Ghana. SCD is a chronic, hereditary illness that has a high incidence and prevalence amongst people of African descent, 25% in Ghana. Brenda's research focuses on the effect of fatigue on children and young people as a result of SCD (Box 7.3).

BOX 7.1
PERCEPTION OF STUDENT LIFE AS PROMOTING MENTAL HEALTH AND WELL-BEING: A STUDY OF FIRST-YEAR STUDENTS IN A NORWEGIAN UNIVERSITY

Through a series of qualitative studies in which students were interviewed in depth, Anne found that:

Support is regarded as important to mental health, and to promote mental health, creating supportive environments is crucial. An inclusive and supportive environment can help students in the *process of finding themselves*. A supportive environment can be created or found in family and peers, financially and psychologically. It can also be found in university staff and how the study programs are organised and in housing arrangements. Conclusively, it will be useful have a broad perspective on where and how students may find support.

During lockdown, the students' need for a sense of belonging and a sense of support became clearer. They also needed to be more thorough in recognising what their needs were, as accessibility to social networks were limited. They also had to be more active in creating a social network. The everyday routines with lecturers and a premade time schedule were diminished, which also gave them an opportunity to reflect on own needs regarding working habits and the need for routines in everyday life as a student. Although lockdown was difficult for many students, it was also an opportunity to accelerate the process of 'finding myself.'

Skoglund, A., Batt-Rawden, K. B., Schröder, A., & Moen, O. L. (2021). Perception of student life as promoting mental health and well-being: A study of first-year students in a Norwegian university. *International Journal of Mental Health Promotion, 23*(4), 487-497. http://dx.doi.org/10.32604/IJMHP.2021.016199.

What these three case studies of research in community nursing illustrate is the global recognition by nurses of the complex health needs experienced in communities that face health challenges and the significant part nursing research can play in highlighting and raising awareness of needs and also in developing evidence-based interventions that can make a difference. These nurses have each made a contribution to the global understanding of health challenges in their ability to hear and understand their communities through research. This is more widely available through their publications and collectively provides strength-based and developing evidence for the value of community nursing, the impact nurses can make

BOX 7.2
ASSESSING KNOWLEDGE AND SELF-MANAGEMENT PRACTICES OF RURAL-BASED PATIENTS WITH DIABETES WHO WERE TREATED WITH INSULIN IN LILONGWE, MALAWI: A PILOT STUDY

The key objective was to strengthen self-management practices among rural-based insulin-treated patients with diabetes.

Following a preintervention amongst people living with insulin-dependent diabetes, the study found that the majority of those surveyed were suffering complications and hospital episodes due to complications of diabetes and missed insulin medication, a lack of information about their condition, misinformation about insulin administration, medication missed due to lack of stock, dietary problems due to lack of food and difficulty with clinic compliance due to lack of transport.

These challenges demonstrate the complexity that is not purely a behavioural issue to be solved. Ellen and her team therefore implemented some interventions to directly support the community, which include:

Focused patient/family teaching and provision of visual-aided information brochures

Provision of resources for self-monitoring of blood glucose levels such as glucometers, blood glucose test strips and lancets

Food and nutritional empowerment through provision of two bags of fertiliser and seed starter packs per participants

Provision of insulin and insulin syringes

Whilst the implementation evaluation phase is still underway, the expected patient outcomes include adherence to all self-management practices, improved glycaemic control and better quality of life.

Ellen and her team (Nkumbule et al., 2021, p. 28) conclude: 'We have found that living with insulin-treated diabetes in rural Malawi is a complex and multifaceted experience; often characterised by enormous challenges. There is a need for multi-factorial approaches at both the community and system levels to improve the livelihoods of people living with insulin-treated diabetes in rural areas'.

Nkambule E., Msosa A., Wella K., Msiska G. (2021).

BOX 7.3
'IT'S LIKE A CAR WITH NO FUEL, IT WON'T MOVE...' FATIGUE EXPERIENCES OF ADOLESCENTS WITH SICKLE CELL DISEASE IN GHANA: A GROUNDED THEORY INQUIRY

The aim of the study was to explore how adolescents with sickle cell disease (SCD) experience and manage living with fatigue in an African context and construct a theory that explains their experiences of fatigue.

Brenda undertook 24 in-depth interviews with young people in Ghana suffering with SCD. Through a process of qualitative analysis using grounded theory, she proposes a conceptual framework where adolescents see their bodies as machines, constructing their fatigue as a car without fuel.

Fatigue was described as a chronic, constant phenomenon of daily life with sickle cell anaemia and recognised as a complex phenomenon that could be influenced by a range of factors: physical activities, pain medication, sickle cell pains, environmental factors, emotions and early school start time. Fatigue impacts the adolescents' overall development, experiences of painful crises and ability to have fulfilling lives.

Brenda's research concludes that there is an urgent need for development and advancement of community health nursing roles in Ghana and Africa to support children with SCD and other chronic conditions Poku et al. (2020).

health and its transformation through PHC and then moved to look at possible futures and its relevance to our world today using community nursing as a case study.

What will a nurse training in 2070 be learning? Will there be a 'global nurse' role? There can be no certainty to these answers, but if we look back to the middle of the last century (1950), the changes we have seen since then could not have been imagined—making real-time calls to someone else with pictures, for example, or holding a search engine to knowledge in our hand. There may be a similar revolution 50 years hence. A young nurse who was asked what he thought would be an innovation in 50 years that would be transformative said he imagined being able to think about an internet search and it would happen and be visible on a nearby wall (Stilwell, 2021). It sounds like science fiction, but in 1950, so did mobile phones.

As nurses, we need to grasp the possibilities and start to think about what we want our role to be. A Google search on 'the vision of nursing for the future'

and the constancy of nursing practice in a changing world.

Looking Ahead

This chapter has taken an exploratory journey through the history of global nursing, its relationship to global yielded 117 million hits—yes, 117 million. Clearly, many people are interested in the future of nursing and sharing their views. The future of global nursing should surely be shaped by those of us practising as nurses now. The use of technology in medicine almost certainly will have transformed treatments and life expectancy. Genetically based diagnoses will surely be commonplace and may be predicative, too. Will climate change be under control or remain a serious threat to health? Will food supplies be secure, and will nutrition needs be met?

Whatever the future holds, it is likely that nurses will remain the largest proportion of the health workforce and will retain a critical role in caring for those who are sick, preventing illness, promoting health and ensuring that individuals, families and communities can thrive. In 2021, ICN published their Vision for Future Health Care toolkit in their series, Nurses: A Voice to Lead (International Council for Nurses [ICN], 2021, p. 34). It says this:

> *Moving forward into the future, it is our hope that the awakening of a widespread consciousness of the work of nurses is positively represented in the media, the public and institutions…In addition, nurses must be respected for their wisdom, knowledge and insight into matters of health. Ongoing discourse between nurses and the public will be required for the promotion of new ways of delivering healthcare and improving health outcomes.*

We pick up ICN's vision for the future of nursing in the final chapter of this book. Before you read it, consider how you can be part of shaping nursing's future where you are.

REFERENCES

All-Party Parliamentary Group on Global Health. (2016). Triple impact: How developing nursing will improve health, promote gender equality and support economic growth. *APPG on Global Health*. http://www.appg-globalhealth.org.uk/reports/4556656050.

Bestsennyy, O., Chmielewski, M., Koffel, A., & Shah, A. (2022). *From facility to home: How healthcare could shift by 2025*. McKinsey and Company. Health Care Systems and Services. Retrieved, December 2022, from https://www.mckinsey.com/industries/healthcare-systems-and-services/how-we-help-clients.

Bryar, R., & Kendall, S. (2006). New challenges and innovations in community health nursing. *Primary Health Care Research & Development, 7*(4), 279–280. doi:10.1017/S1463423606000363.

Crisp, N. (2020). *Health is made at home. Hospitals are for repairs*. Salus.

Dawson, A. J., Nkowane, A. M., & Whelan, A. (2015). Approaches to improving the contribution of the nursing and midwifery workforce. to increasing universal access to primary health care for vulnerable populations: A systematic review. *Human Resources for Health*. Retrieved, December 2022, from https://human-resources-health.biomedcentral.com/articles/10.1186/s12960-015-0096-1.

Dunham, G. C. (1945). Today's global Frontiers in public health: I. A pattern for cooperative public health. *American Journal of Public Health and the Nation's Health, 35*(2), 89–95.

Finkel, M. L., Temmermann, M., Suleman, F., Barry, M., Salm, M., Binagwaho, A., & Kilmarx, P. H. (2022). What do global health practitioners think about decolonizing global health? *Annals of Global Health, 88*(1), 61. http://doi.org/10.5334/aogh.3714.

GAVI. (n.d.). GAVI: The vaccine alliance. https://www.gavi.org/

Girvin, J., Jackson, D., & Hutchinson, M. (2016). Contemporary public perceptions of nursing: A systematic review and narrative synthesis of the international research evidence. *Journal of Nursing Management, 24*(8), 994–1006. https://www.ncbi.nlm.nih.gov/pubmed/27406529.

The Global Fund. (n.d.). *About the global fund*. https://www.theglobalfund.org/en/about-the-global-fund/

Holloway, A., Thomson, A., Stilwell, B., Finch, H., Irwin, K., & Crisp, N. (2021). *"Agents of change: The story of the Nursing Now campaign" Nursing Now/Burdett Trust for Nursing*. Retrieved, November 2022, from https://www.nursingnow.org/wp-content/uploads/2021/05/Nursing-Now-Final-Report.pdf.

International Council for Nurses (ICN) (2021). Nurses: A voice to lead. A vision for future health care. *International Nurses' Day 2021 Resources and Evidence*. ICN Geneva. Retrieved, December 2022, from https://www.icn.ch/system/files/documents/2021-05/ICN%20Toolkit_2021_ENG_Final.pdf.

International Council for Nurses (ICN). (2022). Film series with the BBC. *Caring with Courage*. Retrieved, December 2022, from https://www.icn.ch/what-we-do/projects/caring-courage.

James Lind Alliance. (2021). *Community nursing top 10*. Retrieved, December 2022, from https://www.jla.nihr.ac.uk/priority-setting-partnerships/community-nursing/community-nursing-top-10-priorities.htm.

Khayat, Z. (2019). Sense making conversations: The future of our healthcare. *Video*. https://www.youtube.com/watch?v=QzEzGdq-_tk. Last accessed February 2024.

Koplan, J. P., Bond, T. C., Merson, M. H., Reddy, K. S., Rodriguez, M. H., Sewankambo, N. K., & Wasserheit, J. N. (2009). Consortium of Universities for Global Health Executive Board. Towards a common definition of global health. *Lancet, 373*(9679), 1993–1995.

Lancet Editorial. (2020). The status of nursing and midwifery in the world. Retrieved, February 2024. doi:10.1016/S0140-6736(20)30821-7. Last accessed February 2024.

Malqvist, M., & Powell, N. (2022). Health, sustainability and transformation: A new narrative for global health. *British Medical Journal global health, 7*, e010969. doi:10.1136/bmjgh-2022-010969.

Mathieson, A., Grande, G., & Luker, K. (2019). Strategies, facilitators and barriers to implementation of evidence-based practice in community nursing: A systematic mixed-studies review and qualitative synthesis. *Primary Health Care Research & Development, 20*, E6. doi:10.1017/S1463423618000488.

McKinsey Global Institute. (2020). *Prioritizing health. A prescription for prosperity.* Retrieved, December 2022, https://www.mckinsey.com/~/media/McKinsey/Industries/Public%20and%20Social%20Sector/Our%20Insights/Prioritizing%20health%20A%20prescription%20for%20prosperity/MGI_Prioritizing%20Health_Executive%20summary_July%202020.pdf.

Mikulska, A. (n.d.). *Think globally act locally think globally again. Ideas #8.* Risk Management and Decision Processes Center. Wharton. U. Penn. Retrieved, December 2022, https://riskcenter.wharton.upenn.edu/climate-risk-solutions-2/think-globally-act-locally-think-globally-again/.

Nkambule, E., Msosa, A., Wella, K., & Msiska, G. (2021). This disease would suit better those who have money: Insulin-treated diabetes illness experience in rural Malawi. *Malawi Medical Journal, 33* (Postgraduate Supplementary Iss), 16–22. doi:10.4314/mmj.v33iS.4.

Poku, A., Caress, A-L., & Kirk, S. (2020). "'Body as a machine': How adolescents with sickle cell disease construct their fatigue experiences." *Qualitative Health Research, 30*(9), 1431–1444. doi:10.1177/1049732320916464.

Skoglund, A., Batt-Rawden, K. B., Schröder, A., & Moen, O. L. (2021). Perception of student life as promoting mental health and well-being: A study of first-year students in a Norwegian University. *International Journal of Mental Health Promotion, 23*(4), 487–497.

Stilwell, B. (2020). *Changing the narrative of nursing in nurses: A voice to lead.* Nursing the World to Health; International Council of Nurses. Retrieved, December 2022,. https://www.icn.ch/system/files/2021-07/IND_2020_FINAL_Eng.pdf.

Stilwell, B. (2021). *Personal communication during the Nursing Now campaign.*

Wilson, L., Mendes, I. A., Klopper, H., Catrambone, C., Al-Maaitah, R., Norton, M. E., & Hill, M. (2016). "Global health" and "global nursing": Proposed definitions from the Global Advisory Panel on the future of nursing. *Journal of Advanced Nursing, 72*(7), 1529–1540.

World Health Organization. (n.d.). *Global health workforce network.* https://www.who.int/teams/health-workforce/network

World Health Organization. (1951). World Health Organization Expert Committee on Nursing: Second report. World Health Organization (World Health Organization Technical Report Series, No. 49).

World Health Organization. (1978). *Alma-Ata 1978: Primary health care.* World Health Organization ("Health for All" Series, No. 1).

World Health Organization. (2017). *Nursing and midwifery in the history of the World Health Organization 1948–2017.* Retrieved, December 2022, https://www.who.int/publications/i/item/nursing-and-midwifery-in-the-history-of-the-world-health-organization-(1948%E2%80%932017).

World Health Organization. (2020). *State of the world's nursing 2020.* World Health Organization. https://www.who.int/publications/i/item/9789240003279. Last accessed February 2024.

World Health Organization. (2021). *Global strategic directions for nursing and midwifery 2021–2025.* World Health Organization. https://www.who.int/publications/i/item/9789240033863. Last accessed February 2024.

8

GENDER, NURSING AND GLOBAL HEALTH: WHY DOES GENDER MATTER?

CONSTANCE NEWMAN ■ BARBARA STILWELL

INTRODUCTION AND BACKGROUND

In this chapter, we offer perspectives backed by evidence and theory to better understand the important relationships between gender, nursing and global health.

We will not discuss these perspectives in great detail, as that is far beyond the scope of this chapter, but some theoretical background will be helpful to explain why gender matters to nursing and global health. We aim to answer what we see as the central questions, which are: Which theories and perspectives contribute to understanding a gendered occupation like nursing in a gender-segregated sector like health, with its particular leadership challenges, gender bias and discrimination, inequities in pay and other material conditions under which nurses work? What are the implications for the nursing profession? And how can gender analysis be used to address inequalities in nurse education, development, policy and practice?

THINK BOX 8.1

Of the global nursing workforce, what percentage of nurses are women? Check https://www.who.int/publications/i/item/9789240003279.

- In your country, what percentage of nurses are women?
- What percentage of nurse managers are women?
  Here is a link to global evidence: Delivered by women, led by men: A gender and equity analysis of the global health and social workforce (https://www.who.int/publications/i/item/9789241515467).

- What percentage of health sector managers (e.g. director of a hospital or a department at the ministry of health) in your country or region are women?
- Do you know where to find this information?
  You should be able to find it on the national health workforce database, though it is not consistently collected.

THE SCOPE OF THIS CHAPTER

Gender refers to a complex social system that structures the life experience of all human beings. There are relationships between gender inequality as well as expectations based on gender norms that restrict our roles in society and affect health, well-being, health care delivery and the health workforce (Heise et al., 2019). Individuals born biologically male or female develop into gendered beings whose gender may or may not align with their biological sex. Sexism and patriarchy may intersect with other forms of discrimination, such as racism and homophobia, to influence all kinds of pathways such as careers, health journeys and societal acceptance. Health system actors such as policymakers, service managers and health care providers are not trained to use a 'gender lens' to understand the environments of health care delivery and thus may neglect gender inequalities in health (Hay et al., 2019). Gender has been essential in understanding the experiences of health workers during COVID-19 because it illuminates ingrained inequalities and gendered organisational structures and norms (for example, personal protective equipment was sized for males) (Regenold & Vindrola-Padros, 2021).

NURSING IS A GENDERED PROFESSION

A noted gender theorist (Connell, 2014) wrote that 'global power relations have changed; the old empires have gone, and new formations of power have appeared. It is now necessary to understand gender in the era of transnational corporations, the internet and global neoliberal politics. This requires gender analysis to move beyond states and even regions into "global space"'. Of the 500 largest transnational corporations as of 2012, only just 2.6% had women as chief executives; that is, 97.4% had men. This mirrors the health sector, where globally female workers make up 70% of the health workforce but occupy only 25% of senior management positions (World Health Organization, Global Health Workforce Network and Women in Global Health, 2019). A large majority of those global health workers are nurses and midwives, and globally 90% of nurses are women (World Health Organization, 2020) working at the front lines fighting COVID, HIV/AIDS, tuberculosis, maternal mortality, violence against women and harmful traditional practices—though they are usually not visible in strategic and policy leadership, nor provided with decent working conditions, including protection from occupational hazards (Women in Global Health, 2021).

Evidence from literature scans and global and country studies (Newman et al., 2019; World Health Organization, Global Health Workforce Network and Women in Global Health, 2019) demonstrates that female health workers, including nurses, face particular types of gender bias and discrimination. Nursing as a gendered profession *par excellence* is riddled with stereotypes of femininity that constrain nurses' perceived value and their influence in policymaking arenas such as parliaments and ministries of health (Stilwell & Newman, 2022). Nurses and those developing nursing policy need gender-analytical competencies, alongside leadership and clinical competencies, to identify gender bias, discrimination and the unequal gender power relations that constrain their leadership and limit the influence that nurses can have on shaping the health sector. To begin to address these issues, this chapter will:

■ Discuss and explain gender concepts, theories and perspectives that are relevant to gender structures in global health.

■ Describe the gender segregation of health occupations, of which nursing is a stark example, and consider gender bias, stereotypes and other discriminations that are particularly relevant to nursing.

■ Give an overview of evidence from national and global workforce studies, including a recent global study on nursing leadership, that demonstrate common gender dynamics and their effects on the health workforce.

■ Explore the implications for nursing policy and action.

LIMITATIONS

It is important at the outset to acknowledge some limitations of this chapter. First, because of space constraints, we did not discuss the cross-cultural portability of gender theories.

Second, while we have conducted gender analyses in family planning, reproductive health and HIV service delivery as well as workforce programs in various parts of the globe (USAID, 2011), there has been less focus (by us and others) on collecting data on *sexual and gender minorities* (i.e., LGBT). There are comparatively few large sample surveys or analyses of service quality and access data regarding those who do not identify exclusively as a man or a woman or whose sexual preferences are not exclusively heterosexual. This may be a result of donor and country priorities and inconsistency in category definitions. In addition, most evidence and sociological discussion come from European countries, the United Kingdom or the Americas and cannot be expected to reflect the realities of most societies in the majority of the world. Two exceptions of methodological robustness include a recent population-based study which estimated that 1.4 million adults (0.6% of adults) in the United States identified as transgender (Herman et al., 2022; GLAAD, 2016), and a large-sample Gallup survey conducted in the United States from 2021 that found that 86.7% of Americans identified as heterosexual ('straight') and 5.6% of US adults identified as LGBT, and within that, 3.1% identified as bisexual, 1.4% as gay, 0.7% as lesbian and 0.6% as transgender (Jones, 2021). We recognise the limitations and join the call for better global and country evidence (Colaco & Watson-Grant, 2018). We consider clinical and cultural competence in care to be vital for all health work, so we present the evidence as we know it and encourage readers to reflect on how and if it applies to where you work and how questioning and challenging traditional or hidden assumptions about gender and sexuality could improve quality and reduce harm in health care (Iantaffi, 2020).

FROM CONCEPTS TO THEORY-BASED PERSPECTIVES

Concepts

Concepts of sex and gender are described in many global consensus and national advocacy documents. The United Nations (UN)'s Convention on the Elimination of All Forms of Discrimination Against Women (United Nations, 1979) is one of the core international human rights treaties of the UN and requires member states to undertake legal obligations to respect, protect and fulfil human rights for all women. CEDAW was adopted by the UN General Assembly and came into force as a treaty in 1981. Today, it is one of the most broadly endorsed human rights treaties—having been ratified or acceded to by 187 countries, or about 90% of UN membership. CEDAW defines 'discrimination against women' as 'any distinction, exclusion or restriction made on the basis of sex* which has the effect or purpose of impairing or nullifying the recognition, enjoyment or exercise by women, irrespective of their marital status, on a basis of equality of men and women, of human rights and fundamental freedoms in the political, economic, social, cultural, civil or any other field'. This definition includes not just direct or intentional discrimination but any act that has the effect of creating or perpetuating inequality between men and women.

The following decades of development for women, and then gender, saw a shift in focus to relations between women and men, with expanded definitions and distinctions between gender and sex.

---

*Sex is the classification of people as male or female. Sex is determined at conception. At birth, an infant's sex is established based on a combination of bodily characteristics, including chromosomes, hormones, internal reproductive organs, genitalia and secondary sex characteristics. Sex refers to the biological and physiological reality of being male or female.

THINK BOX 8.2

DISTINCTION BETWEEN GENDER AND SEX
UN Women offers this definition of gender (UN Women Training Center eLearning Campus, n.d.):

Gender refers to the roles, behaviours, activities, and attributes that a given society at a given time considers appropriate for men and women. In addition to the social attributes and opportunities associated with being male and female and the relationships between women and men and girls and boys, gender also refers to the relations between women and those between men. These attributes, opportunities and relationships are socially constructed and are learned through socialisation processes. They are context/time-specific and changeable...Gender determines what is expected, allowed and valued in a woman or a man in a given context. In most societies there are differences and inequalities between women and men *in responsibilities assigned, activities undertaken, access to and control over resources, as well as decision-making opportunities. Gender is part of the broader socio-cultural context, as are other important criteria for socio-cultural analysis including class, race, poverty level, ethnic group, sexual orientation, age, etc.*

Sex (biological sex) is defined as 'the physical and biological characteristics that distinguish males and females'.

What do you think about the distinction between sex being biological/physiological and gender being socially constructed? Is it helpful? Do you think this distinction is commonly understood by people where you live?

A consensus has evolved over the years among global development organisations such as UNICEF (2017), UNFPA (2005) and the World Health Organization (n.d.) regarding definitions. It is now commonly accepted that sex refers to biological and physiological characteristics of males, females and intersex persons, such as chromosomes, hormones and reproductive organs (World Health Organization, n.d.), while gender refers to culturally or socially constructed roles, responsibilities, attributes, behaviours and activities associated with men and women, girls and boys, masculinity and femininity, and males and females, which involves inequalities and discrepancies in opportunities and access and control of resources and decision-making resulting from unequal relations. In many cultures, there are hierarchies in gender relations, and we discuss the effects of hierarchies later in the chapter.

USAID (2021) guidance highlights the importance of analysing gender relations through gender analysis, a social science tool employed to identify, understand and explain gaps between males and females that exist in households, communities and countries and identify the relevance of gender norms and power relations in a specific context (e.g. country, geographic, cultural, institutional, economic). Gender analysis typically looks at:

- Differences in the status of women and men and their differential access to assets, resources, opportunities and services.
- The influence of gender roles and norms on the division of time between paid employment, unpaid work (including subsistence production and care for family members) and volunteer activities.
- The influence of gender roles and norms on leadership roles and decision-making.
- Constraints, opportunities and entry points for narrowing gender gaps and empowering females.
- Potential difference in impacts of development policies and programs on males and females, including unintended or negative consequences (USAID, 2021).

THINK BOX 8.3

- What do you think of the idea of gender relations?
- How can a gender analysis help nurses understand inequalities within their profession or between professions in the health sector?
- How can gender analysis help health managers understand why clients are not able to access health services?

There are multiple social identities and experiences of social marginalisation based on social characteristics such as gender, race or ethnicity, class or caste, and social position that *intersect to* create compounded privilege or disadvantage for people (Hay et al., 2019; World Health Organization, n.d.). This means that gender analyses must explore power and hierarchy in health systems to show ways that make some people more likely to benefit

and be supported and advanced, while others are more likely to be marginalised, excluded or disempowered based on social positioning in health systems.

THEORIES

We believe that relational, structural–materialist approaches drawing from the social sciences have the greatest analytical and explanatory value for gender and nursing in global health, especially its occupational structure and the social–material conditions under which nurses work (Jackson, 2001, 2005). In this part of the chapter, we propose to unpack and explain these theories and discuss why it is important for nurses to understand them.

Based on the definitions given, relational approaches to theorising gender and health make sense. Ridgeway and Correll (2004) defined gender as a *system of social relations* of greater or lesser status and advantage, with cultural beliefs and distributions of resources at three different levels. First is at the levels of organisations (such as a health facility) and societal patterns of behaviour (in the community served by a health facility, for example). Second are the organizational practices at the level where one organisation interacts with another (for example, a hospital and community services, or a ministry and a large hospital), and third is the individual level with perceptions of self and identity. A key feature of gender status and advantage in social relationships is, for example, are women seen as having less authority than men? Or are men assumed to be the 'head of the household'? All these assumptions reflect gender status at individual and societal levels, and gender status may then be carried over into organisational practices.

According to Ridgeway (2006), sex categorisation, the routine social cognitive processes of labelling others as male or female, provides a social framework that organises relations between people based on assumptions of what men and women should do and how they should behave. For example, a common assumption might be that women's priority should be childbearing and men's priority should be paid work, which affects gendered perceptions of sexuality, rights, occupation and behaviour.

A gender system underpins cultural beliefs by which we classify people as male or female, as well as explain to society, and us as individuals, the different behaviours and greater power and privilege ascribed to these categories (Ridgeway & Correll, 2004). As a result, both men and women have deep interest in maintaining a clear and reasonably stable framework of gender beliefs that define 'who' men and women 'are' by differentiating them (Ridgeway, 2006). This is a point to remember, as it implies that gender systems are deeply embedded in social relations, and that people will resist disruptions to the society's basic system of sex labelling that underpins the gender system.

Relational theory is the approach that gives a central place to the patterned relations between women and men (and among women and among men) that constitute gender as a social structure (Connell, 2012). The concept of social structure refers to the large-scale patterns that exist across societal gender orders, such as 'the contrast between masculinity and femininity, the gender division of labour in the home' (Connell, 2012, p. 1677), and which include patterns of everyday social practices in which gender is *enacted* in housework, paid labour, childrearing, sexuality, etc., all of which 'occur in a dense and active social tissue of institutions and sites, such as families, companies, governments and neighbourhoods' (Connell, 2012, p. 1677).

Gender analyses specify how a society handles sexuality, reproduction, child growth, motherhood, fatherhood and all that is socially connected with these processes (Connell, 2012, 2021). According to Connell (2012), the mapping of societal gender orders and institutional gender regimes is a major task of social science research on gender, including gender analysis.

THINK BOX 8.4

- What do you think are the 'social practices' in the health system where you live that are shaped by social relations?

Examples might include fully employed women who are perceived as not fit to be promoted because they have children or women not being allowed to breastfeed at work. It could also mean that men are expected to be the major breadwinner in a home, even though women may lead households or contribute substantially.
- What else can you think of?
- Do you think that people in your society or culture have a strong interest in maintaining a stable framework of who men and women are by differentiating them?
- To what extent would it be easy or hard to disrupt your societal gender framework?

THINK BOX 8.5

'At the core of patriarchal gender orders is the institutionalized control of women's reproductive capacities by men evident in the reproductive rights struggles for autonomy with respect to contraception and abortion worldwide' (Connell, 2014, pp. 1677–1678).
- How far does what Connell says apply where you live? How is your context different?
- How do you think nurses and midwives should be addressing this?

Patriarchy and Hegemonic Masculinity

The concepts of patriarchy and hegemonic masculinity are useful to this discussion of social structure and gender systems.

Patriarchy is a social system that exists in many societies. It is male dominated to the extent that positions of authority—political, economic, legal, religious, educational, military, domestic—are generally reserved for men; male identified to the extent that core cultural ideas about what is considered good, desirable, preferable and normal are associated with how we think about men and masculinity; and male centred so that men and what they do are the primary focus of public discourse and images (e.g. media, film, books) (Johnson, 2014). The idea of a 'patriarchal dividend' refers to the benefits for men in gender-unequal patriarchal social systems and the stakes involved in maintaining an unequal gender order (Connell, 2021). We will return to how the *patriarchal dividend* affects nursing when discussing research findings on the glass escalator later in this chapter.

Hegemonic* masculinity is a term that you might not have come across. It is useful to know this term, as it actually underpins much research on gender, and indeed, it is reflected in societal attitudes, even though it is often not an expressed belief. *Hegemonic masculinity* seeks to explain how and why men maintain dominance over women. It is really about power in society and how perceived masculine traits—such as physical bravery, superior leadership or practical skills—may be the foundation for how society is organised to privilege men as a social group. One example is the role of women in the military—it is only relatively recently

---

*Hegemony refers to the dominance of one group over another, often supported by legitimating norms and ideas.

that women were 'permitted' on the front line of battles because they are not perceived as physically brave. On the other hand, not many men choose nursing, as it is seen as a 'female' and caring occupation. There may be different types of masculinity in a society, but *hegemonic masculinity* is the dominant type. This brings us to one of the core elements in the construction of hegemonic masculinity, which is heterosexuality. To a greater or lesser extent, hegemonic masculinity is constructed as a gender position in a binary system that is as much 'not gay' (i.e. heterosexual) as it is 'not female' (Jewkes et al., 2015).

Gender Binary and Non-binary

The term *gender binary* suggests that in processes of gender differentiation, only two genders are acknowledged—men are masculine and women are feminine to correspond to male and female sex.*
Nonbinary is a term that describes people who may identify or are identified as being both a man and woman, somewhere in between or falling outside these categories (Human Rights Campaign, n.d.). *Nonbinary* identities have been described in Latin America as *travesti* or *metis*, and some Asian and Oceanic cultures embrace forms of a 'third gender' (Jauk, 2016). Muxe refers to a person whose sex at birth is established as male but who dresses and behaves in ways otherwise associated with females in Zapotec cultures of southern Mexico. On the Indian subcontinent, *hijra* are recognised as third gender category which includes eunuchs, intersex people, asexual or transgender people. In Pakistan, a third gender is called *Khawaja Sira* (Azhar, 2017). In Native American culture in the United States, two-spirit people are considered neither men nor women but have a distinct alternate gender status (Carrier et al., 2020).*

Let Us Not Forget That Gender Is About Hierarchy and Structural Inequalities

Increasingly over the last decade, society has started to question the inevitability and naturalness of heterosexuality and the assumption that neither gender

---

*Transgender people are not the same as lesbian, gay and bisexual which are terms that denote an individual's enduring physical, romantic and/or emotional attraction to members of the same and/or opposite sex.

THINK BOX 8.6

- Where you work, is there acknowledgement that some people experience their gender identities as nonbinary?
- To what extent is knowing the gender identity of clients important for nursing practice?

The processes of acquiring a gender identity may differ depending on the type of national culture people live in. Hofstede developed a model with six cultural dimensions (2011), one of which was collectivism versus individualism, which refers to how individuals are integrated into primary groups such as family or clan. In Hofstede's model, national culture can be:

Collectivist: Read this article describing how *becoming a woman* in Malawi is a process of collective conferral of adult female identity through menarche rituals (Bacalja Perianes & Ndaferankehande, 2020).

Individualist: Now take a look at this TEDx talk describing a process of self-recognition and expression of nonbinary gender identity by a person living in the United States, a culture that places high value on individual self-expression and authenticity: https://www.youtube.com/watch?v=OKJjwTEfaKc (Walking Through the World Non-Binary, Jesse Lueck, TEDxRanneySchool)

- In your society, to what extent is gender identity collectively conferred or individually claimed?

---

divisions nor the boundary between heterosexuality and homosexuality/lesbianism are fixed by nature.

These recent considerations have practical consequences for how we analyse gender discrimination and inequalities in the health labour market. Recent analysis pays a lot of attention to gender identity as defined by culture and less on the hierarchical structures that disadvantage women, and so, some may argue, it loses touch with real-world impacts. For example, institutionalised heterosexuality through the marriage contract is an economic relationship in which men can potentially control the reproductive lives of women as well as, in some societies, their financial status, the sexual division of labour and the doubled workload for formally employed women (Jackson, 2001, 2005). These dynamics underlie the problems nurses face as they balance work and family in the absence of childcare (Newman et al., 2019).

The complexities of a postcolonial world, where intersections of gender, ethnicity, race or nationality meet stark and worsening material inequalities, and in which it is often women who are most disadvantaged by global and local exploitation, demand a (gender) analysis of *structural inequalities* (Jackson, 2001). This is particularly true for the nursing workforce that is 90% women globally.

GENDER IN THE HEALTH LABOUR MARKET

There is, by now, ample evidence from country and global workforce studies demonstrating common discriminatory gender dynamics and workforce effects that have emerged from rigorous research. The gender dynamics in Box 8.1 consist of processes of gender differentiations and subordinations that can exclude female health workers from full equality, economic productivity and professional leadership.

A recent paper summarises country and global workforce studies that show that nurses and other female health workers often face exclusion from jobs and leadership on the basis of pregnancy and family caregiving and a 'second shift' of work after formal, paid work hours (Newman et al., 2023). In studies in medical training systems in Mali and Kenya, instructors held female students hostage through coercion and sexual quid pro quo ('sex-based grades' or passing grades for sex). Stereotyping of nurses as vengeful and incompetent emerged in Rwanda, Uganda and Zambia research (Newman et al., 2011b, 2017). In Lesotho, stereotypes of altruistic women willing to work for free rationalised men's absence from sharing the burden of HIV/AIDS community-based care (Newman et al., 2011a). A recent systematic review demonstrated that sexual/sex-based harassment is a problem for nurses (Kahsay et al., 2020), and a study conducted in Uganda documented how professional rewards and sanctions were levied through informal management and supervision practices that required compliance with sexual demands or work-related reprisals for refusal. The abuse of supervisory power in sex-based harassment reinforced vertical segregation, meaning that women did not get promoted as quickly as men if they stayed in these positions, impeding female health workers' career opportunities and economic security. Sexual coercion and unwanted sexual attention toward patients by employees were also documented (Newman et al., 2021). A 2019 global

survey of 2537 practicing nurses from 117 countries about occupational segregation of nursing leadership (Newman et al., 2019) found that discrimination based on pregnancy and family responsibilities was a perceived barrier to leadership jobs. The study also found barriers in pervasive, intense stereotyping, 'prove it again' for female nurses and the *glass escalator* for male nurses.

THINK BOX 8.7

Before diving into the next section, jot down what you think may be happening where you work with regard to gender discrimination and inequality. For example,

- Are there examples of sexual favours in exchange for professional advancement or a good performance evaluation?
- Are there more men in managerial positions?
- Do women earn less than men?
- Does the workforce data that are collected or available to you give this type of analysis?

GENDER SEGREGATION IN THE HEALTH SECTOR: GENDER STEREOTYPING AND HIERARCHY EVERYWHERE

The profession of nursing is buttressed by gender stereotypes and vulnerable not only to a range of biases and discriminations but is also particularly prone to the disadvantages of being typed 'female'.

Analysis of the health sector shows widespread occupational segregation by sex (Boniol et al., 2019). Ninety percent of the global nursing stock is female (World Health Organization, 2020). *Sex segregation* (the term first used) consists of the separation of men and women into different occupations, a pervasive and widely documented form of discrimination that creates rigidity in the types of jobs occupied by women and men in labour markets in which women and men are expected to work in occupational roles dominated by their sex. Gender segregation is a term used later which goes beyond 'sex segregation' to denote jobs that are viewed as somehow requiring female or male attributes. Gender segregation exists at all levels of development, under all political systems and in diverse religious, social and cultural settings. The seriousness

BOX 8.1
DISCRIMINATORY GENDER DYNAMICS IN HEALTH WORKFORCES

Glass ceiling: Invisible barrier to reaching top leadership and management positions, driven by practices such as women's initial placement in relatively dead-end jobs, not getting job assignments that lead to advancement, not being promoted or closer scrutiny of women's performance relative to men's before being promoted and lack of access to informal networks and opportunities for mentoring (Williams, 2015).

Glass escalator: An effect whereby men bring their privileged status in the wider culture to their entry into predominantly female occupations. Men are often accepted and well integrated in the female-dominated profession and work culture and given fair, if not preferential, treatment in hiring and promotion decisions despite their being in a minority (Williams, 1992, 1995). This is an example of a 'patriarchal dividend' (Connell, 2021).

Maternal wall: Refers to practices that use maternity, family responsibilities or childcare as an excuse to not offer opportunities to female employees. For example, passing mothers over for promotion, eliminating jobs during maternity leave or offering a demotion or less desirable assignments after childbirth and at return to work, the 'executive schedule' which requires overtime, marginalisation of part-time workers, and expectations that workers who are 'executive material' will relocate their families in order to take a better job. Often manifests in pregnancy and family responsibility discrimination (Williams, 2015).

Prove it again: Female employees often have to provide more evidence of competence than male employees do to be seen as equally capable, a problem documented in scores of social science studies on double standards, attribution bias, leniency bias, recall bias and polarised evaluations. Linked to the *glass escalator* (Williams, 2015).

Stereotypes: Generalised beliefs or preconception about the attributes or characteristics that are or ought to be possessed by, or the roles that are or should be performed by, members of a particular social group. Gender stereotypes underpin occupational segregation and hold, for example, that women are, by nature, not suited to performing the same jobs or tasks as men and or men are not suited to doing the same jobs or tasks as women (e.g. the concentration of women in nursing because women are believed to be naturally more suited for care work, and the concentration of men at the tops of hierarchies because of greater presumed competence) (Cusack, 2013).

Violence and harassment: Refer to a range of unacceptable behaviours and practices, or threats thereof, whether a single occurrence or repeated, that aim at, result in or are likely to result in physical, psychological, sexual or economic harm, and include gender-based violence and harassment. In the health workforce, it includes physical attack and sexual harassment, bullying and verbal abuse. The term 'gender-based violence and harassment' means violence and harassment directed at persons because of their sex or gender, or affecting persons of a particular sex or gender disproportionately, and includes sexual harassment (ILO, 2019).

Sexual/sex-based harassment: Encapsulates a wide range of behaviours that degrade or humiliate an individual based on their sex and/or gender, including three categories of behaviour: (1) 'gender harassment', referring to sexist verbal and nonverbal behaviours that convey hostility, objectification, exclusion or second-class status about members of one gender. For example, behaviours that demean women and/or femininity or create a hostile work environment but which do not have the goal of sexual cooperation but to enforce gender ideals; (2) 'unwanted sexual attention', or verbal or physical unwelcome sexual advances which can include assault, referring to behaviours such as pressure for dates and unwanted touching. which express a romantic or sexual interest but are unreciprocated and unwelcome; and (3) 'sexual coercion', when favourable professional or educational treatment is conditioned on sexual activity, including behaviours that threaten loss of job, unfavourable work assignments or loss of pay or promised promotion, raises or better assignments in return for sexual cooperation (Newman et al., 2021).

---

of occupational segregation by sex or gender as discrimination has been recognised in International Labour Organization (ILO) Convention No. 111, and the elimination of discrimination is a fundamental right at work under ILO's Declaration on Fundamental Principles and Rights at Work (Anker et al., 2003).

While there may be a decline in sex segregation driven by new laws mandating women's equal workforce participation, gender segregation persists, as it is driven by culture, employer and institutional bias, and people's own perception of 'self' and where they might 'fit' into the workforce, which are shaped by (Charles & Grusky, 2005) the gender stereotypes that are embedded in policies, laws, traditional sayings, educational curricula and the media.

Gender segregation is one of the most enduring aspects of labour markets around the world (Anker et al., 2003), and by pushing women into certain occupations, it depresses female wages and hurts economic security. These trends are also highly racialised in some contexts: women of colour at all education levels are segregated into jobs with lower wages than their White female peers of similar skill levels. These patterns indicate that the persistence of gender segregation results in a significant loss of income for working women and their families, which should be disconcerting to policymakers given the ameliorative effects of lifting women's wages on health, poverty, unemployment and inequality (McGrew, 2016).

The pervasiveness and intractability of gendered occupational structures are sustained by two factors (Charles & Grusky, 2005):

1. *Gender essentialism*, which posits that men and women have *different,* basic unchanging 'essences'. Women are presumed or expected to be emotional and more naturally competent in personal service, nurturance and social interactions characterised by 'niceness', while men are presumed to be more competent in tasks requiring leadership, rationality and decision-making.
2. *Male primacy*, which represents men as naturally dominant and more decisive and status worthy than women.

The workings of gender essentialism and male primacy were illustrated in the study of HIV/AIDS care in Lesotho mentioned earlier (Newman et al., 2011a). Men who took their children to the Under-Fives clinic (a woman's task) were publicly ridiculed. Men who had worked in nursing jobs in the South African mines reported their first aid skills to be something that men did better than women and that gave men superiority (i.e., primacy) over women, as suggested by the following: 'I think men are much better. Women know nothing about "safety" so we are above them', and 'the same example of controlling bleeding applies here. Women do not know blood vessels, so that is where we become better'. Men's skills were associated with saving lives and featured the presumed 'masculine' traits of courage, dignity, bravery, skill and discretion. A belief in male primacy in Lesotho prevented men from crossing into the female-typed social role of caregiver because it involved 'free' (volunteer) labour and low-status female-typed tasks. Women were believed to be naturally altruistic and adept at 'mothering' and the 'dirty work' of HIV/AIDS care (Newman et al., 2011a).

Similarly, in a study from South Africa, many male respondents considered that providing care to sick or disabled relatives was work appropriate only for women. Sick men were cared for by women in the home, but sick women might be left without caregivers if no female caregiver was available. When men did participate in caregiving activities, the care they provided was not considered 'feminine' in nature. They did not provide counselling, bathing or cooking for sick people but, rather, arranged transportation to hospitals, assisted with lifting or offered financial support for illness-related costs. Women shouldered the majority of the physical, psychological and emotional burdens of care, as well as an increased risk of infection and exposure to gender-based violence such as rape (Akintola, 2006, 2008). Research in Jordan (Ahmad & Alasad, 2007) suggested that there were gender essentialist stereotypes about women nurses' ability to 'raise patients' morale' and male nurses' 'ability to avoid (a) panic situation' and to be able to live better with emotional strain than female nurses, the latter finding suggesting that male respondents considered men to be *better suited* than women for nursing because of these (innate) presumably male traits.

The global nurse leadership study (Newman et al., 2019) found that a majority of respondents believed that men and women had specific roles in society and that the attribution or reality of family responsibilities is a 'very important' or 'important' barrier to women obtaining leadership positions. The perception of nursing as a 'nurturing' profession, and nurses as 'submissive', was a consistent finding among male and female nurses and across regions, and female nurses were more likely to be expected to be subservient to doctors than male nurses (67% versus 45%). The relational stereotypes in Box 8.2 seem to suggest that men/doctors have the necessary innate traits to make a good leader (such as assertiveness, decision-making acumen, competence) and are therefore apt at the legitimate exercise of power, while women/nurses do not. Note that gender differentiation and hierarchy are in action here and the limiting effects that gender stereotyping has on nurses and nursing.

The Glass Escalator

It is hard to overlook the effects of male primacy in the *glass escalator* effect for men and the glass ceiling for women in nursing. Reuben et al. (2014) noted that the presumption of greater male competence in science, technology, engineering and math (STEM) subjects has consequences for women's entry into STEM careers: negative sex-based stereotypes of women kept women out of STEM careers, and both male and female subjects were found twice as likely to hire a man than a woman for a STEM job. Furthermore, nursing has not been considered a STEM subject, even though today's nurse has to know and understand a range of STEM subjects. Unconscious gender bias, which is difficult to identify and prevent, remains a significant barrier to women's career advancement, starting with biased evaluations (International Labour Organization, 2017).

Males in the Female-Typed Occupation of Nursing

In many countries, great strides have been made in increasing the number of females working in traditionally male professions, although many women are still held back by material conditions such as unequal access to education and familial obligations such as caring for children and sick relatives and the effect of stereotypical gender roles that are pervasive in employment and educational systems. However, equal strides have not been made in increasing the number of men working in female-dominated professions. Today, despite increasing numbers of male nurses, they are typically in the minority (recall that globally, 90% of nurses are female). This is similarly multifactored: female-dominated professions have historically been undervalued (and stigmatised) and

undercompensated, which makes them less prestigious and less attractive to potential male candidates. Historically, men have engaged in nursing in large numbers under certain circumstances, such as in times of war and necessity when women are not present (e.g. in mining camps; see Burns, 1998).

In a paper reevaluating the notion that it is difficult being a man in nursing, Brown (2009) found that men appear to be well served by a career in nursing; despite their lesser numbers, they are likely to earn more and be promoted into leadership roles more readily. An intersectional gender analysis conducted in the United States (Wingfield, 2009) demonstrated that Black men, Black women and White women waited longer than White men for managerial promotions in female-dominated fields, suggesting the importance of accounting for racial marginalisation 'on the glass escalator'. This has implications for research, policy and management in societies where class or caste may, in addition to gender, be important reasons for exclusion.

The Devaluation of Female-Typed Work

The 2019 global nursing leadership survey and nurse leaders' interviews (Newman et al., 2019) also point to a sense of second-class status among female nurses, as well as an experience of the glass escalator benefitting male nurses. What accounts for the devaluation of this most quintessential of female occupations?

BOX 8.2
RELATIONAL GENDER ESSENTIALIST AND MALE PRIMACY STEREOTYPES

MEDICINE AND NURSING	MASCULINE AND FEMININE
Nursing is inferior to medicine—nurses have 'soft' skills; doctors have 'hard' skills	Men are naturally better leaders
Doctors are leaders; nurses are followers	Men are more competent than women
Nurses are subservient; doctors are served	Men are more decisive
Nurses are less competent than doctors	Women are or should be submissive, obedient
Nurses are not as equipped as doctors with the knowledge and skills to make health/workforce policy	Women are, by nature, gentler, caring, angelic
Nurses do 'dirty', menial tasks (e.g. toileting, bedpans); doctors do the diagnostic/technical tasks	Women's leadership decisions are not legitimate (e.g. 'bossy', 'petticoat power')
There is something wrong with men who want to be nurses	Agentic or assertive women are trying to be men

Source: Newman, C., Stilwell, B., Rick, S., & Peterson, K. (2019). *Investing in the power of nurse leadership: What will it take?* IntraHealth International. https://www.intrahealth.org/resources/investing-power-nurse-leadership-what-will-it-take Last accessed November 2022

First, economic devaluation of work is associated with 'women's work'. Research results strongly support a hypothesis that higher levels of occupational segregation in the labour market level are associated with a significantly increased tendency to devalue women's work roles. Reskin (1988) found evidence that the wage gap is associated with the segregation of men and women into different jobs and that women's occupations pay less, at least in part, because women do them. Men's activities are typically valued above women's, regardless of content (Reskin, 1988, p. 200).

Second, Williams (1995)'s study found that, unlike women who enter traditionally male professions, men's slow movement into female-dominated jobs is perceived by the 'outside world' as a step down in status. Many of the men in her sample identified the stigma of working in a female-identified occupation. According to Williams, men who otherwise might show interest in and aptitude for such careers are likely discouraged from pursuing them because of the negative popular stereotypes associated with the men who work in them. She concluded that for men, the major barriers to integration into female-dominated occupations have little to do with their treatment once they decide to enter these fields, but the social and cultural sanctions applied to men who do 'women's work'. In fact, the men and women interviewed for the most part believed that men were given fair—if not preferential—treatment in hiring and promotion decisions, were accepted by supervisors and colleagues, and were well integrated into the health workplace subculture. Subtle mechanisms seem to enhance men's position in these professions—a phenomenon Williams referred to as the 'glass escalator effect'.

The Glass Escalator

The glass escalator refers to an effect documented in several studies whereby men bring their privileged status in the wider culture to their entry into predominantly female occupations and experience fast-track promotion into leadership and higher salary. Men are given fair, if not preferential, treatment in hiring and promotion decisions despite their being in a minority (Williams, 1992, 1995). To the extent that the glass escalator effect is at work (and it should be subject to assessment in nursing employment and education

contexts), it is an example of a 'patriarchal dividend' (Connell, 2021).

A study in *Nursing Management* (Hader, 2010) collected the demographic and professional attributes of more than 1500 nurse leaders representing every US geographical area, in addition to Saudi Arabia, Canada, China and New Zealand. Not surprisingly, 91.5% of nurse leaders were female, while only 8.5% were male, but although male nurses were poorly represented in nursing leadership positions, it appeared as though they moved into management positions at a younger age than their female counterparts. Men earned greater salaries than women despite no significant difference in the percentage of male nurses holding executive positions within their organisation or attaining a higher level of education. Specifically, 30% of men earned greater than USD$100,000 per year, while only 20% of women earned a six-figure salary. Similarly, Barrett-Landau and Henle (2014) analysed the US Census Bureau's Industry and Occupation Statistics and found that men represented 9% of registered nurses, and at that time, a man's average salary was USD$60,700, as opposed to women, who earned USD$51,100 per year. Even in a gendered, female-dominated occupation such as nursing, the men's advantage was apparent, with men being overrepresented at senior bands compared to their overall proportion in the UK nursing population (Punshon et al., 2019). There also seemed to be an advantage in terms of faster attainment of higher grades from the point of registration. The researchers concluded that reward and remuneration are essential to the workforce, and this work revealed a gender differential towards men in higher-paid nursing work.

It is reasonable to suppose that gender status beliefs that involve male primacy and perceptions of women's lesser worth or inferiority as leaders also—in addition to other material conditions—act as barriers to female nurses in promotion or hiring into positions of policy/strategic nurse leadership, power and authority, all opportunities based on beliefs that men are not only 'different' but 'better', or more competent, than women (Ridgeway, 2006). This calls to mind a male primacy gender status belief that emerged from the 2019 gender and nursing leadership study, where a sense of devaluation and stigma led a respondent to misguidedly recommend increasing the number of men in nursing in order to improve the status of nursing, as if to suggest that if men accepted the profession, then it really couldn't be that bad (Newman et al., 2019).

The research mentioned in this section demonstrates the value of conducting special qualitative and quantitative gender analyses to explore discrimination, segregation and disadvantage, especially since workforce, administrative, census or HR data are not often within the reach or perception of the frontline nurse.

THINK BOX 8.8

- Have you encountered a bias towards you because you are a woman or a man in nursing?
- Are women and men managers given the same respect in your country?
- Do you know if there are effects such as the glass ceiling, the glass escalator or a gender pay gap in the nurse workforce in your country?

Implications for Action and Policies

That nurses face gender bias, discrimination and practical disadvantages as occupational risks in health systems strongly suggests that nurse education and leadership training should include the development of gender analysis skills and a mastery of international labour standards related to gender equality and decent work.

A review of 20th-century reports on nursing in the United States concluded that 'nursing is stuck in a rut' (Gebbie, 2009). Even worse, Gebbie says, it may stay there—the profession has not been willing to make the changes urged on it over many decades. At this point in our observations on gender and nursing, it is worth considering how the occupational segregation of nursing as a female-dominated profession contribute to the barriers to change in the profession and what we can do about it.

THINK BOX 8.9

From your perspective, what needs to change in nursing and how will change be impacted—for better or worse—by the gendered structures in the profession and in health systems?

There is no blueprint for success in bringing about change in nursing; each country has developed its nursing profession from deep roots in society and culture, and this is one of the challenges faced by global

reports and recommendations. What we hope that this chapter might encourage is an honest, shared analysis of the barriers to change in the profession that are underpinned by gender stereotypes. In this section, we discuss where we think gender has a critical influence on the development of nursing and nurses.

- ■ **Most nurses are women in most places**
  The effects on the nursing profession of the place and self-esteem of women in society is something that nurses in most countries have in common (World Health Organization, 2020). Recognising that nursing is a gendered profession means that an initial step to developing leadership in the nursing profession is to change the gender-biased *systems* in which female nurses are seen as unequal and inferior. While gender-transformative strategies are necessary, they are not likely to be sufficient to address outdated societal stereotypes and health professionals' negative perceptions of nurses and nursing. These perceptions influence who chooses nursing as a profession who gets rewarded and why and how effective nurses can be as leaders.

- ■ **Articulating the complexity of nursing**
  As already mentioned, nursing has not typically been included as a STEM occupation despite nurses implementing scientifically based interventions to solve complex health problems—something that has become more evident with the publicity given to nursing care during the global pandemic (Green & John, 2019; Stilwell, 2020). How does this perception of nursing as not scientific affect the way nursing is seen as a profession? An early commentator, sociologist Celia Davies (Davies, 1995), wrote the following:

There is a sense in which nursing is not a profession but an adjunct to a gendered concept of profession. Nursing is an activity, in other words, that enables medicine to present itself as masculine/rational and to gain the power and privilege of so doing. It has clearly had first bite of the cherry in defining its work and…We get closer to the matter in recognising that it is trying to put a conceptual framework around just those aspects of the work of health and healing that are 'left over' after medicine has imposed an essentially masculine vision.

Though this commentary is now old, there remains a grain of truth here. Nursing is still not recognised as a STEM subject, which constrains the funding it can attract as an academic subject. Yet nurses now have to understand a great deal of science, mathematics and technology to be able to do their work, often as the primary patient care manager. When nurses consistently have lower pay than physicians and are not occupying senior management positions in the health sector (World Health Organization, Global Health Workforce Network and Women in Global Health, 2019), it may send a message that nursing is still dominated by medical practice (Newman et al., 2019).

■ **First do no harm**

That men carry gender advantages with them into female-concentrated occupations suggests that in building more robust nursing workforces, health sector policymakers and employers of nurses must hire and promote men in ways *that do not exacerbate existing gender inequalities*. As Anker noted, the choice of occupations 'reserved' for women [is] small, that is, women are excluded from a wide range of occupations, and 'one positive aspect of occupational segregation for women is that it helps protect some women from competition from another large group of workers (men)' and allows them to survive the worst of economic hardship (Anker, 1998). Elsewhere, Anker points out that while there are numerous advantages to decreasing occupational segregation, if the number of men in a female-dominated profession increases, women may be subject to greater and unfair competition for leadership roles and job openings (Anker et al., 2003). This observation gains more importance in light of *glass escalator* research. Because of this, those developing nursing policy and those aiming to desegregate nursing to develop more robust workforces need gender-analytical competencies, alongside leadership and clinical competencies, to identify gender bias, discrimination and the unequal gender power relations in the health workforce. The first lesson of gender policy in nursing and global health must be 'first do no harm', which means assuming a gender lens and *not exacerbating existing gender inequalities*. If gender analysis can act as a tool for nursing policy and planning, then these competencies must become a routine part of professional education, development and practice. Male nurses should join in solidarity to equalise opportunities in the profession.

■ **Legal and policy protections**

What nurses want and what they get are quite different in terms of the way that the profession is regarded and rewarded. Nurses should therefore school themselves in labour standards that bear on gender equality and decent work in their national contexts as well as those stemming from international agreements. For example, based on the earlier evidence from health workforce studies, decent work for nurses might mean getting paid adequately and regularly, working in environments free from sexual harassment and discrimination based on pregnancy and family responsibilities, and having access to vaccinations and personal protective equipment that fits.

There are international labour standards that promote and protect opportunities and rights related to decent work and gender equality that should be operationalised in national and institutional policy. It is important for nurses to know that these exist and to advocate for them. You can check them out at the website of the ILO; search for labour standards and conventions (International Labour Organization, n.d.). Nurses must use power together to change from what nurses get to what nurses want. That will not happen until nurses change their relationship to power.

■ **Nurses and power**

Nurses hold a powerful position in the health sector as the largest profession globally, but they are still not perceived as powerful in shaping policy nor routinely included as high-level decision-makers (Girvin et al., 2016). As we have set out, nursing is a complex gendered profession, and this plays out in nurses feeling disempowered, especially female nurses, and such powerlessness starts to be self-perpetuating when nurses do not feel able to speak out at senior meetings or may not have the resources to succeed in senior roles (Newman et al., 2019). Mary Beard, in *Women and Power* (Beard, 2017), suggests the many ways that power is constructed and conveyed as masculine and makes a compelling case that women are still marginalised from sites of power. Beard goes on to say that while there are many workplace policies—childcare, maternity and paternity leave, family-friendly hours—that can have a positive effect on opportunities for women, there cannot be real change in women's profile and status unless they change their understanding and practice of power.

But there are various sources of power (Eisler, 2015, p. 6): *power over* (associated with hierarchies), *power to* and *power with*, which derive from partnership models rather than hierarchies. It is these partnership models that gave nurses a more powerful voice during the Nursing Now campaign (Holloway et al., 2021). Nurses were globally linked and could articulate together their powerful narratives. This is a different nonhierarchical power structure and one which nurses may be comfortable belonging to but may not easily have access to, though social media now enables global conversations and is a powerful tool for social activism. Used strategically, *power with* can become *power to* change health policies and, eventually, *power over* strategic directions, decisions and resources.

THINK BOX 8.10

- In your context (i.e., where you live and work), do you think that nurses are able to influence policymaking?
- What would make the profession more powerful?
- Do you think that nursing education and professional development should include the understanding and practice of power?

It can only be nurses themselves who articulate the worth of the profession, challenge the pervasive stereotypes around doctor and nurse and men and women and the devaluation of the 'women's work' of care, assert power, and change the professional interactions that constrain nurses' ability to fully and effectively function in multiple service and leadership roles (Newman et al., 2019). To do this may go against the grain of nurses' socialisation, but the time is ripe for asserting the value of nursing and demanding fair pay and decent working conditions as well as equality in opportunities for promotion and senior posts.

THE NEXT GENERATION OF NURSES

The WHO Strategic Directions for Nursing and Midwifery 2021-2025 (WHO, 2021) points out the looming shortfall of millions of nurses by 2030, which means that recruiting young nurses into the profession will be mission critical to have an adequate workforce. But we know that young people now are seeking better work–life balance, interesting and worthwhile employment, decent working conditions and wanting to see the world they see on the internet. Recent research by Deloitte (Agarwal et al., 2018) showed that most companies believe their young employees will be retained for less than 10 years, and there is a similar trend in nursing in some countries, where young nurses are showing a tendency to change jobs within 10 years of qualifying.

The profession of nursing will have to pay attention to what young people are looking for in their careers if enough nurses are to be trained for the future. The contribution of young people to social change in the 21st century is more noticeable (Winston, 2019). One example is the support for climate and environmental concerns: in 2019, in what may be the largest youth-led protest in history, millions of students in 300 cities around the world walked out of school to march for climate action. Greta Thunberg is a notable example of the powerful effect that young people can have as activists.

If young people are to be recruited into nursing, then we suggest that the discriminations, inequalities and disadvantages discussed in this chapter must be eliminated. The future of global health is, to a large extent, nurse dependent. Old attitudes and perceptions of nursing will not attract young people into this profession and will not get nursing out of its rut.

We have shown that gender-influenced stereotypes of nurses still tend to limit the power of nurses as policy influencers, and these stereotypes are not amenable to 'quick fixes'. What is required is a rebranding of nursing that is clear about its value in the 21st-century health system and changing gender-biased social and institutional systems in which nurses are educated and employed. Developing a robust brand image for the 21st century that addressed what has been learned from gender analysis must be part of the nursing research and strategy agendas as a matter of urgency if nurses are to be influential leaders and practitioners.

SUMMARY AND CONCLUSIONS

As we mentioned at the outset, we believe that structural–materialist and relational approaches from the social sciences have the greatest value for explaining the effects of gender on nursing in global health. Gender binaries may be inadequate to understand gender in global health, but gender hierarchy based on the gender dichotomy of masculinity and femininity in heterosexual unions is, in most societies, a central social dynamic, whether in the church, the family or the workplace, with a goal or effect of placing women as a group subordinate to men as a group (Risman, 2004, p. 33) and resulting in social and economic disadvantages. In the earlier part of this chapter, we discussed patriarchy and hegemonic masculinity—these ideas define gender hierarchy, with the powerful attributes of masculinity being perceived as superior to and dominant over feminine traits.

Policymakers are wise to not underestimate the ubiquitous and seemingly inflexible gender systems and structures of patriarchal, hegemonic masculinity that are created through human cognition and reproduced through social relations and interaction. In the next section, we look more closely at how these play out in nursing.

REFERENCES

Agarwal, D., & Bersin, J. (2018). *Catch the wave: From careers to experiences; new pathways*. Retrieved, November 2022, from https://www2.deloitte.com/insights/us/en/focus/human-capital-trends/2018/building-21st-century-careers.html.

Ahmad, M. M., & Alasad, J. A. (2007). Patients' preferences for nurses' gender in Jordan. *International Journal of Nursing Practice, 13*, 237–242.

Azhar, M. (2017). Pakistan's traditional third gender isn't happy with the trans movement. *The world*. Retrieved, November 24, 2022, from https://theworld.org/stories/2017-07-29/pakistans-traditional-third-gender-isnt-happy-trans-movement.

Akintola, O. (2006). Gendered home-based care in South Africa: More trouble for the troubled. *African Journal of AIDS Research, 5*(3), 237–247. doi:10.2989/16085900609490385.

Akintola, O. (2008). *Towards equal sharing of aids caring responsibilities: Learning from Africa*. Retrieved, November 24, 2022, from https://www.researchgate.net/publication/241613895_Towards_Equal_Sharing_Of_Aids_Caring_Responsibilities_Learning_From_Africa.

Anker, R. (1998). *Gender and jobs: Sex segregation of occupations in the world*. International Labour Organization.

Anker, R., Melkas, H., & Korten, A. (2003). *Gender-based occupational segregation in the 1990's*. International Labour Organization.

Barrett-Landau, S. B., & Henle, S. (2014). Men in nursing: Their influence in a female dominated career. *Journal for Leadership and Instruction*. Retrieved, November 2022, from https://files.eric.ed.gov/fulltext/EJ1081399.pdf.

Bacalya Perianes, M. & Ndaferankhande, D. Becoming Female: The Role of Menarche Rituals in "Making Women" in Malawi. In: The Palgrave Handbook of Critical Menstruation Studies (Internet). Singapore: Palgrave MavcMillan; 2020. Chapter 33. Accessed February 2024: https://pubmed.ncbi.nim.nih.gov/33347188.

Beard, M. (2017). *Women and power. A manifesto*. Profile Books.

Boniol, M., McIsaac, M., Xu, L., Wuliji, T., Diallo, K., & Campbell, J. (2019). *Gender equity in the health workforce: Analysis of 104 countries*. World Health Organization. Retrieved, November 2022, from https://apps.who.int/iris/handle/10665/311314.

Brown, B. (2009). Men in nursing: Re-evaluating masculinities, re-evaluating gender. *Contemporary Nurse, 33*(2), 120–129. doi:10.5172/conu.2009.33.2.120.

Burns, C. (1998). "A man is a clumsy thing who does not know how to handle a sick person": Aspects of the history of masculinity and race in the shaping of male nursing in South Africa, 1900–1950. *Journal of Southern African Studies, 24*(4), 695–717. Special Issue on Masculinities in Southern Africa.

Carrier, L., Dame, J., & Jennifer, L. (2020). Two spirit identity and indigenous conceptualization of gender and sexuality: Implications for nursing practice. *Creative Nursing, 26*(2), 96–100.

Charles, M., & Grusky, D. B. (2005). *Occupational ghettos: The worldwide segregation of women and men*. Stanford University Press.

Colaco, R., & Watson-Grant, S. (2018). A global call to action for gender inclusive data collection and use. *Policy brief*. 2021. RTI Press. Retrieved, November 2022, from https://www.rti.org/rti-press-publication/gender-inclusive-data-collection/fulltext.pdf.

Connell, R. (2012). Gender health and theory: Conceptualizing the issue, in local and world perspective. *Social Science and Medicine, 74*, 1675–1683.

Connell, R. (2014). The sociology of gender in Southern perspective. *Current Sociology Monographs, 62*(4), 550–567.

Connell, R. (2021). *Gender in world perspective* (4th ed.). Polity Press.

Cusack, S. (2013). *Gender stereotyping as a human rights violation*. UN Office of the High Commissioner. Retrieved, November 2022, from https://www.esem.org.mk/pdf/Najznachajni%20vesti/2014/3/Cusack.pdf.

Davies, C. (1995). *Gender and the Professional Predicament*. Open University Press.

Eisler, R. (2015). Human possibilities: The interaction of biology and culture. *Interdisciplinary Journal of Partnership Studies, 1*(1), 1–39.

Gay and Lesbian Alliance Against Defamation (GLAAD). (2016). *GLAAD media reference guide* (10th ed.). Retrieved, November 2022, from https://www.glaad.org/reference/transgender.

Gebbie, K. (2009). 20th century reports on nursing and nursing education: What difference did they make? *Nursing Outlook, 57*(2), 84–92.

Girvin, J., Jackson, D., & Hutchinson, M. (2016). Contemporary public perceptions of nursing: A systematic review and narrative synthesis of the international research evidence. *Journal of Nursing Management, 24*(8), 994–1006.

Green, C., & John, L. (2019). Should nursing be considered a STEM profession? *Nursing Forum.* https://doi.org/10.1111/nuf.12417. Last accessed February 2024.

Hay, K., McDougal, L., Percival, V., Henry, S., Klugman, J., Wurie, H., Raven, J., Shabalala, F., Fielding-Miller, R., Dey, A., Dehingia, N., Morgan, R., Atmavilas, Y., Saggurti, N., Yore, J., Blokhina, E., Huque, R., Barasa, E., Bhan, N., ... Raj, A. (2019). Disrupting gender norms in health systems: Making the case for change. *Lancet, 393,* 2535–2549.

Hader, R. (2010). Nurse leaders: A closer look. *Nursing Management, 41*(1), 25–29.

Heise, L., Greene, M. E., Opper, N., Stavropoulou, M., Harper, C., Nascimento, M., & Zewdie, D. (2019). Gender inequality and restrictive gender norms: Framing the challenges to health. *Lancet, 393,* 2440–2454.

Herman, J. L., Flores, A. R., & O'Neill, K. (2022). *How many adults identify as transgender in the United States?* UCLA School of Law. Williams Institute. Retrieved, November 2022, from https://williamsinstitute.law.ucla.edu/publications/trans-adults-united-states/.

Hofstede, G. (2011). Dimensionalizing cultures: The hofstede model in context. Unit 2 Theoretical and Methodological Issues. *Subunit 1 Conceptual Issues in Psychology and Culture.* Article 8. Retrieved, November 2022, from https://scholarworks.gvsu.edu/orpc/vol2/iss1/8/.

Holloway, A., Thomson, A., Stilwell, B., Finch, H., Irwin, K., Crisp, N. (2021). *"Agents of change: The story of the nursing now campaign" Nursing Now/Burdett Trust for Nursing.* Retrieved, November 2022, from https://www.nursingnow.org/wp-content/uploads/2021/05/Nursing-Now-Final-Report.pdf.

Human Rights Campaign. (n.d.). https://www.hrc.org/resources/transgender-and-non-binary-faq.

Iantaffi, A. (2020). Increasing gender awareness to reduce harm in health care. *Creative Nursing, 26*(2), 83–87.

International Labour Organization. (2019). *Violence and harassment convention 190.* Article 1. Retrieved, November 2022, from https://www.ilo.org/dyn/normlex/en/f?p=NORMLEXPUB:12100:0::NO::P12100_ILO_CODE:C190.

International Labour Organization. (2017). Breaking barriers: Unconscious gender bias in the workplace. *Research note.* Bureau for employers activities. Retrieved, November 2022, from https://www.ilo.org/actemp/publications/WCMS_601276/lang--en/index.htm.

International Labour Organization. (n.d.). *Decent work.* Retrieved, November 2022, from https://www.ilo.org/global/topics/decent-work/lang--en/index.htm.

Jauk, D. (2016). Transgender movements in international perspective. In Naples, N. A. (Ed.), *The Wiley Blackwell Encyclopedia of gender and sexuality studies* (1st ed.). John Wiley & Sons.

Jewkes, R., Morrell, R., Hearn, J., Lundqvist, E., Blackbeard, D., Lindegger, G., Quayle, M., Sikweyiya, Y., & Gottzén, L. (2015). Hegemonic masculinity: Combining theory and practice in gender interventions. *Culture Health and Sexuality, 17*(sup2), S112–127.

Jackson, S. (2001). Why a materialist feminism is (Still) possible and necessary. *Women's Studies International Forum, 24*(3–4), 283–293.

Jackson, S. (2005). The social complexity of heteronormativity: Gender, sexuality and heterosexuality. *Lecture.* International Conference "Heteronormativity-a fruitful concept?" Trondheim. Retrieved, November 2022, from https://scienceandsexuality.files.wordpress.com/2015/10/jackson-gender-sexuality-heteronormativity.pdf.

Johnson, A. G. (2014). *The gender knot: Unraveling our patriarchal legacy.* Temple University Press.

Jones, J. M. (2021). LGBT identification rises to 5.6% in latest U.S. Estimate. Retrieved, November 2022, from https://news.gallup.com/poll/329708/lgbt-identification-rises-latest-estimate.aspx.

Kahsay, W. G., Negaandeh, R., Dehghan, N. D., & Hasanpour, M. (2020). Sexual harassment against female nurses: A systematic review. *BMC Nursing, 19,* 58.

McGrew, W. (2016). *Gender segregation at work: Separate and equal or inefficient and unfair?* Washington Center for Equitable Growth. Retrieved, November 2022, from https://equitablegrowth.org/gender-segregation-at-work-separate-but-equal-or-inequitable-and-inefficient/.

Newman, C., Nayebare, A., Gacko, N. M. N. N., Okello, P., Gueye, A., Bijou, S., Ba, S., Gaye, S., Thiam, N. C., Gueye, B., Dial, Y., & N'doye M. (2023). Systemic structural gender discrimination and inequality in the health workforce: Theoretical lenses for gender analysis, multi-country evidence and implications for implementation and HRH policy. *Human Resources for Health, 21,* 37. https://doi.org/10.1186/s12960-023-00813-9.

Newman, C., Nayebare, A., Neema, S., Agaba, A., & Akello P. L. (2021). Uganda's response to sexual harassment in the public health sector: from "Dying Silently" to gender-transformational HRH policy. *Human Resources for Health,* 1–19. Retrieved, February 2024, from https://human-resources-health.biomedcentral.com/counter/pdf/10.1186/s12960-021-00569-0.pdf.

Newman, C., Stilwell, B., Rick, S., & Peterson, K. (2019). *Investing in the power of nurse leadership: What will it take?* IntraHealth International. Retrieved, November 2022, from https://www.intrahealth.org/resources/investing-power-nurse-leadership-what-will-it-take.

Newman, C., Chama, P. K., Mugisha, M., Matsiko, C. W., & Oketcho, V. (2017). Reasons behind the current gender imbalance in senior global health roles and the practice and policy changes that can catalyze organizational change in gendered organizations. *Global Health, Epidemiology and Genomics, 2,* e19.

Newman, C., Fogarty, L., Makoae, N. L., & Reavely, E. (2011a). Occupational segregation, gender essentialism and male primacy as major barriers to equity in HIV/AIDS caregiving: Findings from Lesotho. *International Journal for Equity in Health, 10,* 24.

Newman, C., de Vries, D., Kanakuze, J., & Ngendahimana, G. (2011b). Workplace violence and gender discrimination in

Rwanda's health workforce: Increasing safety and gender equality. *Human Resources for Health, 9*, 19.

Punshon, G., Maclaine, K., Trevatt, P., Radford, M., Shanley, O., & Leary, A. (2019). Nursing pay by gender distribution in the UK – does the glass escalator still exist? *International Journal of Nursing Studies, 93*, 21–29.

Reskin, B. (1988). Bringing the men back in: Sex differentiation and the devaluation of women's work. *Gender & Society, 2*(1), 58–81.

Reuben, E., Sapienza, P., & Zingales, L. (2014). How stereotypes impair women's careers in science. *Proceedings of the National Academy of Sciences, 111*(12), 4403–4408.

Ridgeway, C. L., & Correll, S. J. (2004). Unpacking the gender system: A theoretical perspective on gender beliefs and social relations. *Gender and Society, 18*, 510–531.

Ridgeway, C. L. (2006). Gender as an organizing force in social relations: Implications for the future of inequality. In Blau, F. D., Brinton, M. C., & Grusky, D. B. (Eds.), *The declining significance of gender?* (pp. 265–287). Russell Sage Foundation.

Risman, B. J. (2004). Gender as a social structure: Theory wrestling with activism. *Gender and Society, 18*(4), 429–445.

Regenold, N., & Vindrola-Padros, C. (2021). Gender matters: A gender analysis of healthcare workers' experiences during the first COVID-19 pandemic peak in England. *Social Sciences, 10*, 43.

Stilwell, B., & Newman, C. (2022). Nurses learning to be powerful leaders: What will it take? *Creative Nursing, 28*(1), 23–28.

Stilwell, B. (2020). A new narrative of nursing. In *nursing the world to health, international council of nurses toolkit for international nurses' day 2020* (PP. 18–19). International Council of Nurses. Retrieved, November 2022, from https://2020.icnvoicetolead.com/wp-content/uploads/2020/03/IND_Toolkit_120320.pdf.

UNICEF. (2017). Gender equality. *Glossary of terms and concepts*. UNICEF regional office for South Asia. Retrieved, November 2022, from https://www.unicef.org/rosa/reports/gender-equality.

UNFPA. (2005). *Frequently asked questions about gender equality*. Retrieved, November 2022, from https://www.unfpa.org/resources/frequently-asked-questions-about-gender-equality#:~:text=Author%3A%20UNFPA%20What%20is%20meant%20by%20gender%3F%20The,a%20matter%20of%20different%20biological%20and%20physical%20characteristics.

UN Women Training Center eLearning Campus. Gender Equality Glossary. (n.d.). Retrieved, November 2022, from https://portal.trainingcentre.unwomen.org/unw-catalog-mobile/.

United Nations. United Nations Human Rights. Office of the High Commissioner. Convention on the elimination of all forms of discrimination against women. (1979). Accessed February 2024: https://www.ohchr.org/en/instruments-mechanisms/instruments/convention-elimination-all-forms-discrimination-against-women.

USAID. (2021). Automated directive system 205. 3.2. *ADS Chapter 205: Integrating gender equality and female empowerment in USAID's program cycle. What is gender analysis?* Retrieved, November 2022, from https://www.usaid.gov/sites/default/files/documents/205.pdf.

USAID. (2011). *A summary report of new evidence that gender perspective improves reproductive outcomes*. Retrieved, November 2022, from http://www.prb.org/igwg_media/summary-report-gender-perspectives.pdf.

Williams, J. C. (2015). The 5 biases pushing women out of STEM. *Harvard Business Review, 93*(6), 22–23.

Williams, C. L. (1992). The glass escalator: Hidden advantages for men in the "female" professions. *Social Problems, 39*(3), 253–267.

Williams, C. L. (1995). *Still a man's world: Men who do "Women's work."*. University of California Press.

Wingfield, A. H. (2009). Racializing the glass elevator: Reconsidering men's experience with women's work. *Gender and Society, 23*(1), 5–26.

Winston, A. (2019). Young people are leading the way on climate change, and companies need to pay attention. *Harvard business review*. Retrieved, February 2024, from https://hbr.org/2019/03/young-people-are-leading-the-way-on-climate-change-and-companies-need-to-pay-attention.

Women in Global Health. (2021). *Fit for women? Safe and decent PPE for women health and care workers*. Retrieved, November 2022, from https://womeningh.org/our-advocacy/fitforwomen-report/.

World Health Organization. (n.d.). *Gender and health*. Retrieved, November 2022, from https://www.who.int/health-topics/gender#tab=tab_1.

World Health Organization, Global Health Workforce Network and Women in Global Health. (2019). *Global health: Delivered by women, led by men: A gender and equity analysis of the global health workforce* (p. 76). (Human Resources for Health Observer Series No. 24) (who.int) Retrieved, February 2024, from https://www.who.int/activities/value-gender-and-equity-in-the-global-health-workforce.

World Health Organization. (2020). *State of the world's nursing 2020*. World Health Organization. Retrieved, November 2022, from https://www.who.int/publications/i/item/9789240003279.

World Health Organization. (2021). *Global strategic directions for nursing and midwifery 2021–2025*. World Health Organization. The WHO Global Strategic Directions for Nursing and Midwifery (2021–2025). Retrieved, February 2024, from https://www.who.int/publications/i/item/9789240033863.

Section 3

NURSES FINDING A GLOBAL VOICE

SECTION OUTLINE

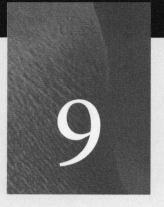

9

UNRAVELLING THE COMPLEXITIES OF GLOBAL NURSE MIGRATION

FRANKLIN A. SHAFFER ■ THOMAS D. ÁLVAREZ

INTRODUCTION

The migration of nurses is not a new phenomenon. Since the early days of the profession, nurses have crossed international borders to practice, study and live. In the 21st century, the global mobility of persons broadly is not only a norm but is exploding in numbers due to transportation and communications technology, advancements in credentials evaluation and portability, economic and financial opportunities, as well as more sinister factors, including climate change, natural disasters, war, conflict and economic and political turmoil. Nursing is not immune to these trends; today, one in eight nurses globally lives and works in a country other than their place of birth or education.

The benefits of nurse migration are enormous. Receiving countries gain many economic benefits from immigrant workers, including taxes paid and money spent in local economies. Hospitals and health systems benefit from internationally educated nurses (IENs) in the form of culture, language, diversity and the alleviation of critical workforce shortages. Though sending countries lose professionals in their workforces, they gain economic compensation through remittances or money sent home from a migrant; in many common sending countries of nurses, remittances make up significant portions of their gross domestic product (GDP). Finally, the benefits for the individual nurses themselves are invaluable; through their migration, nurse migrants often gain better pay, benefits, working conditions, professional and educational opportunities and the ability to support themselves and their families better.

Though the benefits of nurse migration are many, several drawbacks should be considered. Stakeholders are increasingly grappling with the ethics of nurse migration, that is, the individual nurse's right to practice their profession and live and work in their country of choice versus protecting health systems and workforces in vulnerable regions. Similarly, the ethical recruitment of nurses worldwide is being increasingly considered and protected by governments, policymakers and advocates.

This chapter will attempt to unravel the many complexities of global nurse migration, particularly in the context of increased global mobility and workforce shortages in nearly all countries. The chapter begins with an overview of the history of international nurse migration, including current contexts and future trends. Ethical considerations, that is, the delicate balance between the individual's right to migrate versus protecting health systems in vulnerable regions, will be examined. Several leading initiatives and mechanisms for managing nurse migration will be highlighted, including multilateral agreements, codes of ethics and domestic policies. The chapter concludes by identifying the nurse leader's role in this conversation, including suggestions for policy options for management.

To complement these dense, often abstract topics, several case studies will be presented throughout the chapter that feature different journeys by nurse migrants worldwide. Case Study 9.1 follows a typical trajectory of a Filipino nurse seeking work in the United States, while Case Study 9.2 overviews the immense challenges faced by refugee nurses (one from Ukraine and one from Syria) seeking employment without access to their credentials. The final case study follows a border nurse who experienced mobility challenges because of border shutdowns in the early days of the COVID-19 pandemic.

THINK BOX 9.1

- Do you know any nurses who are migrants to your country?
- Have you noticed any particular challenges they face?
- Do you know any nurses who have migrated to another country?
- What have you heard about their experience?

THE PAST, PRESENT AND FUTURE OF GLOBAL NURSE MIGRATION

The mobility of persons is a defining characteristic of the 21st century and is not expected to vanish anytime soon. For as long as humans have roamed the Earth, people have crossed borders as workers, students and tourists, contributing to their destination countries' economic and cultural growth while often benefitting their home countries through earned remittances, skills and education. Increased transportation infrastructure, communication technology and freer trade agreements have facilitated and promoted the migration of persons in all sectors. Regarding nursing and health care, nurse migration is the movement of nurses educated in one country (i.e., source country) across borders to live, work or study in another country (i.e., destination country) and is a significant component of the global health care workforce. Depending on the country and context, these labour migrants are commonly referred to as foreign-educated nurses, IENs or nurse migrants (Sherwood & Shaffer, 2014). This section will attempt to unravel the complexities of global nurse migration by acknowledging the history, looking at current trends and examining future shifts.

A Brief History of Global Nurse Migration

Today, health care migrants represent a significant component of the global labour market and economy, and their contributions to systems worldwide are rightfully being recognised. Still, a brief overview of the history of global nurse migration is essential for understanding current contexts and future predictions.

Following the European Age of Exploration and Discovery, the world witnessed a significant blending of peoples, cultures, diseases and even medicinal practices; the same is true for nursing practice. Throughout the 17th and 18th centuries, European religious missionaries brought nurses and educators from the Global North to developing countries and territories in the Global South to improve health issues, and they founded schools of nursing and introduced Western approaches to caring for the sick (Yeates, 2011). European and American missionaries transported nursing traditions to Korea and China in the late 1800s (Shin et al., 2002), while the United Kingdom transferred its nurses and health workers to posts throughout its colonies (Solano & Rafferty, 2007). Even following the era of colonisation, the United Kingdom recruited nurses and health workers from its commonwealth to address workforce shortages back home (there is more on decolonising nursing in Chapter 6 of this book). Similarly, the United States's military presence throughout Asia during World War II and the Cold War inadvertently brought Western methods of health care and nursing to its occupied territories in Japan, Korea, Vietnam and, most notably, the Philippines (Shaffer & To Dutka, 2013). In the context of global nurse migration, the latter example is worthy of further examination.

Today, the Philippines is the world's largest exporter of nurses and health care workers; of its 2.2 million overseas workers, over 25% are nurses (Caulin, 2018). The Philippine nursing economy can be traced back to the turn of the 20th century, specifically, the end of the Spanish-American War. The Treaty of Paris of 1898 saw the transfer of several Spanish territories to the United States, including Puerto Rico, Guam and the Philippines, thus marking the entrance of Washington into the Pacific region (US Library of Congress, 2011). Under American rule, Filipinos were assimilated into American culture through education and English language instruction. Amid the Philippine malaria and cholera epidemics in the early 1900s, local Filipino females were recruited to volunteer as auxiliary contract nurses. Shortly after that, the first Filipino nurse migrants travelled to the United States per the US Pensionado Act, legislation that enacted a scholarship program for Filipinos to attend school in North America.

In the early 1970s, amidst a global and domestic economic crisis, the Philippines government adopted a national policy of producing and exporting nurses as an economic development strategy. This set the stage for a Filipino diaspora in the United States and eventually other high-income countries, further fuelling American Dream mentalities in the Philippines. Fast forward to today—there are over 200 Philippine schools of nursing that have graduated more than 20,000 nursing graduates per year since 1999, a number well above the domestic health system's ability to absorb into its workforce (Lorenzo et al., 2007). Over time, the increasing number of nursing schools and the lack of investment in the domestic work economy illustrate an underlying national approach to training a health care workforce for exportation and as a tool for socioeconomic development (Ortiga, 2017).

As a result, the Philippines became strategically positioned to profit from its nurse export industry. Beyond the United States, Filipino nurses began immigrating to new lands, seeking new opportunities in Saudi Arabia, Germany, the United Kingdom, Ireland, Japan and Singapore. Nurses in other countries noted the many benefits—educational, professional and economic—they could gain from migrating abroad for work.

In the late 1970s, amidst a high failure rate of IENs sitting for the US National Licensure Examination (NCLEX), the Commission on Graduates of Foreign Nursing Schools, later renamed CGFNS International, Inc., was founded by the American Nurses Association (ANA) and the National League for Nursing (NLN) to create a qualifying predictor exam for IENs to determine whether they could pass the RN State Licensure Exam prior to migrating to the United States. Since its founding in 1977, CGFNS has continued to serve IENs by helping them realise their dream to migrate successfully to the United States (and later to Canada and New Zealand) while ensuring ethical recruitment practices and patient safety through evidence-based credentials evaluation (O'Day, 2007).

THINK BOX 9.2

Thinking about the role of CGFNS described earlier, what might be the effects of having a global equivalent where nurses could have an internationally recognised qualification and be able to work in any country?

Global Nurse Migration: Current Context

Before the COVID-19 pandemic, global migration was robust and increasing. In 2020, more than 280 million people resided outside their country of origin, a notable increase from 221 million in 2010 and 173 million in 2000 (United Nations Department of Economic and Social Affairs [UN DESA], 2020). While numbers stalled during the pandemic, we can expect a continued rise in global migration due to a range of issues from climate emergencies and natural disasters, war, and conflict, socioeconomic inequality, as well as increased opportunities in labour, education and technology (Shaffer et al., 2022a).

The World Health Organization's (WHO) 'State of the World's Nursing Report 2020' (SOWN) highlighted, for the first time at this scale, the current situation of the global nursing workforce, exposing dire nursing workforce shortages in most regions of the world. At the time of the report, the global shortage of nurses and midwives was estimated at 5.9 million, the majority of which were in low- and middle-income countries (World Health Organization [WHO], 2020). Follow-up research by the International Centre on Nurse Migration (ICNM) estimated a much higher shortage, due in large part to the pandemic, reaching upwards of 7 million (Buchan et al., 2022); these findings were supported by the WHO, which updated its estimated nurse shortage to 9 million or higher by 2030 (World Health Organization [WHO], 2022).

Regarding the global nurse migration landscape, we know today that one in eight nurses in the world is a migrant; that is, they are working in a country other than that in which they were born, educated or trained. Of this cohort, nearly three-quarters of these nurses are females, and the average age is around 30 years old. While nursing shortages exist in all regions of the world, many OECD countries are among the highest recipients of IENs. For example, IENs comprise around 8% of the Canadian nursing workforce, 15% in the United States and the United Kingdom, and upwards of 20% to 25% in Australia, Switzerland and New Zealand (Organisation for Economic Co-operation and Development [OECD], 2020). Filipino nurses comprise more than half of the US IEN workforce, followed by Canada, Kenya, India and Nigeria (CGFNS International, Inc. [CGFNS], 2022). While circumstances and immigration barriers may vary, the United

States is often used as an example to examine the state and trends of the world's nurse migrant workforce.

While global nurse migration has changed over the years, many of the typical 'push' and 'pull' factors remain the same. Though nurses migrate for a plethora of reasons, they typically are motivated by a standard set of 'push' factors, including lack of educational and professional opportunities, low pay, burnout, unsafe working conditions, lack of resources such as personal protective equipment, political instability, corruption, violence and the overall absence of safe and secure conditions. On the opposite end, there are many drivers among specific receiving countries, or 'pull factors', that encourage nurses to migrate, including better working conditions, higher wages, job security and advancement, educational opportunities, avenues to improve skills and remittances for families back home. The typical flow of labour is from lower-income developing countries to higher-income developed countries; however, recent shifts have been observed apart from typical 'south–north' patterns, including 'south–south' and even 'north–south' nurse migration flows (Shaffer et al., 2020).

As with all industries, the COVID-19 pandemic disrupted health care, nursing and global nurse migration. The pandemic both demonstrated and exacerbated a dire global demand for nurses and health care workers. In response to the COVID health emergency, governments, health systems and recruitment firms worldwide sought to increase nurse migration to fill gaps and shortages, particularly in high-income, developed countries. However, to stop the virus spread, much of the world closed its borders and focused efforts domestically. Following the WHO declaration of coronavirus as a pandemic in March 2020, nearly 110,000 mobility restrictions were enacted globally; at the same time, many exceptions were issued for nurse and health care migrants, demonstrating both the demand for the IEN workforce and also the fragility of the global nurse migration landscape (Shaffer et al., 2022b).

A few examples can be given to illustrate this fragility, particularly in times of crisis. The first is basic border shutdowns, as witnessed during the early days of the pandemic, as a response to global crises. In 2020, for example, 91% of the world's population resided in countries with travel restrictions, and 40% of the world lived in countries with borders that were closed

entirely (Shaffer et al., 2022b). The Republic of India, which comprises one of the most significant portions of IENs throughout much of Europe and the United States, restricted domestic travel within the subcontinent and banned all international flights to prevent the spread of the virus. In this situation, Indian nurses, even those who were granted work visas, though not explicitly targeted, were physically unable to migrate abroad and begin their contracts. A more targeted approach could be seen when Philippine President Rodrigo Duterte issued an executive order barring all domestically educated nurses from leaving the country in response to critical shortages and workforce concerns in the Philippines. Though this ban was short-lived and has since been lifted, an additional annual cap of 6500 Filipino nurse emigrants was enacted, a shocking decrease from the typical 17,000 Filipino nurses who travelled abroad in 2019 (Shaffer et al., 2022b). Despite a worsening global nursing shortage and the subsequent reliance on nurse recruitment and migration to fill gaps in health workforces, the delicacy of the global nurse migration framework should be noted, particularly as it relates to political movements and global emergencies.

Apart from the pandemic, several global movements are worth noting, as they, too, are likely to impact global nurse migration flows. The first is the seeming global political shift towards nationalism; this has been witnessed in all corners of the globe, including the United States under President Trump, Brazil under Bolsonaro, the United Kingdom and Brexit, and authoritarian shifts in Modi's India and Duterte's Philippines. The antiimmigrant sentiments and policies that often come from these governments could disrupt common nurse migration flows in the future or halt them altogether (as seen in the example earlier, though for a short time, in the Philippines).

The rise in global crises, from climate disasters to pandemics and global conflict, should be noted, as they relate to forced migration trends globally. Today, amidst the Russia-Ukraine conflict, the ongoing COVID-19 pandemic and increased climate emergencies, there are over 100 million forcibly displaced persons worldwide, one of the highest numbers ever recorded. Concerning nurses and nurse migrants, these groups should be considered in discussions around forced migration and refugee situations, as they not only care for these populations but are increasingly refugees themselves.

The Future of Nurse Migration

Today, one in seven people, or one billion, is a migrant. Though it slowed during the COVID-19 pandemic due to physical border shutdowns, global migration, including labour and nurse migration, is only expected to rise in years and decades. Similarly, the demand for health care workers will only rise in light of increased health emergencies and pandemics, ageing populations, particularly in the Global North, and nurse retention issues, which all signal a looming tsunami of global health care worker migration. Considering this anticipated tsunami, several issues impacting migration trends should be examined, including the evolving role of technology and security in health worker migration and advancements in credential evaluation processes and regulations.

As in most sectors of our world today, the rapid evolution of technology will undoubtedly disrupt the future of nurse migration. Increased transportation and communication technology facilitates increased migration and abilities to work and live in new lands. More specifically, technological advancements will shift the regulatory norms of nurse migration, particularly evaluating and transporting one's academic and professional credentials. One notable example was experienced during the pandemic when the collection and submission of primary source documents by migrating health care professionals (e.g., diplomas, transcripts, curriculum, licensure, registration) presented significant challenges due to unplanned closures of schools, government agencies and licensing regulators. In practice, the lag time between requesting, mailing and receipt of paper documents has resulted in delays for migrating nurses and other health care workers.

The digitisation of credentials has become increasingly essential and utilised to overcome common challenges with paper documentation and traditional 'snail mail' processes, as experienced during the COVID-19 pandemic. Digital credentials are easy to share and difficult to misplace, they protect the integrity and validity of documents, and they cut the typical costs of packaging and postage. Using CGFNS International, Inc. as an example, its new Digital Credentials Exchange provides an initial method for authorised agencies to submit documents for applicants. The standard methodology to verify primary-source documents requires the recording of qualified persons to submit materials on behalf of students/applicants. This is a burdensome method due primarily to turnover in primary source institutions which necessitates constant interaction and contact to maintain the current roster of acceptable administrators to submit the required documents. The development and implementation of a digital portal eliminate the constant update of personnel from agencies of interest while guaranteeing that documents come from their primary source. Similar methods and models, including utilising blockchain as a secure holding place for digital credentials, are increasingly becoming the norm among regulatory bodies, educational institutions and credential evaluation organisations worldwide, enabling more unrestricted flows of labourers and nurse migrants around the world.

The future and evolution of credentials evaluation processes for nurse and health care migrants broadly should be noted. Currently, policies and regulations governing the movement of nurses from one country to another safeguard the public by ensuring educational comparability and competence. The global movement of nurses and other health care workers calls for quality and safety competencies that meet national and global standards. With the broadening diversity of nurse migration worldwide, state boards of nursing and regulatory bodies have relied on credential evaluation to determine whether a nurse migrant meets the regulatory and education requirements in their country of destination. Additional factors to consider include the impacts of nurse migration on the domestic nursing workforce, issues determining educational comparability of nursing programs between countries, quality and safety concerns and strategies to transition and integrate nurse migrants into the workforce in their destination countries.

Furthermore, anticipating the future of credential evaluation requires consideration of educational program comparability versus equivalency, determinative assessment versus advisory assessment, the possibility of fraudulent documentation and customised credential evaluation reports. For a credential evaluation to serve its purpose and yield consistently reliable and valid results, attention needs to be directed not only to the character of the assessment but also to its content and methodology. Regulatory authorities and credential evaluation organisations must work closely to continually refine assessment processes and tools to achieve this shared goal. Still, further advancements are necessary—increased digitisation, cultural considerations and language requirements—to meet the demands of an increasingly complex yet interconnected, globalised world.

ETHICAL CONSIDERATIONS: THE DELICATE BALANCE BETWEEN THE RIGHT TO MIGRATE AND PROTECTING HEALTH SYSTEMS IN VULNERABLE REGIONS

The issue of global nurse migration is complex and delicate, particularly when considering the ethics of the topic. There are several competing interests and trade-offs concerning migration and nursing workforces, both at national and international levels, including the individual's right to migrate versus more significant ethical concerns, both within sending and receiving countries, regarding international recruitment. This section will attempt to untangle the complexities of nurse migration, international recruitment and ethics for the IENs themselves and the countries from which and to which they are migrating.

Today, it is commonly understood that an individual *nurse* has the right to live and work in their country of choice. Economic opportunities and workforce shortages have created mechanisms that allow for this mobility; nurse migration is only expected to increase in decades to come. For the individual nurse, there are many benefits gained from seeking work across borders. Firstly, working abroad has enormous personal economic and financial benefits. In many countries, particularly in the Global South, there are insufficient job opportunities for the actual supply of registered

nurses and nurse graduates. Beyond job opportunities, salary, career mobility and educational opportunities are significant drivers for nurses. In turn (and as mentioned earlier in the chapter), nurse migrants often send money back home to their families or communities, known as remittances, which contribute greatly to the economy of the sending country. The Philippines, the world's largest supplier of nurses, received upwards of USD $35 billion in remittances in 2020 and 2021, a number equivalent to 10% of the country's entire GDP (Shaffer et al., 2021; World Bank, 2021).

Stakeholders in high-income developed regions—the common receiving countries of nurse migrants—should consider several ethical concerns. Health care administrators, chief nursing officers and other executives have historically grappled with workforce sustainability and the temptation to rely on foreign-educated nurses as quick-fix solutions to shortages in their health systems. During the COVID-19 pandemic, amidst physical border shutdowns in the United States and around the world, US health systems were reminded of the dangers of overrelying on IENs as nurse immigration into the United States reached record lows. Instead, health systems should diversify their workforce to create sustainable models that leverage domestic and foreign-trained health care workers. The pandemic highlighted the dire need for strategic planning around health workforce sustainability amidst predicted future demands and fluctuations (Shaffer et al., 2022a).

THINK BOX 9.4

- What are the challenges to sustainable health workforce planning, especially for nurses?
  Think of the labour market model that draws our attention to recruitment, attrition and retirement within the context of national policies.
- In your country, what do you think the strengths and weak points are?

Despite the enormous financial and professional benefits for the individual nurse migrant and their families as well as the economic and cultural benefits for receiving countries, stakeholders in lower-income developing regions (i.e., typical heavy suppliers of nurses and health care workers) are also grappling with their own need to maintain health care workforces versus their lack of capacity to offer decent work to their nurses. Their citizens' right to migrate and the workforce issues associated with emigration are being weighed against the enormous economic contributions (i.e., remittances) that sending countries benefit from. For many countries in the developing world, remittances sent home by their migrant workers abroad make up considerable amounts of their economy's GDP.

At the international multilateral level, governments, policymakers and advocates must equally grapple with the individual nurse's right to migrate and the reality that nurse migration is only increasing and also think about brain drain and other issues around ethical international recruitment. In this context, several initiatives, namely, the UN Global Compact for Migration (GCM) and the WHO Global Code of Practice on International Recruitment of Health Personnel, sought to mitigate the possible adverse effects of migration, namely, unsafe, irregular and unethical migration and recruitment of nurse and health care migrants. Additionally, the WHO regularly identifies countries with critical health workforce shortages and encourages

countries, through its code, to not recruit from said countries as a matter of public health and safety.

CASE STUDIES

To better understand the complexities of global nurse migration, it is helpful to examine some case studies highlighting the individual journeys that different nurses take to leverage their educational and professional experience to work across borders. These three case studies will overview three varying situations of nurse migration. The first follows a commonly understood story of a Filipino nurse, Angelo, wishing to work in the United States. The second case study examines the challenges faced by nurses from turbulent regions or who were forced to migrate. This case study will follow two nurses, Natasha, a Ukrainian nurse refugee forced to flee her home in Kyiv due to the Russian invasion, and Fatima, a Syrian nurse refugee currently residing in the UNHCR refugee camp outside of Beirut, Lebanon. The final case study will look at a border nurse, Charlotte, who crosses the US–Canada border daily for work.

CASE STUDY 9.1

The Journey of a Filipino Nurse Migrant

Angelo, 30 years old, is a registered nurse who lives in Manila. He and his wife of 3 years, a US business consultant stationed in the Philippines, recently decided to move back to New Jersey, United States, to be closer to her family and ageing parents. Though he's never left his home in the Philippines, Angelo is eager to begin his new life in the United States.

For as long as he can remember, Angelo has always wanted to follow in his mother's footsteps and become a nurse. After much hard work, he completed his nursing education at a reputable nursing school in Manila. Since graduating, he's worked as an ICU nurse in a local hospital. He knew he wanted to continue working as a nurse in his new home.

To work in the United States, Angelo applied for an evaluation of his academic and professional credentials (e.g., diploma, transcripts, licensure, certifications), which was a requirement to sit for the NCLEX and gain licensure by the New Jersey State Board of Nursing.

Angelo's school was reputable; many of its graduates had successfully migrated abroad, securing work in Europe, North America and the Persian Gulf region. Given this, the evaluation process was relatively straightforward. The recruitment firm he worked with had years of experience with this process and quickly facilitated the secure transfer of his documents from their primary source to the credential evaluation organisation. Angelo's credentials were verified within a few weeks, and he was deemed comparable to a US-educated nurse.

Upon moving to New Jersey with his wife, Angelo soon after sat for the NCLEX examination, which he passed on his first try, securing him nursing licensure with the state and enabling him to return to practice in the ICU as a registered nurse. Given his easy access to documents, fluency in English and recruiter's familiarity with the typical Filipino nurse migration journey, Angelo was able to move to the United States and secure licensure relatively quickly.

CASE STUDY 9.2

Nurse Migration in Times of Crisis: Nurses Who Have Lost It All

It is not always the case that the nurse migration journey is as smooth as experienced by Angelo. His nursing education in the Philippines was primarily designed to migrate abroad and, therefore, easily transferable. His English language skills were strong. There were many resources in the Philippines and the United States to ensure his safe travel, stable employment and integration into the workplace and society. Above all, his government, professional nursing associations and educational institutions were fully functioning and willing to supply the necessary documentation to support his migration efficiently.

Nurses educated and trained in countries impacted by natural disasters, political instability or full-out war face great difficulties leveraging their well-earned credentials to work abroad. For some, the reliability of their professional and educational institutions to provide primary-source documentation (e.g., diplomas, transcripts, licensure, registration), which is a requirement for credential evaluation and migration, is either lacking or nonexistent. This case study will examine two stories, that of Natasha, a Ukrainian nurse refugee seeking work in the United States, and Fatima, a Syrian nurse refugee attempting to work in Lebanon, drawing similarities, differences and challenges faced by nurses who have lost it all.

NATASHA: A UKRAINIAN NURSE REFUGEE

Before the war, Natasha was a highly educated and relatively advanced nurse in her home in Kyiv. After earning her *Bakalavr* (bachelor's degree in nursing equivalent), Natasha continued to earn a *Magistr* (master's) in nursing science, becoming the first in her family to earn a postgraduate level of education. She has practiced nursing for nearly 20 years and worked as a nurse manager in her local hospital.

Following the Russian invasion of Ukraine in February 2022, Natasha made the difficult decision to leave her home and seek safety elsewhere in Europe or North America. Having extended family in Philadelphia, Pennsylvania, United States, she secured temporary refugee ('parole') status in the United States and made the journey across the world to her new home in Pennsylvania. Due to the rapid escalation of the conflict, Natasha left her home before being

able to secure some of her physical documents, most notably her two nursing diplomas and her licensure.

Upon arriving in the United States, Natasha vowed to do all she could to practice again as a nurse. To do this, she would be required to provide primary source documentation from her educational institution and licensing authority as hard evidence of her comparability to the US-educated and trained nurse. Unfortunately, she learned that her school of nursing, located on the outskirts of Kyiv, was severely damaged by shelling and could not deliver the documentation; the state of her documents remains unclear, as they were physically located in the school. Amazingly, she secured her proof of registration from her nursing council, which did not cease operations despite the conflict.

Natasha turned to CGFNS International, the primary credentials evaluation organisation for IENs seeking to work in the United States, to see if there was anything that could be done. To help those impacted by the war, CGFNS was waiving primary-source documentation requirements and, for the first time, accepting secondary or corroborative evidence, which would then be backed against an educational database and recognised seals and signatures.

After months of stress, Natasha's credentials were verified, and she secured Pennsylvania state licensure and was again able to practice as a registered nurse in her temporary home in Philadelphia. Though she hopes to return home someday, in the meantime, she can leverage her skills and competencies and support the US nursing workforce.

FATIMA: A SYRIAN-EDUCATED NURSE REFUGEE

Fatima shares a very similar story to Natasha. She, too, has been a practicing nurse for many years, nearly 15. After earning her baccalaureate and master's level of nursing education from the top university in Syria, she earned her doctorate in nursing and worked as a practicing nurse and nurse educator at her local academic hospital in Damascus. Fatima was among the top in her field and eager to bring her nurse leadership to international realms within the Middle East and North Africa region and beyond. Her plans quickly fell apart in March 2011 when her home, Syria, collapsed into a violent civil conflict.

Continued

Fatima was one of the lucky ones, or so she thought, as her university hospital in Damascus remained largely untouched during the early years of the conflict. Though the situation across the country was turbulent, she remained able to care for patients and provide education to the next generation of nurses. Finally, however, after a particularly violent week, her hospital and neighbourhood were critically damaged, forcing her and her family to leave Damascus, seeking refuge west in neighbouring Lebanon or Jordan.

Having ample time to prepare, Fatima was lucky in that she possessed the original copies of all her educational diplomas, transcripts and licensure documents. Having them with her, she hoped to return to work in her new place of refuge quickly. Upon arriving to Lebanon as a UNHCR refugee, Fatima was surprised to learn that refugees were only permitted to work in three low-skilled sectors, none of which included health care or nursing. Although she possessed the required documents for credentials evaluation and licensure abroad, Fatima could not practice in her new host country.

Given her inability to practice nursing in Lebanon because of her refugee status, she is seeking opportunities to move to Western Europe or North America to regain her right to practice. However, despite receiving her education from one of the top nursing schools in the region, public perceptions of Syrian refugees are less than favourable, especially in comparison to other groups such as Ukrainian refugees, only further challenging the process.

Though sharing a similar circumstance as Natasha, Fatima's experiences are vastly different, representing the range in disparity and privilege among IENs.

CASE STUDY 9.3

Border Nurses

While most migrating nurses reside in the countries where they practice, this is not the case for those from border towns and cities, such as between Canada and the United States. The case of Charlotte, a Canadian-educated nurse, will be used to demonstrate the journey of a border nurse.

Charlotte has lived in Windsor, Ontario, her entire life, though, given the proximity to Detroit, she has friends, family and colleagues on both sides of the border. After 4 years at a local Windsor University, she earned her baccalaureate degree in nursing, which qualified her for the NCLEX, a mandatory registration exam required for all nursing graduates wishing to practice in Canada and the United States.

Given better pay and career opportunities, Charlotte decided to work for a Detroit hospital, though she chose to remain at home in Windsor. Instead, like many border nurses, she would commute daily across the border for work. As per the 1994 North American Free Trade Agreement (NAFTA), since renamed the United States-Mexico-Canada Agreement, Charlotte is permitted to freely live and work in the United States with a specific 'TN visa'. On a daily basis, nearly a quarter of a million people and USD $1.5 billion in goods cross the United States–Canadian border (Coletta & Scruggs, 2020).

When COVID-19 was declared a pandemic in March 2020, Charlotte grew somewhat worried about the risks associated with working in a hospital setting; however, she remained committed to her patients and colleagues and vowed to support the fight against the virus in any way she should. This decision was often challenged, as she faced harsh stigma in her hometown, which had relatively low recorded cases of COVID compared to its neighbouring city of Detroit.

Unexpectedly, the United States and Canada announced the closure of their 5500-mile border to prevent the virus's spread. In an instant, Charlotte and thousands of other professionals, including health care workers, were seemingly stripped of their ability to work and care for their patients. Though nurses and health care workers were ultimately exempt from this border shutdown, daily commuters still faced many difficulties and confusion around the rules and requirements to cross and inconsistent interactions with different border agents.

Though Canadian and US nurses were ultimately unimpacted by the closure of their border, this was not the case for all nurse migrants. Particularly nurses educated outside of the United States faced many challenges travelling to and entering the United States during this period, even though they had immigrant work visas. Though many exceptions were made for health care and other essential workers, the pandemic and subsequent swift immigration and travel changes demonstrate the fragility of the current global nurse migration landscape and highlight additional barriers IENs face in practicing their profession.

MECHANISMS FOR MANAGING NURSE MIGRATION: ENSURING SAFE, ORDERLY AND REGULAR MIGRATION FOR ALL

In a world where increased health workforce shortages are only worsening due to ageing populations, health emergencies and workforce sustainability and retention issues, coupled with an anticipated increase in global migration flows, mechanisms for managing safe, ethical and regular migration of people, particularly nurses and health care workers, should be highlighted. This section will examine several noteworthy top-down, multilateral initiatives, such as the UN GCM and the WHO 2010 Code of Global Practice on the International Recruitment of Health Care Personnel (WHO Code), as well as bottom-up, grassroots initiatives, such as the CGFNS Alliance for Ethical International Recruitment Practices (the Alliance). Critical strategies for developing sustainable health care workforces will be noted to mitigate severe shortages and prevent dire demands of foreign-educated health care workforces as quick fixes. This, in turn, can ensure safe staffing levels, patient safety and sustainable health worker migration flows.

At the international level, several preexisting mechanisms can better manage the flow of health worker mobility and ensure safe and ethical migration. More broadly, the UN Global Compact for Safe, Orderly, and Regular Migration was built around global commitments to migrants and refugees as formalised in the 2016 UN General Assembly Resolution 71/1, *New York Declaration for Refugees and Migrants* (Shaffer et al., 2019; United Nations [UN], 2018; United Nations General Assembly [UNGA]). The compact, signed in 2018, was the first intergovernmentally negotiated agreement specifically addressing migration. The GCM stresses the importance of migrant empowerment and calls for efforts to ensure 'safe, orderly, and regular' migration for all. The 23 objectives and commitments of the document include the following:

- supporting vulnerable groups within migrant populations
- combatting human trafficking
- improving migrant documentation
- combatting xenophobia
- leveraging migrants' skills and experiences

Since its signing in 2018, the UN Global Compact has entered its national implementation phase through which federal governments and stakeholders are advocating for the domestic policy implementation of the goals and objectives laid out in the compact.

More specifically, to ensure safe and ethical *nurse* migration, multilateral efforts by the health care sector have been vital in fighting for international ethical recruitment. The WHO Code is a primary example (World Health Organization [WHO], 2010). The WHO Code is a multilateral mechanism attempting to manage the flow of nurse and health worker migration by ensuring safe and ethical recruitment. WHO Member State signatories of the code pledged to follow the code and report on their progress every 3 years. If correctly implemented and executed, the WHO Code serves as an effective response to the looming nurse and health worker migration tsunami (Shaffer et al., 2022a), though an evaluation of the impact of the code by Tam et al. (2016) found that it had not produced the tangible improvements in health worker flows it aspired to achieve. Tam et al. suggest several actions to improve the effectiveness of the code, including a focus on developing bilateral codes (i.e., between countries) and linking the code to topical global priorities.

Whereas the UN GCM and the WHO Code are top-down, multilateral initiatives, bottom-up and grassroots initiatives to manage safe and ethical nurse migration are equally as important. The Alliance is a worthy example of ethical international nurse recruitment in the United States. In 2008, amidst heightened international recruitment efforts to counter workforce shortages in the United States, many recorded unethical practices were carried out by unscrupulous actors in the recruitment realm. As a result, a multistakeholder task force comprised of recruitment firms, employers, nursing associations, union and credential evaluation organisations was assembled to address the situation and establish a voluntary code of practice for safe and ethical recruitment practices. In 2008, the Health Care Code for Ethical International Recruitment & Employment Practices (Alliance Code) was written, and the Alliance, now a division of CGFNS International, Inc., was established to advance its principles. Today, the Alliance Code has been adopted by dozens of the top recruitment firms in the United States, representing a large majority of the IENs and health care professionals currently being recruited to work in the United States (Alliance for Ethical International Recruitment Practices [Alliance], 2017).

Though the Alliance Code is voluntary and not administered or monitored by the government, the Alliance has developed a monitoring, remediation and verification process to certify that recruitment firms and organisations are adhering to the code and meeting ethical standards and practices. Every 2 years, certified firms must undergo a recertification assessment through which they report on their practices and commitments to the code. On the health professional's side, the Alliance provides internationally educated health care professionals and health care organisations with accurate and timely information on safe and ethical practices to ensure responsible decisions when considering working with a particular recruiter. Additionally, internationally educated health care professionals can contact the Alliance with questions or concerns about their contracts or relationships with the recruitment firm, through which the Alliance would carry out an investigation on behalf of the health care professional to ensure ethical practices. This dual model has proven successful in guaranteeing the ethical recruitment of health personnel in the United States and should be considered and replicated in other regions of the world.

While different in functionality and reporting, the two codes support each other and work harmoniously.

The WHO Code provides the international framework and principles for international cooperation and multilateralism, while the Alliance Code provides tangible guidelines for individual employers, recruitment firms and health care migrants to ensure ethical recruitment practices at all levels (Shaffer et al., 2016).

THINK BOX 9.5

Can recruiting nurses from low- to high-income countries ever be ethical?

Managing Nurse Migration Through Domestic Policies and Considerations

In addition to these initiatives to address and manage regular, safe and ethical migration, particularly as it pertains to the recruitment aspect of migration, other mechanisms work to manage nurse migration by ensuring safe and sustainable domestic staffing and workforce levels, educational capabilities and health workforce retention that decrease the extreme need for nurse migrants as short-fix solutions. Some of the most impactful domestic policies and considerations to ensure safe and sustainable health workforces include supporting older nurses, combatting nurse burnout, improving retention and diversifying workforces.

A 2020 report by the ICNM, a partnership between CGFNS International and the International Council of Nurses (ICN), focused on interprofessional ageing and policies to better support older nurses at work. The report highlighted that, globally, one in six nurses is over 55 and expected to retire in the next 10 years; health crises such as the COVID-19 pandemic threaten to shorten this time dramatically. It is estimated that around 5 million new nurses will have to be educated and trained to replace those retiring nurses; this number is in addition to the 7 million nurses already needed to meet growing demands. To address this, the ICNM proposed a 10-point plan for supporting older nurses to lessen the burden on them, maintain their experiences in the workforce and lessen future shortages of nurses (Buchan et al., 2020). This is one of many strategies that can be taken domestically to reduce deficits and the dire need for foreign-educated health care recruitment.

ICNM's 10-Point Plan for Supporting Older Nurses

1. Understand the workforce profile and employment needs of older nurse by conducting surveys, focus groups and nurse labour market analysis.
2. Avoid age bias in recruitment and employment practices.
3. Provide flexible working opportunities that meet older nurses' requirements.
4. Ensure that older nurse have equal access to relevant learning and career opportunities.
5. Ensure that occupational health and safety policies enable staff well-being.
6. Support job redesign to reduce heavy workload and stress and support job enrichment to optimist contribution of older nurses.
7. Maintain a pay and benefits system that meets older nurses' needs and rewards experience.
8. Support older nurses in advanced and specialist practices and mentorship and preceptor roles.
9. Maintain succession planning to enable knowledge transfer and leadership development.
10. Provide retirement planning options and, where appropriate, flexible pension provisions.

In additional to supporting older nurses and to slow increasing rates of retirement within the profession, additional retention strategies were suggested by ICNM in their 2022 report, 'Sustain and Retain in 2022 and Beyond: The Global Nursing Workforce and the COVID-19 Pandemic'. This report had the hindsight of the pandemic, during which time the nursing profession experienced high levels of burnout, mistreatment and retention issues. The report predicted the future global nursing shortage not at 5.9 million, as previously predicted before the pandemic, but upwards of 7 million or higher. In response to enormous pressures on the nursing profession as intensified by the COVID-19 pandemic, this report laid out a set of long-term policy responses at national and international levels that should be taken to ensure workforce sustainability (Buchan et al., 2022).

National Policy Responses

Act	Plan
Commit to support safe staffing levels, including consistent application of staffing methods, necessary resource allocation and health system good governance	Review and expand the capacity of the domestic nurse education system
Commit to support early access to full vaccination programs for all nurses	Assess and improve retention of nurses and the attractiveness of nursing as a career through fair pay and benefits, structured career opportunities and access to continuing education
Commit to regular nurse workforce impact assessments to develop a better understanding of pandemic impact on individual nurses and the overall nursing workforce	Implement policies to enable the nursing workforce contribution to the pandemic response to be optimised (e.g., supporting advanced practice and specialisation, skills mix and working patterns, teamworking and provision of appropriate technology)
	Monitor and track domestic nurse self-sufficiency to determine the level of reliance on foreign-born and trained nurses

Continued

International Policy Responses

Act	Plan
Support and immediate and regular update of the WHO's SOWN data and analysis	Commit to early access to full vaccination programs for all nurses in all countries
	Implement and evaluate effective and ethical approaches to managed international supply of nurses through collected approaches framed within a fuller implementation of the WHO Global Code of Practice on the International Recruitment of Health Personnel
	Support regular and systematic nurse workforce impact assessments, particularly in resource-constrained countries
	Invest in nurse workforce sustainability in small states, lower-income states and fragile states, those most vulnerable to nurse outflow and those most impacted by the pandemic

The dual urgent action items and long-term visions are necessary to ensure sustainable health care workforces beyond the COVID-19 pandemic. Though not in direct reference to nurse migration, mechanisms that focus on nurse retention, supporting older nurses and national self-sufficiency will ensure stable supply and demand of IENs, in turn stabilising global nurse migration flows and trends. While foreign-educated health care professionals can serve as a piece of the puzzle in addressing health workforce shortages, over-reliance on this group as 'quick-fixes' jeopardises both the sustainability and longevity of health workforces in both sending and receiving countries.

THE ROLE OF NURSE LEADERS: DESIGNING OUR FUTURE

Since the beginning of the profession, nursing has maintained an active role at the global level, be it in international education, policy or practice. For centuries, nurses have migrated worldwide, carrying their educational and professional competencies to new lands and workforces. Concerning global policy, nursing's position has been equally as robust. Since the founding

of the United Nations in 1945 and the WHO in 1948, for example, nursing has proactively advocated for nursing-centric policies, elevating the profession's status and ensuring a seat at decision-making tables. This leadership has only been encouraged and advanced during the 21st century; today, nurses are at the forefront of global health care and policy. Nurse leaders should leverage the profession's years in the advocacy and policy spheres and its recent recognition by governments and the public to advance nursing-positive policies at local, national and global levels.

To do this effectively, we, as a profession, must train the next generation of nurses to be global citizens, leveraging their local knowledge, skills and experience and taking them to the international policy level. A nurse of the future must be able to contextualise their local work at the bedside within more significant global initiatives and issues. As a profession, we should disrupt commonly assumed norms, pushing beyond a basic seat at the table and ensuring our active involvement and consultation in policy as stakeholders, board members and government representatives. There are several worthy initiatives aiming at this that are worth mentioning. The Nurses on Boards Coalition aims to ensure significant nursing representatives are on boards and strives for a meaningful impact on nursing leadership (Nurses on Boards Coalition, n.d.). Globally, the ICN's Call to Action to establish government chief nursing officers within all WHO member states and WHO regions is an admirable initiative for ensuring nursing engagement and participation in policy at the global level and all areas of the world (International Council of Nurses [ICN], 2020).

Regarding nurse migration, several specific policy considerations are worth thinking about with regard to nursing leadership and our profession's role at national and global policymaking tables. It is undeniable that the COVID-19 pandemic only exacerbated the worldwide demand for nurses in nearly all regions of the world; the global shortages of nurses and health care professionals are not likely to let up but, rather, intensify due to an array of factors such as educational limitations of nursing schools, workforce demographic changes (e.g., retiring nurses, burnout, high turnover rates) and public demographic shifts (e.g., increased pandemics and illnesses, ageing populations). Historically, in times of workforce shortage, particularly in the Global North, international recruitment of nurses and health personnel skyrockets, raising several concerns that future generations of nursing leaders should consider.

Firstly, while nurse migrants bring various economic and cultural benefits to workforces and economies, international recruitment is a short-term solution to workforce shortages. Though internationally educated health care workers bring enormous benefits, their recruitment should not be the sole solution to addressing health workforce shortages; international recruitment should be coupled with investments in domestic workforces, educational systems and strategies to retain and sustain. Additionally, an overreliance on nurse migration and international recruitment can lead to severe shortages in typical sending countries, often in underdeveloped regions, creating an ethical dilemma. In terms of ethics, not only should the state of sending countries' workforces be considered when recruiting but a commitment to safe and ethical recruitment models and practices should be enforced; both top-down and bottom-up codes of ethical standards, such as the WHO Code and CGFNS Alliance Code, should be leveraged and furthered (Shaffer et al., 2022b).

CONCLUSION

This chapter highlighted the importance of nurse migration for individual nurses and sending and receiving countries as well as the ethical considerations and dangers of overreliance on IENs. Managing health worker migration is crucial to balancing the supply of nurses with increasing demand. As the WHO's 2020 SOWN report made clear, one in eight nurses works outside of their country of birth and education. Nursing is a globally sourced profession that requires proactive and multistakeholder management to ensure the safe and ethical migration and recruitment of nurses and health care workers.

Though this topic is complex and ever changing, several key conclusions can be drawn:

- Global migration, including nurse migration, is on the rise and is only expected to increase; today, one in seven people globally is a migrant, and one in eight nurses works abroad.
- Nurses migrate abroad due to a variety of push factors, including lack of educational and professional opportunities, low pay, burnout, unsafe working conditions, lack of resources (e.g., personal protective equipment), political instability, corruption, violence and the overall absence of safe working conditions, and pull factors, including better working conditions, higher wages, job security, educational opportunities, avenues to improve skills and remittances for families back home.
- There are several competing interests and trade-offs concerning migration and nursing workforces, both at national and international levels, including the individual's right to migrate versus more significant ethical concerns regarding safe staffing levels, brain drain and ethical international recruitment.
- To ensure the safe and ethical migration of nurses, there are several noteworthy examples, including multilateral efforts such as the UN GCM and the WHO Code, as well as domestic efforts such as the Alliance and its health care code.
- Though not in direct reference to nurse migration, mechanisms focusing on nurse retention, supporting older nurses and national self-sufficiency will ensure a stable supply and demand of IENs, stabilising global nurse migration flows and trends.

- While foreign-educated health care professionals can serve as a piece of the puzzle in addressing health workforce shortages, overreliance on this group as 'quick fixes' jeopardises both the sustainability and longevity of health workforces in sending and receiving countries.
- The nursing profession is strategically positioned to leverage its years in the advocacy and policy spheres and its recent recognition by governments and the public to advance nursing-positive policies at local, national and global levels.

THINK BOX 9.6

Imagine you take on the following roles. What will the perspective be of international nurse migration from each player?

1. A minister of health in a recruiting country
2. A nurse in a recruiting country with severe shortages
3. A minister of finance in a 'sending' country
4. A nurse manager in a 'sending' country
5. The CNO at WHO Geneva

This exercise shows how systems thinking is critical in considering the complexities of global nurse migration.

IDEAS FOR FUTURE READING

The global nurse migration landscape is increasingly complex and evolving. Given both the rise in global migration in general and the global shortage of nurses and health care professionals, global nurse migration is a topic that will increasingly become visible and relevant for the nursing community in all regions of the world. For this reason, it's important to remain abreast on current and future trends in nurse migration, including shifts in commonly assumed flows, the role of evolving technology and ethical considerations associated with this topic. You may find the following reports and publications particularly helpful to take deeper dives into the topics of nurse migration, human resources for health and ethical international recruitment practices.

The *ICNM*, a collaboration between the ICN and CGFNS International, is the leading resource and repository for research and reporting on global nurse migration and human resources in nursing. ICNM regularly features news, resources and publications on this topic that are relevant for policymakers, planners and practitioners alike. Two reports of interests include:

- Buchan, J., Catton, H., & Shaffer, F. A. (2020). *Ageing well? Policies to support older nurses at work*. International Centre on Nurse Migration. https://www.icn.ch/sites/default/files/inline-files/Ageing%20ICNM%20Report%20December%209%202020.pdf
- Buchan, J., Catton, H., & Shaffer, F. A. (2022). *Sustain and retain in 2022 and beyond: The global nursing workforce and the COVID-19 pandemic*. International Centre on Nurse Migration. https://www.icn.ch/sites/default/files/2023-04/Sustain%20and%20Retain%20in%202022%20and%20Beyond-%20The%20global%20nursing%20workforce%20and%20the%20COVID-19%20pandemic.pdf

For the most timely and comprehensive data on global nurse migration, readers should look to the WHO, including its momentous 'State of the World's Nursing Report 2020: Investing in Education, Jobs, and Leadership'. The WHO has committed to revisiting this document and updating the data on a regular basis. The next 'State of the World' report will be published in 2025. It is important to contribute to data collection when you can.

REFERENCES

Alliance for Ethical International Recruitment Practices (Alliance). (2017, *revised*). *Health care code for ethical international recruitment and employment practices*. Retrieved, December 01, 2022, from https://www.cgfnsalliance.org/wp-content/uploads/2019/03/Health-Care-Code-for-EIREP-Sept-2017_FINAL.pdf.

Buchan, J., Catton, H., & Shaffer, F. A. (2020). *Ageing well? Policies to support older nurses at work*. International Centre on Nurse Migration. Retrieved, December 1, 2022, from. https://www.icn.ch/sites/default/files/inline-files/Ageing%20ICNM%20Report%20December%209%202020.pdf.

Buchan, J., Catton, H., & Shaffer, F. A. (2022). *Sustain and retain in 2022 and beyond: The global nursing workforce and the COVID-19 pandemic*. International Centre on Nurse Migration. Retrieved, December 1, 2022, from https://www.icn.ch/resources/publications-and-reports/sustain-and-retain-2022-and-beyond.

Caulin, V. (2018). How the Philippines created a global network of nurses. *Culture Trip [Blog]*. Retrieved, December 1, 2022 from https://theculturetrip.com/asia/philippines/articles/why-are-there-so-many-filipino-nurses/.

CGFNS International, Inc. (CGFNS). (2022). In: Bakhshi, M., Álvarez, T. D., & Cook, K. (Eds.), *CGFNS nurse migration report: Trends in healthcare migration to the United States*. Retrieved, December 1, 2022, from www.cgfns.org/2022nursemigrationreport.

Coletta, A., & Scruggs, G. (2020). Americans, Canadians scramble to get home before border shuts down. *Washington post*. Retrieved, December 1, 2022, from https://www.washingtonpost.com/world/the_americas/americans-canadians-scramble-to-get-home-before-border-largely-shuts-down/2020/03/20/bd997a20-6a4e-11ea-b199-3a9799c54512_story.html.

International Council of Nurses (ICN). (2020). Government chief nursing officer (GCNO) positions. *ICN briefing*. Retrieved, December 1, 2022, from https://www.icn.ch/system/files/documents/2020-01/ICN%20briefing_GCNO_ENG.pdf.

Lorenzo, F. M. E., Galvez-Tan, J., Icamiina, K., & Javier, L. (2007). Nurse migration from a source country perspective: Philippines country case study. *Health Research and Educational Trust, 42*(3), 1406–1418.

Nursing on Boards Coalition. (N.d.). Nursing on boards coalition: Make the most trusted, your trustee. *Website*. Retrieved, December 1, 2022, from https://www.nursesonboardscoalition.org/.

O'Day, V. (2007). A brief history of the commission on graduates of foreign nursing schools: Shaping policy through collaboration. *Journal of the New York State Association, 38*(1), 6–8.

Organisation for Economic Co-operation and Development (OECD). (2020). *Contribution of migrant doctors and nurses to tackling COVID-19 crisis in OECD countries*. OECD Brief. Retrieved, December 1, 2022, from https://www.oecd.org/coronavirus/policy-responses/contribution-of-migrant-doctors-and-nurses-to-tackling-covid-19-crisis-in-oecd-countries-2f7bace2/.

Ortiga, Y. Y. (2017). The flexible university: Neoliberal education and the global production of migrant labor. *British Journal of Sociology of Education, 38*(4), 485–499, doi:10.1080/01425692.2015.1113857.

Shaffer, F. A., & To Dutka, J. (2013). Global mobility for internationally educated nurses: Challenges and regulatory implications. *Journal of Nursing Regulation, 4*(3), 11–16.

Shaffer, F. A., Bakhshi, M., To Dutka, J., & Philips, J. (2016). Code for ethical international recruitment practices: The CGFNS alliance case study. *Human Resources for Health, 14*(Suppl 1), 113–119.

Shaffer, F. A., Bakhshi, M., Farrell, N., & Álvarez, T. (2019). The role of nurses in advancing the objectives of the global compacts for migration and on refugees. *Nursing Administration Quarterly, 43*(1), 10–18.

Shaffer, F. A., Bakhshi, M. A., Farrell, N., & Álvarez, T. D. (2020). The recruitment experience of foreign-educated health professionals to the United States. *American Journal of Nursing, 120*(1), 28–38.

Shaffer, F. A., Bakhshi, M. A., Cook, K. N., & Álvarez, T. D. (2021). The contributions of immigrant nurses in the U.S. During the COVID-19 pandemic: A CGFNS international study. *Nurse Leader, 19*(2), 198–203.

Shaffer, F. A., Alvarez, T. D., & Stievano, A. (2022a). Guaranteeing dignity and decent work for migrant nurses and health care workers beyond the COVID-19 pandemic. *Journal of Nursing Management, 30*(8), 3918–3921.

Shaffer, F. A., Bakhshi, M., Cook, K., & Álvarez, T. D. (2022b). International nurse recruitment beyond the COVID-19 pandemic: Considerations for the nursing workforce leader. *Nurse Leader, 20*(2), 161–167.

Sherwood, G. D., & Shaffer, F. A. (2014). The role of internationally educated nurses in a quality, safe workforce. *Nursing Outlook, 62*, 46–52.

Shin, S. R., Shin, K. R., & Li, C. Y. (2002). Nursing education systems in Korea, China and the United States of America and its future directions. *Journal of Korean Academy of Nursing, 32*(7), 949–959.

Solano, D., & Rafferty, A. M. (2007). Can lessons be learned from history? The origins of the British imperial nurse labour market: A discussion paper. *International Journal of Nursing Studies, 44*(6), 1055–1063.

Tam, V., Edge, J. S., & Hoffman, S. J. (2016). Empirically evaluating the WHO global code of practice on the international recruitment of health personnel's impact on four high-income countries four years after adoption. *Globalization and Health, 12*, 62.

United Nations (UN). (2018). *Global compact for safe, orderly and regular migration*. Retrieved, December 1, 2022, from https://refugeesmigrants.un.org/sites/default/files/180713_agreed_outcome_global_compact_for_migration.pdf.

United Nations General Assembly (UNGA). (2018). *Resolution 71/1, New York declaration for refugees and migrants 2016*. Retrieved, December 1, 2022, from. https://www.un.org/en/development/desa/population/migration/generalassembly/docs/globalcompact/A_RES_71_1.pdf.

United Nations Department of Economic and Social Affairs (UN DESA). (2020). *International migration 2020 highlights*. Retrieved, December 1, 2022. https://www.un.org/development/desa/pd/sites/www.un.org.development.desa.pd/files/undesa_pd_2020_international_migration_highlights.pdf.

US Library of Congress. (2011). Treaty of Paris of 1898. *The world of 1898: The Spanish American War*. [Website]. Retrieved, December 1, 2022, from https://www.loc.gov/rr/hispanic/1898/treaty.html#:~:text=The%20islands%20of%20Puerto%20Rico,signed%20on%20December%2010%2C%201898.

World Bank. (2021). Personal remittances received (% of GDP)—Philippines. *Webpage*. Retrieved, December 1, 2022, from https://data.worldbank.org/indicator/BX.TRF.PWKR.DT.GD.ZS?locations=PH.

World Health Organization (WHO). (2010). *The WHO global code of practice on the international recruitment of health personnel*. Sixty-third World Health Assembly—WHA63.16. Retrieved, December 1, 2022, from https://www.who.int/publications/m/item/migration-code.

World Health Organization (WHO). (2020). *State of the world's nursing 2020: Investing in education, jobs, and leadership*. Retrieved December 01, 2022, from, https://www.who.int/publications/i/item/9789240003279.

World Health Organization (WHO). (2022). Nursing and midwifery. Retrieved, May 6, 2022, from https://www.who.int/newsroom/fact-sheets/detail/nursing-and-midwifery.

Yeates, N. (2011). Ireland, transnationalism and the global nursing crises. In: Murch, R., & Fanning, B. (Eds.), *Globalization, migration, and social transformation: Ireland in Europe and the world*. Ashgate.

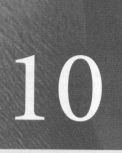

10

NURSES FINDING A GLOBAL VOICE. 1. BECOMING INFLUENTIAL LEADERS THROUGH ADVOCACY

ELIZABETH MADIGAN ■ GRETA WESTWOOD ■ EMILY MCWHIRTER ■ RUTH OSHIKANLU ■ BARBARA STILWELL

INTRODUCTION

For many years, nurses have been working to take their rightful place at leadership tables. There is prepandemic evidence of the barriers to this important contribution to global health, including being a female-predominant workforce (Daly et al., 2015). The historical views of nursing show it being less socially desirable or softer as a career, and a profession closely related to the roles of females in their personal lives (Nursing Now, 2019). The COVID-19 pandemic showed the world, often in new ways, the contributions of nurses to the health care workforce and that without nurses, there was no one to provide the care needed by the ill and dying, give lifesaving vaccines or do health promotion/disease prevention for the world's population. Although we will not know the full impact of the pandemic on nursing for a number of years, reports confirm that thousands of nurses died from COVID-19 through occupational exposure (World Health Organization, 2021). The revelations of the pandemic about the failures of the health systems to support nurses at a time when nurses were essential to every part of the care pathway are indefensible. These failings, combined with the historical barriers to nurse leadership, have brought the nursing profession to a moment that requires strong action on their part to step up and step into leadership positions to become more effective advocates for themselves and their colleagues.

What will nursing leaders of the future have to do to be more successful than their past colleagues? This chapter will provide some of those answers, recognizing that the future is always uncertain, especially as the world moves into its new state following COVID-19. The overarching theme for this chapter is nurses as advocates. While nurses have always learned how to be advocates for their patients and clients, the next phase of nursing leadership will require nurses to advocate for themselves within their organizations, with their political and governmental leaders and within their communities for support and action. For nurses who have been in the profession for any period of time, the need for advocacy for one's self and other nurses runs counter to the humility that many nurses portray in their daily work. Terms such as 'just' a nurse' or 'it's my job' are often used by nurses when describing what they do (Salvage & Stilwell, 2018) which resonates with some studies that have shown nurses to have low self-esteem (Serafin et al. [2022] is a good discussion of the role of self-esteem in nursing competence; see also Chapter 8 in this book for further discussion). The result of not being heard professionally is that the contribution of nursing to patient care is not articulated or recognized as important. When nursing's essential work is recognized, as it was during the pandemic, then nurses are called out as 'superheroes' rather than being recognised for their professional technical competence delivered with empathy and comfort in times of physical and mental pain.

THINK BOX 10.1

In your country, what do you think is the image of nursing held by (1) the public, (2) other professions such as medicine or pharmacy, and (3) the media? You may want to ask some of your friends and family to respond to this, too.

- How can your image be changed?
- What would need to happen?

Cardoso and colleagues examined 1271 health-related news items in the Portuguese media in 2011, finding that nurses were the source of information in only 6.6% of those news items (Cardoso et al., 2014). The Woodhull Studies, conducted in the United States in 1998 and 2018, found that the proportion of nurses cited in the US media fell from 4% in 1998 to 2% in 2018 (Mason et al., 2018). When 'experts' were cited during the pandemic, they were often physicians, and they were even talking about nursing issues and nurse staffing (Mason, 2020). There are a number of reasons for this, including nurses' discomfort with interacting with public media and restrictions by employers on what nurses can say about their jobs. While the latter is more challenging, nurses have experience with talking with the lay public in their professional roles and can undertake media training to become more effective advocates for their work, the profession and the people they care for. This is not the usual type of advocacy that nurses think about, but it can be persuasive when making a case for change, especially with the public.

Nurses as advocates: Florence Nightingale was a tireless advocate for nursing, using her connections to high levels in government to influence policymakers to invest in nursing and health care. She spoke and wrote about the importance of standards of care, discipline and cleanliness, and used her position and influence to highlight the need for females to 'understand the fundamental needs of the sick and the principles of good nursing'. Her 'Notes on Nursing, What It Is and What It Is Not', first published in 1860, were used to inform and educate females about both the art and science of nursing.

What is often forgotten about Florence Nightingale is that her notes were backed up by data and evidence. She was the first female member of the Royal Society of Statistics and was greatly respected for her use and presentation of data. She advocated for basic amenities, though at that time, the importance of clean, well-ventilated environments, the need for regular observation of a patient's clinical condition and the benefit of healthy food to support healing were not widely known or accepted. Hospitals were dangerous places, dirty and full of infection; wealthy people opted to be nursed at home (Wyatt [2019] discusses conditions in relation to the development of nursing). But Nightingale's effective advocacy meant

that her voice was heard by those who were building institutions and organisations to care for the sick, and many of her recommendations were adopted. Her role as an advocate for the hygienic care of patients has influenced generations of nurses and others with responsibility for health care.

Florence Nightingale has far more to teach nurses today than is usually attributed to her. She was, above all, a brilliant communicator visually and verbally, adept at presenting data in a graphic form to show her audience where they needed to act. She understood the power of statistics to change minds (Rafferty, 2020; Rouleau et al., 2019). In other words, what Nightingale did was to create a bridge between nursing and policymakers so she could give evidence to policymakers in a way they understood. The Nursing Now campaign (Holloway et al., 2021) also used bridging techniques to influence governments and policymakers and, like Nightingale, used connections that the campaign had with high-level health policymakers and influencers. The Nursing Now report presents the stories of what happened as a result of nurses becoming high-level influencers, notably that several governments increased their investment in nursing during the campaign.

THINK BOX 10.2

Can you think of ways that you might connect with a high-level policymaker or influencer in your country?

Maybe one of your ministers has a relative who is or was a nurse—for example, President Jimmy Carter's mother was a nurse, and he has been a great advocate for, and supporter of, nurses. The Nursing Now campaign had a well-known actor as an advocate, as she had experienced the importance of nursing first hand. Identifying such a person in your community can help to get nursing messages out.

SPEAKING UP—FOR OTHERS AND OURSELVES

Our early lessons as student nurses teach us the importance of promoting patient-centred care, ensuring that patients are empowered to choose, be informed and be in control of their health care. This type of advocacy has become a normal process for many nurses around the world as we seek to speak up for vulnerable patients who are unable have a voice of their own. The concept of advocacy goes beyond the provision of good nursing practice to ensuring that patients, families and others providing care are kept well informed.

Nurses have a key role as educators for patients. Giving information about illness and disease and advice around treatment options and medication choices are types of advocacy that build trust and confidence in nurses. Patient education is a core skill required of all nurses. Presenting balanced, clear information in a way that the patient will understand and accept is a skill that builds the reputation of the profession as honest and ethically trustworthy. Year after year, nurses have been recognised as the most trusted profession (Ipsos Veracity Index, 2022), in part due to the role we play as advocates for those we care for.

This is particularly important in the care and support of marginalised and fragile communities. Nurses play an essential role in advocating for vulnerable groups, and the potential to use their voice to influence is an important tool in the development and improvement of health services around the world. In many countries, nurses play a critical role in supporting vulnerable patients to seek treatments for diseases that may be stigmatised (Rouleau et al., 2019). By advocating for gender equity, human rights and access to health services, nurses may enable patients to access medical care for diseases such as HIV, mental health disorders and certain cancers, where there is fear of abuse or stigma. This kind of advocacy can also play a powerful role in influencing health care policy to create accessible services for people who may be anxious to come forward for treatment, by creating demand and highlighting the issues.

THINK BOX 10.3

In your present role, are you an advocate for individuals for whom you are caring or for their families?

Jot down the things that you do that you consider to be advocacy.

Nitzky (2018) proposes six ways in which nurses advocate for patients:

- **Ensure safety.** Ensure that the patient is safe when being treated in a health care facility and, when they are discharged, by communicating with case managers or social workers about the patient's need for home health or assistance after discharge so that it is arranged before they go home.
- **Give patients a voice.** Give patients a voice when they are vulnerable by staying in the room with them, while the doctor explains their diagnosis and treatment options, to help them ask questions, get answers and translate information from medical jargon.
- **Educate.** Educating patients on how to manage their current or chronic condition to improve the quality of their everyday life is an important way nurses can make a difference. For example, patients undergoing chemotherapy can benefit from the nurse teaching them how to take their antinausea medication in a way that will be most effective for them and will allow them to feel better between treatments.
- **Protect patients' rights.** Protect patients' rights by knowing their wishes: this might include communicating those to a family member who disagrees with the patient's choices.
- **Double check for errors.** Everyone makes mistakes. Nurses can catch, stop and fix errors and flag conflicting orders, information or oversights by physicians or others caring for the patient.
- **Connect patients to resources.** Help patients find resources inside or outside the hospital to support their well-being. Be aware of resources in the community that you can share with the patient such as financial assistance, transportation, patient or caregiver support networks or helping them meet other needs.

Developing skills to advocate in any setting or at any level requires training. Whilst many of us may be comfortable speaking up and confident when presenting a well-balanced argument, advocacy requires a measured and considered perspective, best learnt from experts and fine-tuned by practice (Souders, 2020). Successful advocates are those who present evidence using reliable sources of data and are clear about their messages and purpose. Whether talking to a patient or a politician, they adapt their messages to their audience, using techniques that will strengthen their argument or emphasise a key point.

In clinical settings, nurses will often adapt their approach to a situation depending on their task. Persuading a child to accept a vaccination requires gentle, clear and subtle advocacy to ensure they understand why it is good for them, but in contrast, influencing a hospital management team to purchase new equipment may require a presentation requiring detailed data analysis and robust evidence. Both use similar skills around influence but in very different ways. Understanding how to structure an argument to influence and advocate is an important skill to acquire when developing competencies for leadership.

THINK BOX 10.4

As a nurse leader, when might it be important to speak up about concerns related to the quality of care that patients are receiving?

One example from the United Kingdom is the relationship between the number of qualified nursing staff and the quality of care in a facility—whose business is this? Who would need to be persuaded (advocacy) that action was needed?

The article by Tomajan (2012), cited in this chapter, helps answer these questions.

INFLUENCING PUBLIC POLICY— ADVOCATING FOR SYSTEMIC CHANGE

Cullerton et al. (2018) discuss the complexities of influencing public policy, especially for poorly resourced advocates—which often include nurses. They developed a conceptual model to show key steps for those wishing to influence policymakers. This model was developed specifically for nutritionists, but it is worth exploring and adapting for nurses, too. In this section, we present some key steps from that and other models and relate them to nursing knowledge so that nurse leaders can become better leaders in advocacy for public policy.

What's in Our Toolbox?

As we develop and learn new skills through nurse training and through clinical experiences, we acquire additional professional tools which strengthen our ability to advocate successfully. Advocacy is a complex process that requires a combination of skills which nurses often learn as part of nursing practice, so

becoming aware of how good your skills are in these areas is important for leadership (Tomajan, 2012).

1. **Understanding the context**

   Nurses who want to be health care policy influencers must have knowledge of the national and local systems in which health care is delivered. This will include financing of care and wider health workforce issues, such as migration or the education system, as well as epidemiology and demography. This combination of knowledge is part of political know-how, and nurses do not routinely understand the political scene (Salvage & Stilwell, 2018). But to be an effective advocate to policymakers, understanding the political context is vital so as to be able to identify and use windows for change.

   Part of understanding context is understanding where power lies and where responsibility for decision-making lies, too (Cullerton et al., 2018). Mapping the stakeholder landscape is a good foundational step for advocacy to identify where efforts can best be directed for change, as it is not always obvious.

THINK BOX 10.5

- Where is the power to make decisions held in your organisation?
- What gives the power?
- Is it holding a budget or being connected to policymakers?

2. **Problem-solving**

   What problem or issue are you trying to address? Sometimes this step is missed, and there is no specificity of what is being addressed. For example, trying to advocate for improving care in a health facility involves finding the individual causes—for example, too few staff, staff not qualified to deal with health issues, or no medicines available—and advocating for each to be changed.

   It is likely that you will have to approach a decision-maker or budget holder with a request for change or action, so think about what the request will be and what evidence you have that action is needed. Present evidence in a compelling way—so make it short, easy to read, hear or understand, and attractive to look at. You may not be successful the first time—and may require a series of actions over time and with others in order to achieve a desired outcome. Persistence is key.

3. **Build relationships**

If you take the time to make a stakeholder map* of those involved in any decision you want to influence, you will see a network of people with whom you should be building relationships. This is not to manipulate but, rather, to learn about their vested interests and to develop trust between you on the issues that you will be trying to change or solve.

Nurses are consistently the most trusted profession, as we have said earlier, but interestingly, they are not often sought by media to give expert opinions (Mason, 2020). To be really influential, nurses need to change this. Managing up—towards those top bosses—is just as important as managing your team, but it's not nearly as often discussed in leadership training. Building relationships with stakeholders can also help identify your allies for any particular change so that you can collaborate to be more powerful. Collaboration means working with other individuals or groups to achieve a common goal rather than working together (cooperating) to achieve individual goals.

Collaboration, like most of the strategies for advocacy, is built on trust, mutual respect and credibility. The end result of groups collaborating to achieve a common goal can be greater than that which each group could accomplish independently.

4. **Develop communication skills**

Successfully communicating for advocacy requires both heart and mind—facts and figures that make your case but also any human stories that show the need for change through results of poor care or lack of resources. It is these stories that will frequently be left in the mind of the listener. The data-based evidence can be left with them in graphic form.

Nursing provides access to a wide range of real-life experiences, and these experiences provide an authentic viewpoint that is both genuine and truthful. Using authentic narratives to advocate for vulnerable groups strengthens the evidence for change and is an important source of data. Combining these tools with data, evidence, education and our own experiences presents us with powerful options when addressing the complex issues around health care and service delivery.

It is worth considering preparing a brief, practiced speech when you want to introduce an issue and advocate for a solution (Tomajan, 2012). Distributing a one-page fact sheet or brochure is an excellent way to close the speech and ensure that the listener is walking away with the key points (Amidei, 2010).

THINK BOX 10.6

Practice a 60-second speech—60 seconds is a long time to hold attention and, at the same time, demands discipline in conveying information. Here's a way to practice:

- Think of an issue you would like to address.
- Tell a story related to the issue that will get the attention of your listeners.
- Prepare an evidence-based one-page handout to back up your case that could be left with someone you want to influence.

5. **Influence**

Influencing others means being able to sway their decisions by using evidence as well as human stories to make a case for the solution you are focused on. Individuals, government and corporate decision-makers may all be the target for influence, and tactics will be adapted accordingly. All influence is built on credibility and trustworthiness—which nurses have as a trusted profession. Honesty and trust are powerful tools. Nursing authority—derived from navigating paths through health care—is a respected asset and provides us with a platform from which to speak.

Remembering the vested interests of those involved in the situation will enable you to target

---

*If you are not sure how to develop a stakeholder map, enter that term into a search engine, or ask a librarian. Many tools will pop up, some of them free. Stakeholder mapping is a great way to understand the context in which you are making decisions.

arguments, stories and evidence. For example, if you are trying to influence a budget holder, facts about return on investment of a proposed strategy will be important.

INTERNATIONAL ADVOCACY AND THE PANDEMIC EFFECTS

Advocating for high-quality patient care and safe health services remains a core function for nursing leaders around the world. Political advocacy is a key function of many national and international organisations such as national nursing associations, the International Council of Nurses and health care advocacy groups.

Raising awareness and presenting evidence and data is an established method used by organisations to inform and influence policy and guidance. Forums varying from protests and rallies to congresses and assemblies, written statements and face-to-face meetings all present opportunities for nurses to advocate for changes in legislation and practice. A strategic approach is essential to take advantage of different policy windows (see earlier discussion and toolbox), as actions have to suit the level of governance and the people being targeted. For example, in the Nursing Now campaign, there was a season of advocacy in 2021 when nurses were encouraged to write a manifesto for change in their country and present it to the minister of health all on the same day. It was both a local request adapted for the country but with global resonance, as many countries participated (Holloway et al., 2021).

Since the onset of the COVID-19 pandemic, advocacy has become more important and urgent than ever before. During the pandemic, as patients became ill with COVID-19, they also became isolated. Across the world, lockdown and periods of quarantine and isolation meant that families were unable to care for their loved ones when they became sick. In many countries, patients were isolated, and visitors were not permitted in hospitals. Nurses were often the only advocates for patients in hospitals, providing not only critical information and education but compassion and care for patients who were away from their loved ones. Nurses were frequently supporting families from afar, as they became the connecting link between the patient and their loved ones.

The pandemic has shone a spotlight on the work of nurses around the world, and in doing so, it has provided an opportunity for the nursing voice to grow louder, expand its sphere of influence and engage with the wider issues that impact the health of our global populations.

The nursing profession has been affected deeply by the impact of the pandemic. As a result of working under pressure in often distressing environments without adequate resources and equipment, many nurses have opted to leave their jobs. The effects of this on a workforce already short of staff will have devastating and potentially catastrophic consequences on global health if there are insufficient nurses to deliver the services that are required (Buchan et al., 2022).

Nurses, particularly those in leadership positions, have opportunities to use their advocacy skills to influence government, policymakers and leaders of health care organisations. By emphasising the need for improved working conditions, including fair pay, access to education and training, counselling and psychological support and essential safety equipment, it is possible to influence the development of recruitment and retention strategies to support nurses who are considering leaving the profession.

Using the skills required for effective advocacy, we must draw on the tools in the toolbox. Our credibility, authenticity and authority, combined with unbiased evidence and data from global sources such as the World Health Organization, International Council of Nurses and International Labour Organization, provide weight and credibility to support discussion and debate.

WHEN ADVOCACY GOES WRONG

In any role where advocacy plays a part, there is a risk that messages may be misheard, misinterpreted or ignored (Nsiah et al., 2019). Passionate or emotional actions may be ill timed or poorly executed, resulting in a mixed or discredited message. This can result in a loss of trust, which may, in turn, lead to a negative outcome.

It is possible to avoid these situations by using the tools of advocacy discussed earlier whilst, at the same time, considering the context within which the message is received and heard. It is worth also reading the article referenced in this chapter by Nsiah et al. (2019) which describes the results of a research study that identified barriers to patient advocacy. There are useful stories from nurses in South Africa that highlight what can doom advocacy efforts to failure. Culture, gender and hierarchy all play a part in the exchange of information, and taking account of these issues may strengthen an argument, support discussion and dialogue, and influence the timing of when the message is released.

Nurses are known for acting with kindness, compassion, respect and dignity. Nursing leaders who display these qualities in their actions will build on the image of the trusted professional, opening opportunities for successful advocacy.

THINK BOX 10.7

Think of a time when you advocated for your profession. Consider the questions here and write a reflective statement about your experience.

- Who was I advocating for?
- What was my message?
- Why was it important?
- Why was it important to me?
- Who was my audience?
- What would strengthen my message?
- Did I have good data and evidence?
- How did I know if I was being heard?
- What would have helped me achieve a good outcome?
- What would I do differently next time?

TIPS FOR SUCCESS

- ■ Advocate for the issues you believe are important.
- ■ Draw on your own experiences to present an authentic story.
- ■ Know your data and evidence and ensure it is from reliable sources.
- ■ Practice advocacy—give speeches, write reflective notes and seek feedback in safe spaces.
- ■ Don't give up—nurses' voices need to be heard.

ADVOCATING FOR INTERNATIONALLY EDUCATED NURSES AND MIDWIVES

This section provides a real-world and important example of nurses using the skills of advocacy.

The example is that of internationally educated nurses and midwives (IEN&Ms) who have migrated from their home countries to work overseas, the part they have played in the destination workforce and the impact they have made in advocating for their own international nursing and midwifery associations and their diaspora groups.

The need to recruit and retain an adequate health and care workforce is the greatest challenge currently facing the nursing and midwifery professions worldwide. The global shortage of nurses has recently been emphasised in the WHO 'State of the World's Nursing' report (2020). The predicted worldwide nursing shortage is estimated to be 6 million by 2030, and 'The State of the World's Midwifery Report' (UN/WHO, 2021) declares a 1.1 million shortage of midwives. To fill these gaps, developed countries will continue to recruit IENs. Many experts deem the 'brain drain' of health care workers as disastrous (World Health Organization, 2010), arguing that recruiting nurses and midwives from low-income settings results in a scarcity of health care professionals in those places and contributes to poor health outcomes for the local population. In contrast, the recruitment of health care professionals for high-wage positions abroad might induce more nurses and midwives to invest in their own education rather than seek opportunities to migrate, leading to a 'brain gain' (Cortés & Pan, 2014). The pull to migrate from low- to high-income countries is strong: salaries and working conditions are likely to improve with job security, professional development, access to better health care technologies and enhanced opportunities for professional development. In lower-income settings; some nurses may face long working hours, poor and irregular salaries, stigma against the profession, especially during the pandemic, and a lack of autonomy and dignity in the workplace, all of which contribute to push factors that influence decisions to migrate (Buchan et al., 2022).

The issue is therefore one of retaining enough nurses in low-income settings with attractive working conditions so that they do not migrate and, in high-income settings, training and retaining enough indigenous nurses so that overseas recruitment is not necessary. But we are a long way from that point (Buchan et al., 2022). As a consequence, the professional nursing and midwifery registers in all higher-income countries include both in-country-trained and internationally trained nurses and midwives. For nurses who are working outside of the country where they trained, this presents many challenges. As well as all the challenges of relocation, which may include loneliness, language difficulties and cultural isolation, they also may not be able to get on to the nursing register immediately, as their qualifications may not be recognised, and that usually means working in a lower-paid job until they can qualify.

In this section of the chapter, we take UK case studies of challenges for nurses who are migrating from Africa, India and the Philippines and hear their accounts of why and how they have advocated for themselves and others.

ADVOCATING FOR OURSELVES AND OTHER NURSES

The latest data (September 2021) released from the UK Nursing and Midwifery Council (NMC) identifies that of the 744,929 registrants, 13.7% (102,220) are from outside the European Economic Area (EEA), and 3.9% (29,420) are from the EEA. Therefore, the number of non-UK registrants is now 17.6% (131,640) of the total UK registrar. NMC data indicate 5.2% (38,558) of UK registrants trained in Philippines, and 32,576 (4.4%) trained in India. These two groups make up 70% of all registrants who trained from outside the EEA. There are estimates that 6-16% (168,000 to 480,000) nurses in the US were educated in another country. The actual numbers are difficult to determine because of the state-based registration for nurses (NYU, 2020). These data demonstrate that our nursing and midwifery teams are culturally diverse; they include IENs and midwives. This highlights the need for cultural advocacy, and while case studies here come from the United Kingdom, the principles enshrined in them are much more widely applicable.

THINK BOX 10.8

- What do you understand by cultural advocacy?
- What information might you need to be a cultural advocate?
- Can you see how to use cultural advocacy in your practice situation?

CULTURAL ADVOCACY AND WHY IT MATTERS

Supporting people in a way that considers their unique cultural needs is crucial to good advocacy. Many IENs require support to adapt to life in a new country: understanding their cultural experiences and beliefs in relation to diet, language, community support and spiritual needs is critical to prevent social isolation. It is important to use a collaborative 'done with' rather than a 'done to' approach, and examples of this are given in case studies later. Also pivotal is understanding IENs' sense of community and belonging and what they need to feel safe and happy and adapt to life and work in the new country. This will improve both performance and retention of IENs (Souders, 2020).

Many organisations have developed cultural competence training programmes to support nursing staff to understand, appreciate and interact with their colleagues from cultures or belief systems different from theirs. Such programmes can be helpful, but cultural humility is always essential. Cultural humility (Tervalon & Murray-García, 1998) is a dynamic and lifelong process that focuses on self-reflection and self-critique to acknowledge one's own biases and areas of ignorance. This can help address power imbalances where people from a different culture feel unsafe when they feel they have lost their cultural identify. This can of course be true of anyone—patients, colleagues or neighbours. People will feel culturally safe when they are in an environment where there is no challenge to their identity and where their needs can be met. Racism, discrimination, othering, bullying and oppression can significantly impact health and well-being and result in systemic inequities—such as being held back from promotion or denied senior roles. (See the case studies for examples of this.) Health care organisations and their employees need to be held accountable for providing culturally safe care, as defined by IENs, and measured through progress towards achieving equity.

THINK BOX 10.9

Look at the details about Mary's migration journey. If you were her manager, what steps might you take to better understand her situation and provide culturally competent management?

CASE STUDY 10.1

Mary Arrives From an African Country

Mary (not her real name) is a nurse from one of the African countries. She had practiced in her home country for 10 years prior to migrating to the United Kingdom as an infection control specialist nurse and was a district manager for the ministry of health in her home country. Mary chose to come to the United Kingdom to utilise her expertise, positively contribute to nursing and health care in the United Kingdom and improve the quality of life for herself and family.

Mary arrived in the United Kingdom recruited via an agency who charged her employer £12,000 for a 3-year contract with an NHS Trust. She had to leave her husband and three young children behind, moving into shared temporary accommodation provided by her employer. Separation from her family, isolation, the cold climate and the initial shock of the unmet expectations were huge sources of anxiety. Within 3 months of commencing employment, she passed her Objective Structured Clinical Examination (OSCE) and was admitted to the Nursing and Midwifery Council register. Upon becoming a registered nurse, the trust refused to promote her to a Band 5 nurse (the minimum level a registered nurse holds in the United Kingdom). Mary wanted to leave her employer due to lack of progression but was advised she would have to repay the recruitment fee due to a breach of contract, causing undue distress.

Mary Was Unfairly Treated in Comparison with Colleagues Who Were Educated in the United Kingdom, including some Black and Brown nurses. She was accused of being disruptive and was put on a 'no conflict action plan'. She involved the trade union and, instead of the issues being addressed, was moved to another department, and the unfair treatment worsened. As a result, Mary became extremely depressed and had to be signed off work for several months with work-related stress. She was terrified that she could lose her right to remain in the United Kingdom if she became unemployed.

The case study shown here highlights the complexity of the challenges for nurses recruited to work in high-income countries from LICs. Many of these

nursing professionals are not prepared for the experiences they may face living and working in the new country. Let's now focus on two areas where advocacy to support the nurse will make a difference to their experience: individual advocacy and collective advocacy.

Individual Advocacy for Mary

Individual advocacy involves providing advocacy support to someone with a particular problem. Sometimes the focus is on helping them to help themselves, or it may be to assist them with an issue they haven't been able to solve alone. In Mary's case, the many issues she was facing were becoming overwhelming, especially for her mental health and certainly for her future as a nurse in the United Kingdom.

Mary was provided with individual coaching support sessions designed for IENs and midwives delivered remotely via telephone, WhatsApp or Zoom. The coaches delivering the programme were from historically marginalised backgrounds and had an understanding of the challenges IENs face. Active listening skills were used to build rapport and trust while finding out what her greatest challenges were. The nurse was provided with information that was used to get suitable accommodation and for bringing her children over from her home country. She was assisted with getting a grant from a nursing charity for nurses facing financial hardship, which was used to pay a deposit for accommodation and airline tickets for her children to come to the United Kingdom.

Mary was signposted to a diaspora nursing and midwifery organisation for pastoral support and provided with a pack containing details of a local buddy, housing, banking, salary arrangements, phone contract support, transportation, help to get utilities, food and locations of faith organisations and places of worship. She was supported with writing an email to her manager to get a Band 5 nursing post and was subsequently given interview preparation; she successfully obtained a Band 6 post a year after arriving in the United Kingdom. Feedback obtained from Mary was shared with permission to her diaspora nursing and midwifery organisation and the chief nursing officer for England's Black and Minority Ethnic Strategic Advisory Group (CNOBMESAG) to develop a programme of support for other IENs.

THINK BOX 10.10

- What do you think might be the benefits of individual advocacy over other advocacy strategies?
- Do you have examples of individual advocacy where you work?

Thinking about the people you care for, how might individual advocacy work in a care setting for patients?

COLLECTIVE ADVOCACY BY AND FOR INTERNATIONALLY EDUCATED NURSES AND MIDWIVES

International educated nurses and midwives are now acting as advocates for other IEN&Ms, and many are developing collective and powerful voices within their diaspora groups. This is collective advocacy where people with a common concern or interest come together to explore issues and find solutions. The advocates in the group draw on their knowledge of, and connection to, their community's social, cultural, spiritual and gender issues. There are several examples of collective advocacy relating to IEN&Ms described in this chapter.

Bespoke advocacy programmes have been developed by diaspora nursing and midwifery organisations for nurses recruited from their home countries. Support provided includes welcoming newly arrived IEN&Ms to the new country, linking them with a buddy and the provision of pastoral support to prevent isolation and support with settling into the new country. These organisations run regular listening events to hear the experiences of IENs, share good practice and collect narratives of poor experiences. Several representatives of the diaspora organisations are also members of the CNOBMESAG and report directly the concerns and challenges IEN&Ms face to the Chief Nursing Officer for England in order to be actioned. Concerns include poor treatment, discrimination, poor induction/orientation and lack of training or career progression.

Diaspora organisations have worked closely with nursing unions to develop a comprehensive guide for IEN&Ms considering coming to the United Kingdom to live and work. They enlist the support of the unions to call out employers who exploit IEN&Ms. For example, many internationally recruited nurses are tied into contracts through early exit fees and, in some cases, intimidated by their employers into repaying them through threats of deportation. These fees (reported to be as high as £14,000) may pressure workers to remain within contracts despite poor treatment.

They also run regular workshops to prepare IEN&Ms for life in the United Kingdom, including advice on immigration, language requirements, obtaining nursing licensure, how to avoid rogue recruitment agencies and how to deal with culture shock. The diaspora organisations also run regular well-being sessions and celebration events to enable IEN&Ms to feel a sense of belonging and community and inspire one another.

We have read Mary's story earlier, and now there is a selection of lived experiences from Filipino nurses, the largest group of international nurses in the United Kingdom. They highlight some outstanding advocates who seek always to represent the voices of their colleagues and promote rewarding careers.

CASE STUDY 10.2

Jen, International Recruitment and Ethnic Minority Nurse Advisor, England

Jen arrived in England in 1999 with 34 other nurses from across the Philippines to work in a hospital that had never employed IENs before. Those nurses had big dreams and high hopes and were excited about starting a new life in a new country.

'Being able to integrate into the organisation is critical to ensuring a positive work experience. I had a positive experience back then. We had Bev, our lead nurse for overseas nurses; she was Jamaican. She became like our second mom, taking care of us, teaching us what we needed to know about nursing and life in the United Kingdom.

I have had supportive managers who have given me the opportunity to deliver and excel in the roles I've had. But not everyone is as lucky as I have been. As a lead nurse, I started a vascular access service. I led in improving standards across my trust, published articles and was awarded *British Nursing Journal* (BJN) "IV Therapy Nurse of the Year" in 2016. I had found my niche.

Continued

But in 2018, it came to my attention that internationally recruited nurses from India and Philippines were struggling with their new life in the United Kingdom. I kept hearing stories about their problems with accommodation, the need for clarity in their role and their need for information and pastoral support. It was clear that they were not having a good experience and they had just arrived. It brought back memories for me. As a result, I started "Project KINs: How Are We Doing?", an initiative to improve the experiences of newly arrived international educated nurses, and my role was to escalate issues to senior management. I was going beyond my comfort zone. When one is working in a specialty for so long, it is so easy to be siloed and just focus on your craft. It took courage from within me to speak to senior managers, hoping that they will listen because they have the power and authority to improve these nurses' working conditions. I was full of self-doubt in the early years of my career, but I realised I am good enough, that I can be my authentic self, live my values and be an advocate for others. It is both liberating and empowering. I have tried to fit in and mirror English ways as I look up to role model managers, but there is that discomfort within me that I am not being true to myself. After almost two decades of working in the United Kingdom, I found my voice!

My advocacy and passion for staff support turned into a post during the pandemic because of its disproportionate impact of COVID-19 on our staff from historically marginalised groups. I was seconded as the Chief Nursing Officer for England (CNO)'s Ethnic Minority (EM) Nurse Advisor supporting the CNO EM action plan for COVID-19, with an initial focus on the Filipino issues. I became the voice for the concerns of my fellow Filipinos and represented the international nurses' perspective and experience.

Due to the increased number of Filipino deaths in the first wave of the pandemic, we started to reflect and tried to understand what was happening to us. As a community, we started to also find our voice and come together to make this stronger. A milestone, January 2022, was the inclusion of Filipino as a category on our electronic staff record. We needed to self-identify so that our needs and experiences can be understood. To be counted is to be visible, to be recognised for the contributions that we have brought to British society and to the NHS for so many years now.

Of the nearly 39,000 NMC registered Filipino nurses, more than 17,000 working within the NHS England, there are only 38 senior and very senior Filipino nurses. We learned that it takes 20 years for Filipinos to get to a senior role! These senior Filipino nurses have now come together and formed the Filipino Senior Nurses Alliance, United Kingdom, and are committed to have a collective voice and purpose to advocate for the Filipino health care workers in the United Kingdom.

As International Recruitment and Ethnic Minorites Nurse Advisor, I am leading work at the International Nursing Association, which aims to support the collective voice and advocate for our nursing workforce from historically marginalised groups. I aspire to be a role model of inclusive and compassionate leadership at a national level, and I also want to promote the positive contribution of the Filipino workforce within NHS/United Kingdom because for the last 20 years, we've never really had a seat at the table and had a voice.

In all of these, I can say that my advocacy gives me a higher purpose, and that has given me the ability to use my voice to benefit others'.

THINK BOX 10.11

Read Jen's account of her migration experience and all she has done as an advocate for herself and for other Filipino nurses in the United Kingdom.

Prepare a 60-second speech for Jen using the guidelines earlier in this chapter. If you are reading this chapter with others, share your efforts and critique them.

The next case studies are the perspectives of a clinical academic nurse and then young nurses from Kenya and Zimbabwe. As you read them, think about what you have read in this chapter—the competencies of advocacy in clinical practice, advocating for patients, advocating for other nurse colleagues and advocating at different levels for change. Can you see principles of advocacy reflected in these accounts? How is collective advocacy used and who for?

CASE STUDY 10.3

Louie, Senior Intensive Care Nurse

In 2001, Louie created a pastoral nursing group, most of them from the Filipino community. The group discussed work challenges, using a supportive, rather than a formal, leadership discussion.

'I started encouraging Filipino, Indian, African and other nurses from historically marginalised backgrounds to do the same. There was a lot of continuous encouraging initially, as most IENs do not think they have it in them to be promoted. I went to gatherings and would discuss how leadership roles can be accessed. I talked with them about their career aspirations. I started giving interview techniques (how I would do it, nothing formal). I would signpost them to good articles about how to speak in public and how to network within their workplace.

Due to the increasing support I have been giving to the community, I pushed and applied for leadership courses so that I can equip myself in my pastoral role outside of my work. Those I mentor are also mentoring others, and we hold a monthly pastoral induction for every cohort of Filipino nurses arriving in the United Kingdom.

I am pushing for a bespoke mentoring programme for IENs by IENs, as we are the ones who truly understand the need to navigate cultural support, the language barrier, assertiveness challenges and the many other complex issues when mentoring someone from a historically marginalised background'.

CASE STUDY 10.4

Oliver, Senior Nurse, England

'I have worked with mindful, motivational and transformational mentors and leaders who saw the value of 'individuals' to cohesively work as a collective vision. I have been greatly supported by my line managers and mentors and who saw the best in me and allowed me to trust in my capacity and capability, which has helped me to build my confidence to step up on the ladder of leadership and management. I am now in position to pay this forward and have been advocating, mentoring and 'coaching' colleagues, both locally and nationally, to progress in their career. I enable them to believe in and unlock their potential to be their best'.

CASE STUDY 10.5

Francis, Executive Nurse, Advocate and Influencer

During the COVID-19 pandemic, Francis has influenced grant giving charities, UK Parliament and the Chief Nursing Officer for England to support the Filipino Nurse community. He secured financial grants for the families of those who affected by the pandemic. He raised concerns of the high and disproportionate numbers of Filipino nurses and health and care workers dying from COVID-19 with the national media. He founded the Filipino Nurses Association UK (FNA-UK) in July 2020. He has advocated for and supported other international nurse associations in the United Kingdom to establish their own associations, including the British Indian Nurses Association UK, the Malawian Nurses Association UK and the Spanish Nurses Association UK. He cofounded the Filipino Senior Nurses Alliance UK in 2021 and publicly advocates for increased numbers of Filipino nurses in very senior roles. The alliance enthusiastically celebrates each promotion into a senior position through social media channels. On 8 December 2020, May, a matron and officer of the FNA-UK, became the first person in the world to administer a COVID-19 vaccine to a patient outside of clinical trials. She was watched by millions across the world.

'I lead a national initiative of mentoring and coaching for more than 150 of my Filipino nurse

Continued

colleagues in the NHS. There is a lot of enthusiasm, interest and genuine offers of pro bono support from national, regional and local health, care, private, charity and academic leaders.'

It is evident Jen, Oliver, Louie and Francis are absolute champions and advocates for IEN&Ms working in the United Kingdom, providing their lived experiences and offering support to set standards for the future through a range of advocacy initiatives, including collective and individual advocacy.

THINK BOX 10.12

- Who are the most vulnerable of your colleagues?
- They may be immigrants or possibly those who are of a historically marginalised group. How do you support them?
- How could you advocate for them?

  Using the examples given, think about what role good nursing workforce data collection plays in advocacy.

Earlier in this chapter, we suggested ways of influencing those in power to listen to our concerns as nurses. It is clear from the powerful case studies that we have important stories to tell, but they can only be influential if they are *heard*—and that means that nurses everywhere have to become more powerful advocates—with the leadership in advocacy skills in this chapter.

CASE STUDY 10.6

Navigating Through Advocacy as a Clinical Academic Nurse, by Jonathan Bayuo, Ghana

Advocacy is at the core of nursing practise. In fact, not a single day goes by without nurses having to mediate between other members of the health care team and patients regarding treatment recommendations and patients' beliefs and concerns. The central role of nurses within the health team and direct contact with patients and their families' places nurses at the fore of advocacy. Patients are often vulnerable, and this may be worsened by the paternalistic nature of some health care systems suggesting that the voices of patients often go unheard. Nurses are well positioned to act and speak on behalf of patients as they deliver care. Advocacy can occur spontaneously without even knowing, and at other times, there may be a need to consciously prepare for an advocacy role. Patient education remains a core nursing duty which serves to empower patients to be able to participate actively in their care as much as practically possible.

Beyond clinical care, advocacy also deals with institutional policies which are not favourable to patient care in given instances. For example, policies regarding visiting hours can occasionally be overruled based on the patient circumstances to enable family members to spend more time with their loved one. Financial issues can also trigger discharge against medical advice in our setting, and it

is often the nurses who advocate for other alternatives such as stepping down from the intensive care unit to the general ward as soon as the patient's condition permits it.

As a clinical academic nurse who is actively involved in clinical research and education, the notion of advocacy extends beyond the immediate clinical care. Patients are vulnerable not only in the clinical scenario but also regarding their participation in research. Patients need to understand the nature of a research project to make an informed decision regarding their participation. Research nurses often need to support the process to ensure that patients and their families understand their responsibilities and rights as research participants. Nurses are driven by ethical principles such as beneficence and nonmaleficence to ensure that patients who are not fit to participate in a research project are duly protected from harm.

The reach of a nurse's advocacy is further expanded as nurses support each other as well as students in clinical placement. Challenging working conditions can often spark advocacy so as to improve the situation. Overall, the advocacy roles played by nurses is all encompassing. Although this may not always be visible or 'loud', its subtle power demonstrates nursing's commitment to a culture of safety.

CASE STUDY 10.7

Advocacy from Young Nurses and Its Importance, by Zipporah Iregi, Kenya

Advocacy for the nursing and midwifery professions is really important. The raised profile of nursing and midwifery can go a long way in ensuring that nurses and midwives step up to make their contributions towards achieving good health and well-being. However, more often than not, most of the nurses and midwives look to their unions, professional associations, senior colleagues and other leaders for advocacy for the profession, hardly ever to the early career nurses and midwives. This is influenced by a number of things, such as early career nurses and midwives having less experience in the profession, the lack of trust by more senior nurses and midwives, or the fact that they do not hold leadership positions. The truth is that these young nurses and midwives have a lot that they can offer, a fresh perspective, curiosity and, to top it all off, understanding the use of technology.

Advocacy is geared towards building a strong workforce and improving health as we look to the future. Early career nurses and midwives will be the leaders of that future. Are we then not to involve them in that conversation now? How then do we go about this? Education, mentorship and coaching. This needs to begin at the very first point of nursing and midwifery education. Thankfully, the curriculum already teaches nurses and midwives to be advocates for their patients. We can then build on these and train student nurses and midwives on the role they play in the health care system and how they can leverage this to build better systems and consequently improve health. The education ought to be learner centred and focused on problem-solving, equipping the students with skills in leadership, critical thinking and research, using their technological know-how and advocacy. Moreover, mentorship should be readily provided to these early-career nurses and midwives. Mentoring will give them an opportunity to learn from those who are already advocating at the front lines. Early-career nurses and midwives can also be given exposure through debates, exchange programs or even sit-downs with their leaders in health early in their careers to watch advocacy in action.

Looking ahead to the future, the young nurses and midwives will take up space at every level of health care and in every area of expertise. Having inculcated the principles of advocacy in them shall cause them to be drivers of change and advocates in their small spaces of influence. They shall be well equipped to lead wherever they are and cause a ripple effect towards the improvement of health and building a stronger workforce. Ultimately, nurses shall find a global voice and take their seats at the decision-making tables! Early career nurses are the leaders of tomorrow; that future is in their hands.

CASE STUDY 10.8

Advocacy Begins From a Deep Awareness and Understanding of One's Social Environment, by Munashe Nyika, Zimbabwe

As a nurse, I take inspiration from Florence Nightingale, who changed nursing by creating a new awareness of the effects of the environment on the care of patients that transformed nursing care. Our current awareness of environment as nurses has extended from bedside to include the sociostructural, economic, geopolitical and climate environments in which we provide care for our patients today—the social determinants of health. Our environments include our local, regional, national and international community spaces. As a nurse, I have taken advocacy to be for myself, my community and patients I care for, beginning with an awareness of the environment in which I am delivering care.

Through being aware of challenges faced in our environments, we are then best placed to provide solutions that improve health and well-being of our communities. I have found that advocating for issues I am passionate about keeps me motivated to keep advocating and find new approaches for advocating. As a nurse, health for our communities, particularly those that are most vulnerable, forms the basis of our

Continued

advocacy. We need nurses in senior leadership positions, where decisions are made, to engage in discussions that affect our practice, our environments and the health of the people we care for. As the largest group of health care professionals, together with our closeness to the people we serve, our voices are paramount in any conversation towards achieving universal health coverage and the well-being of communities worldwide.

Over the years, I have challenged myself to reflect more and more on the challenges and issues in society to which the nursing voice can provide solutions. The nursing voice can impact advocacy, not only for health but for other global challenges, with a focus on how these macrosocial challenges have a direct impact on health. I am motivated by nurses tackling key issues such as climate change and global politics

and the impact the nursing voice can bring to more of the global development goals. There needs to be a greater emphasis on training in advocacy and awareness of social determinants of health through nursing education.

As with any other discipline, advocacy requires practice and work. It requires commitment, a sense of community and constant persistence towards achieving a common goal. Connecting with others and creating partnerships and communities creates a powerful medium for effective advocacy. It requires effective planning and preparation—advocacy is organised. It requires creating a collective message that is clear and concise to produce the best results. Through resilience and advocacy, we are able to create lasting change, dynamic communities and develop lifelong friendships and partnerships.

THINK BOX 10.13

All of these case studies from practitioners, young nurses and nurses who have migrated away from their home countries tell powerful stories of the way that nurses think about their role in advocacy.

- Do you see yourself in any of these stories?
- Can you see an area where you are not currently involved in advocacy but would like to be involved?
- What would you do to become an effective advocate in this area?
- Can you write your 60-second speech?

SUMMARY AND CONCLUSION

There is no doubt that the skills required to advocate must be part of a wider set of key competencies for nursing leaders. Learning the skills for advocacy starts at the onset of nurse training because nurses are advocates for their patients, but those skills have to be developed and integrated throughout a nurse's career, regardless of the setting where nursing is practiced.

Nurses have always advocated for the safety and well-being of their patients, but as we reflect and learn lessons from the global pandemic, it is clear that nursing must use its higher profile to advocate for the profession itself. Nurse education, workforce, service delivery and leadership are essential components of a

strong and healthy workforce. As we face the unprecedented challenges around strengthening global nursing, our leadership and our skills as advocates are essential, not only for those we care for but also for the health of our fragile planet.

Nursing advocacy, as described in this chapter through both background and examples, is how nursing's contributions to world health and better lives for all will be made possible. As noted several times, nurses learn early in their education and careers how to effectively advocate for their patients and those that they care for. It is now time for nurses to use those same skills to advocate for changes in their communities, whether local, regional, national or global, and in the health care systems in which care is provided. Addressing issues of inequity is one of nursing's core principles, yet many nurses do not see themselves as leaders or as persons who are in a position to effect change. Without the nursing voice representing more than half the world's workforce, it will be impossible to make progress on the many problems facing the world. The time is now for all nurses to identify the advocacy role that they are going to assume.

REFERENCES

Amidei, N. (2010). So You Want to Make A Difference. OMB Watch.
Buchan, J., Catton, H., & Shaffer, F. A. (2022). *Sustain and retain in 2022 and beyond: The global nursing workforce and the COVID-19*

pandemic. International Centre on Nurse Migration Commissioned paper. Retrieved February 2024, from https://www.intlnursemigration.org/commissioned-papers/.

Cardoso, R. J., Graveto, J. M., & Queiroz, A. M. (2014). The exposure of the nursing profession in online and print media. *Revista Latino-Americana de Enfermagem, 22*(1), 144–149. doi:10.1590/0104-1169.3144.2394.

Cortés, P., & Pan, J. (2014). Foreign nurse importation and the supply of native nurses. *Journal of Health Economics, 37*(Issue C), 164–180.

Cullerton, K., Donnet, T., Lee, A., & Gallegos, D. (2018). Effective advocacy strategies for influencing government nutrition policy: A conceptual model. *International Journal of Behavioral Nutrition and Physical Activity, 15*, 83. doi:10.1186/s12966-018-0716-y.

Daly, J., Speedy, S., & Jackson, D. (2015). *Leadership and nursing: Contemporary perspectives* (2nd ed.). Churchill Livingstone.

Holloway, A., Thomson, A., Stilwell, B., Finch, H., Irwin, K., & Crisp, N. (2021). Agents of change: The story of the nursing now campaign. *Nursing Now/Burdett Trust for Nursing*. Retrieved November 2022, from https://www.nursingnow.org/wp-content/uploads/2021/05/Nursing-Now-Final-Report.pdf.

Ipsos Veracity Index. (2022). Retrieved November 2022, from https://www.ipsos.com/en-ie/ipsos-veracity-index-2022.

Mason, D. (2020). Nurses lack representation in media: Recognize them for the leaders that they are. (June 26, 2020). *Opinion USA Today*. Retrieved February 22, 2024 from https://www.usatoday.com/story/opinion/2020/06/26/nurses-leaders-medicine-but-overshadowed-media-column/3223242001/.

Mason, D. J., Nixon, L., Glickstein, B., Han, S., Westphaln, K., & Carter, L. (2018). The woodhull study revisited: Nurses' representation in health news media 20 years later. *Journal of Nursing Scholarship, 50*, 695–704. doi:10.1111/jnu.12429.

Matthews, J. (2012). Role of professional organizations in advocating for the nursing profession. *The Online Journal of Issues in Nursing, 17*(1), 3.

Nightingale, F. (1969). *Notes on Nursing – What it is and what it is not*. Dover Publications, Inc.

Nitzky, A. (2018). Six ways nurses can advocate for patients. *Oncology Nursing News*. Retrieved November 2022, from https://www.oncnursingnews.com/view/six-ways-nurses-can-advocate-for-patients.

Nsiah, C., Siakwa, M., & Ninnoni, J. P. K. (2019). Barriers to practicing patient advocacy in healthcare setting. *Nursing Open, 7*(2), 650–659. doi:10.1002/nop2.436.

Nursing Now. (2019). *Investing in the power of nurse leadership: What will it take?* Retrieved February 2024, from https://www. intrahealth.org/resources/investing-power-nurse-leadership-what-will-it-take.

NYU. (2020). *Hospitals with internationally trained nurses have more stable, Educated Nursing Workforces*. Retrieved February 2024, from https://www.nyu.edu/about/news-publications/news/2020/february/internationally-trained-nurses.html.

Rafferty, A. M. (2020). The influence and legacy of a nursing icon. Retrieved February 22, 2024 from https://www.kcl.ac.uk/the-influence-and-legacy-of-a-nursing-icon.

Rouleau, G., Richard, L., Côté, J., Gagnon, M. P., & Pelletier, J. (2019). Nursing practice to support people living with HIV with antiretroviral therapy adherence: A qualitative study. *Journal of Association of Nurses in AIDS Care, 30*(4), e20–e37.

Salvage, J., & Stilwell, B. (2018). Breaking the silence: A new story of nursing. *Journal of Clinical Nursing, 27*(7–8), 1301–1303.

Serafin, L., Strząska-Kliś, Z., Kolbe, G., Brzozowska, P., Szwed, I., Ostrowska, A., & Czarkowska-Pączek, B. (2022). The relationship between perceived competence and self-esteem among novice nurses—a cross-sectional study. *Annals of medicine, 54*(1), 484–494.

Souders, B. (2020). The science of improving motivation at work. *Positive Psychology.com*. Retrieved November 2022, from https://positivepsychology.com/improving-motivation-at-work/.

Tervalon, M. & Murray-Garcia, J. (1998). Cultural humility versus cultural competence: a critical distinction in defining physician training outcomes in multicultural education. *Journal of Health Care for the Poor and Underserved, 9*. doi: https://doi.org/10.1353/hpu.2010.0233.

Tomajan, K. (2012). Advocating for nurses and nursing. *The Online Journal of Issues in Nursing, 17*(1), 4.

United Nations Population Fund/WHO. (2021). *The state of the world's midwifery*. Retrieved February 2022, from https://www.unfpa.org/publications/sowmy-2021.

World Health Organization. (2010). *WHO global code of practice on the international recruitment of health personnel*. World Health Organization. Retrieved November 2022, from http://apps.who.int/gb/ebwha/pdf_files/WHA63/A63_R16-en.pdf.

World Health Organization. (2020). The state of the world's nursing report—2020. Retrieved November 2022, from https://www.who.int/publications/i/item/9789240003279.

World Health Organization. (2021). *The impact of COVID-19 on health and care workers: A closer look at deaths*. World Health Organization. Retrieved February 2024, from https://apps.who.int/iris/handle/10665/345300.

Wyatt, L. (2019). *A History of Nursing*. Amberly Publishing.

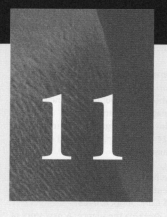

11

THE INFLUENCE OF NURSING NOW AS A GLOBAL SOCIAL MOVEMENT: LESSONS FOR NURSING'S FUTURE

BARBARA STILWELL

INTRODUCTION

This chapter will tell the story of how the Nursing Now campaign became an influential global social movement. Global connectedness has become possible through technological advances, and it allows us all to share experiences, knowledge and challenges. This chapter is included in the book because such sharing can create a sense of global solidarity over important issues: think of the climate change activists or the Black Lives Matter campaign as examples. Until the Nursing Now campaign, there had not been a global nursing social movement, although the International Council of Nurses (ICN) links professional nursing associations around the world, and there are several organisations that bring nurses together for conferences and specialist events. Nursing Now was different in that it offered platforms for informal conversations between nurses in many countries through web-based events and by linking Nursing Now groups with each other, politicians and the media. The importance and potential impact of these new global connections in the future of health care will be explored in this chapter.

THE NURSING NOW CAMPAIGN

Nursing Now was a campaign initiated and, at first, led by a British lord—Lord Nigel Crisp—who was so convinced that strengthening nursing was the key to universalhealth coverage that he persuaded colleagues from many sectors to support a campaign focused on nurses, which would run from 2018 to 2020 (Stilwell, 2021). Lord Crisp had been head of the

British National Health Service for several years and now has a seat in the House of Lords, which is the upper chamber of the British parliamentary system. The cochair of the board was Dr Sheila Tlou, a professor of nursing from Botswana who has also held senior positions in the United Nations and was minister of health in the government of Botswana. The global network of individuals who were willing to join the Nursing Now board was impressive and diverse; half of the board were nurses, and half were not. Board members came from every region of the world. The campaign was run in association with the World Health Organization (WHO) and the ICN, with the aim of improving health globally by raising the status and profile of nursing (Holloway et al., 2021).

The Nursing Now campaign aimed to achieve its goal by influencing policy globally and supporting action locally. The Nursing Now partners, WHO and ICN, were well placed to be high-level influencers, and local Nursing Now groups could be linked not only with WHO and ICN but also with the Nursing Now board. The campaign, through its activities and connections at local, regional and global levels, acted as a bridging network, connecting groups and people that might not previously have known about each other. Bridging networks can be important mechanisms for change, as they give access to new knowledge and people, allowing the different networks to hear novel ideas (Battilana & Casciaro, 2013).

It was internet connectivity and social media that were pivotal to the campaign's success, as those technologies attracted young nurses, offered global reach and, when the COVID pandemic locked down the world in 2020, allowed the campaign to continue online with minimum disruption. Internet-based communications also enabled the campaign to communicate regularly with Nursing Now groups in all regions of the world and for groups to share their activities with each other.

By the time the campaign ended in 2021, there were over 700 Nursing Now groups in 126 countries (Holloway et al., 2021), and it was estimated that these groups represented over 1 million nurses, many of whom worked at the facility level. There was a tremendous enthusiasm from nurses globally to advocate for the Nursing Now campaign and for better investment in nursing, even though nurses are often not political activists (Wilson et al., 2022). Some commentators have asserted that there has been a lack of unity within nursing, so nurses are more inclined to fight amongst themselves than to unite to influence politics. Political behaviour by nurses has not been considered appropriate by some; this is evident now in the United Kingdom as nurses strike for better pay and are having to defend their right to strike (RCN News, 2022; Salvage & White, 2019; Wilson et al., 2022). The Nursing Now campaign was not a political campaign, but it had its roots in the British Parliament, as it derived from a parliamentary paper (All-Party Parliamentary Group, 2016) and was designed to encourage nurses to engage with policymakers and politicians in order to influence political thinking about health and the place of nurses in the health workforce.

Undoubtedly, 2020 and 2021 saw the status and profile of nurses rising, and while some of that increased visibility could be attributed to the activities of the campaign, it is impossible to separate the effects of the pandemic from those of the Nursing Now campaign. In the final appraisal of what the Nursing Now campaign had achieved, it was noted that 42% of groups confirmed government investment in nursing during the campaign (Holloway et al., 2021, p. 43). Though subjective, this assessment showed that where the groups were large and numerous, investment in nursing was more likely.

THINK BOX 11.1

- Did you have a Nursing Now group in your country?
- Does it still exist?
- What do you think it achieved?
- What action did it take?

NURSING NOW AS A SOCIAL MOVEMENT

The Nursing Now campaign was not designed to be a social movement, but looking back at how it developed and what drove it, the role of networks and connections in its success is undeniable. The Nursing Now campaign was described in its appraisal as a 'rich tapestry of stories' (Holloway et al., 2021, p. 59). Individuals and groups brought their stories together, especially during the pandemic, and individual experiences were then seen as common to many.

Social movements are said to have three defining characteristics.

1. Those in them engage in collective action that will bring about social change, possibly in opposition to others, though this is not always the case.
2. Those in the social movement use strong networks to coordinate goals and exchange resources.
3. The movement has a collective identity which links people and leads to a common purpose and shared commitment to a goal (Della Porta & Diani, 2020).

The Nursing Now campaign demonstrated all of these characteristics in that those involved had the goal of changing societal perceptions of nursing, shared a collective identity (nurses, members of Nursing Now groups) and were linked as an informal network through social media. Social movements related to health are usually focused on 'collective challenges to medical policy and politics, belief systems, research and practice that include an array of formal and informal organisations, supporters, networks of cooperation and media' (Brown & Zavestoski, 2005, p. 682). Examples include groups that campaigned for female reproductive rights, especially in the United States in the 1960s, though with Roe v Wade* being overturned in 2022, new social movements have quickly developed to assert females' rights over their own bodies.

---

*Roe v Wade was the landmark piece of legislation that made access to an abortion a federal right in the United States. The decision dismantled 50 years of legal protection and paved the way for individual states to curtail or outright ban abortion rights.

THINK BOX 11.2

- Can you identify any health-related social movements in your country or neighbourhood?

They could include, for example, healthy eating campaigns such as campaigning for a farmer's market or campaigns for more exercise facilities, such as in parks and playgrounds.

- Do you know how successful they have been?

Nurses have tended to be on the periphery of social movements in the past, probably because, as noted earlier, nurses are not usually involved in politics (Wilson et al., 2022). During the COVID-19 pandemic, nurses were seen campaigning in several countries for more personal protective equipment (PPE) for their own safety and for patients, too (Levin & Bekiempis, 2022; watch a clip of nurses campaigning at Ghana Registered Nurses and Midwives Association, 2020). The effects of the pandemic—with inadequate PPE, increased stress, staff shortages and the constant threat of infection with COVID-19—has resulted in attrition of nurses from the workforce (Buchan et al., 2022; see also Chapter 5 by Sharplin et al. in this book on the survey of nurses about their COVID experiences). In the United Kingdom in 2022, nurses have voted for strike action for the first time ever, having been offered a low pay raise in 2021. Strike action is a form of social mobilisation usually associated with the labour movement, and this form of social activism is rare in nursing. However, the Royal College of Nursing (RCN)—the biggest nurses' trade union in the United Kingdom—points out that nurses have long been involved in the labour movement (RCN Bulletin, 2022).

Two examples from recent history in the United Kingdom are the RCN Raise the Roof campaign, which led to nurses publicly campaigning for a pay increase for the first time. It resulted in a 22% increase. Five years later, nurses marched to Downing Street and demonstrated outside Parliament, and the RCN held talks with the government based on their report, 'The State of Nursing'. They threatened unprecedented action from their members despite not yet being a union. Their call for an independent inquiry into nurses' pay was agreed, and the result was an average 30% rise. These UK examples show the potential power of social movements in nursing, though they are used infrequently. A strike is the most common form of collective action in a social movement. For nurses, there are challenges in managing strikes, or other industrial action, in that victims of disruption are likely to be the public, who may then lower their opinion of, and trust in, nurses.

In Kenya, nurses were on strike for 150 days in 2017 when the government did not sign a collective bargaining agreement with their union as had been agreed. The medical doctors also came out on strike for 100 days at the same time and for the same reason, but their dispute was settled first, which was perceived as unfair by the nurses. After 150 days of strike action, the nurses agreed to return to work when the government increased pay and improved conditions for them, even though the collective bargaining agreement had not been signed. Such a long strike by nurses (and doctors) is unusual, and it certainly influenced the ability of the health system to function (Waithaka et al., 2020). When doctors and nurses did go on strike, the doctors' collective bargaining agreement was signed, but the nurses' collective bargaining agreement was not. Such background conditions and, in particular, feelings of unfairness between cadres have also triggered nurses' strikes in Ghana and Nigeria (Waithaka et al., 2020).

As Wilson et al. (2022) write, the historical development of nursing, rooted in service and religion, has contributed to the nursing voice not being heard (Salvage & Stilwell, 2018). Chapter 8 in this book discusses at some length the historical and social factors behind this reality, especially with regard to nursing being a gendered occupation. Nursing is a highly stereotyped as a female profession with feminine-associated values, which are not valued as much as the more scientific medical roles (Newman & Stilwell, Chapter 8 in this book). Perhaps because of this feminine stereotyping, political behaviour by nurses has not been considered appropriate (Salvage & White, 2019). However, when nurses do come together around an issue, they can be powerful—maybe because it is an unusual occurrence. Take a look at the discussion in Chapter 8 about nursing and power.

POWER AND SOCIAL MOVEMENTS

The Nursing Now campaign enabled nurses to form a collective identity around their shared concerns and have a platform from which to influence policymakers at national, regional and global levels, facilitated by social media. Although social movements differ in size, they result from a spontaneous coming together of people whose relationships are not defined by rules and procedures but who share a common outlook. This was the nature of both the campaign (not rule defined or procedure governed) and of the groups (spontaneous and each one responding to its wider environment). Nursing Now groups were informal, self-funding and self-governing, and their level of engagement was a unique and critical factor in the reach and influence of the campaign. In effect, the activities of these groups focused on advocacy and disruption more akin to such groups as Black Lives Matter or #MeToo, though stopping short of civil disruption.

Looking at how nursing has developed over decades, discontent in the profession has been demonstrated by strike action described earlier or voiced in letters to nursing journals and even in longer papers and books. Nursing Now took the discontent and allowed it to be shared globally, and then it became a social movement for change in nursing. The campaign offered a way to organise around a common message, which is that to improve health, it is essential to raise the profiles and statuses of nurses globally. Members of the campaign could connect with each other through websites and social media. Nursing Now flourished globally because of internet connectivity. It is almost impossible to imagine such a movement forming and coalescing prior to the internet (Holloway et al., 2021).

Coalescing into a social movement gave nurses a new kind of power: 'power with'. There is much more on power in nursing in Chapter 8, and it is an important subject for us to consider in global nursing given that 90% of nurses are female (World Health Organization, 2020) and females make up 70% of the health workers but occupy only 25% of senior management roles (World Health Organization, 2019). It is males who hold the decision-making power in health systems. According to Eisler (2015, p. 6), 'power with' derives from a partnership model and offers a different non-hierarchical power structure, one in which nurses are more comfortable than in hierarchical models which are competitive, and in life and health care, it is frequently males and physicians who assume the power

in a health hierarchy (Beard, 2017; World Health Organization, 2019). It is partnership models that gave nurses a more powerful voice during the Nursing Now campaign. They were globally linked and could articulate together their powerful narratives effectively as a social movement. Used strategically, power with can become powerful, as social movements are, and can disrupt the status quo and change health policies and strategic directions, decisions and resources. In the final Nursing Now report (Holloway et al., 2021), there are many examples and descriptions of what was achieved by local and international action.

BUILDING BRIDGES TO THE MEDIA: WHY BOTHER?

The Nursing Now campaign caught a moment, even before the 2020 pandemic, when nurses in many places were becoming more aware of their value to health systems and also their lack of visibility in media briefings and in high-level decision-making (Mason, 2020). There is a global shortage of nurses (Buchan et al., 2022) that has been noted for decades (World Health Organization, 2020) but has not resulted in investment in pay and conditions for nurses that would attract and retain them. Consequently, despite the growing need for nurses, the shortage continues to grow, largely due to the retirement of an aging workforce (more than half are over age 50), lack of nursing faculty, high job stress, which was amplified by the pandemic, and high turnover (Buchan et al., 2022). Media and public images of nurses are largely outdated and do not portray nursing as an attractive science-based profession. The nursing profession has struggled to communicate a brand image that conveys its complex role in a changing health care landscape (Godsey et al., 2020), and so, others are able to portray other images (for example, a female caring role which assists other health professionals), which may be based on their own agenda.

THINK BOX 11.3

- What do you think the public image is of nurses and nursing as a profession in your location?
- Do you get attention from the media?
- Has it changed since the pandemic?

While nursing is often cited as the most trusted profession, nurses struggle to be viewed as influential or autonomous (Godsey et al., 2020). Findings from a systematic review by Girvin et al. (2016) found images of nurses influencing important decision-making to be absent from media portrayals of nursing. The Nursing Now campaign offered a bridge between networks of nurses and the media.

Networks were vital at a high level for global influence, and the campaign was a platform for nurses to connect with each other, creating a new global network of nurses who were involved in nursing practice, education and research. Once the Nightingale Challenge was launched with its focus on young nurses, another network was created and linked. Nursing Now brought the voices of national and local groups closer to the international arena in a way that had not previously been done at such a scale, through bridging networks (Stilwell, 2022).

Linking nurses to the media to address issues of global concern is important because, in general, there is scant media attention on nursing. Nurses are seldom asked to give their views in health news stories, even though they may be germane to the topic and can add important perspectives (Mason et al., 2018). Mason et al.'s US-based study found that nurses were identified as the source of only 2% of quotes in health-related stories, while physicians provided 21% of quotes. Journalists admitted to not understanding the roles or education of nurses, and they said that they often have to justify to editors their use of nurses as sources for stories.

While the COVID-19 pandemic made nurses and nursing highly visible, nurses were not consulted by the media for expert opinions (Mason, 2020). When they were depicted, their image was one of caregiver, not scientist, and this is important, as media portrayals of health issues and health professionals influence the public's perceptions of the leadership of each profession. While nurses see themselves rightly as well-trained professionals, the public views nursing as a low-status profession and is oblivious to the different levels of education and professionalism involved in nursing (Ten Hoeve et al., 2014). The absence of nurses from media briefings and interviews during the pandemic adds to the perception that nursing lacks scientific knowledge and value.

Nursing Now successfully used its position as an advocacy campaign to create bridges between networks, bringing together nurses, international health experts, politicians and policymakers. Nurses have not historically demonstrated great capacity to build bridges between nursing and policy. For example, only 4% of hospital boards in the United States include a nurse member (Mason, 2020), and not all countries yet have a chief nurse in post, even though the largest proportion of the health workforce is made up of nurses. The less that nurses are involved in policy and are not seen as prominent leaders, the weaker their networks with policymakers will be and the more difficult it will be to be noticed and recruited. It is a cycle of failure.

THINK BOX 11.4

- Can you prepare a press release—perhaps on the role nurses have played in infection prevention throughout the pandemic?
- Would you feel comfortable giving a press interview?
- What would make it difficult for you?
- Have you ever been offered media training?
- What preparation would you plan for nurse leaders of the future to change the current image of nursing held by global media?

SOCIAL MEDIA PRESENCE

The Nursing Now campaign had several ways of creating network bridges to give new opportunities to nurses to have their views heard and shared. As already described, having campaign board members who were not nurses was an immediate link to other professional worlds, including politics, which was illuminating for both nurses and board members (Holloway et al., 2021). Social media also proved to be an essential tool in the campaign—and not only because of the pandemic. Nurses are familiar with social media and use it. As an example, the assessment of the use of Twitter by Nursing Now showed how much it is used by nurses. In 2018, tweets from Nursing Now received, at best, 54,000 impressions, and by 2021, on several occasions, there were more than 1 million impressions,* showing the reach of the campaign and the use of X (previously known as Twitter) (Holloway et al., 2021).

---

*High impressions are associated with higher engagement (retweets and likes), meaning more people have seen and reacted to the tweet.

Being a social media presence can be an effective bridge from nursing to the media—newspaper, radio and television reporters look at social media and pick up stories from there. Social movements have used social media to great effect. Think of the social activism created by hashtags such as #MeToo, which served to uncover females' shared stories of sexual harassment, and #BlackLivesMatter, whose 'mission is to eradicate white supremacy and build local power to intervene in violence inflicted on Black communities by the state and vigilantes' (Black Lives Matter, 2024). You may also remember the 2014 #IceBucketChallenge which raised funding for the US charity, the Amyotrophic Lateral Sclerosis (ALS) Foundation. The #IceBucketChallenge resulted in over 17 million people uploading over 10 billion videos viewed by over 440 million people internationally, leading to donations of over USD $220 million.

Social media can be used by nurses to engage with the public, the media and policymakers, and indeed, it already is being used that way, though there is huge potential to expand its use and reach. During the Covid pandemic, nurses used social media to share information about COVID-19 and to support each other. Nursing Now contributed to this process. It was also possible for nurses to show their working conditions and depict the effects of stress (Glasdam et al., 2022). For example, a powerful picture of a nurse in Italy that showed the bruises on her face caused by wearing a protective mask revealed the emotional and physical effects of caring for COVID-19 patients. Social media—which includes X (previously known as Twitter), Facebook, Instagram, LinkedIn, blogs and web presence, Wikipedia and YouTube—provides nurses a way to engage with the public as well as the media and build a nursing brand which reflects modern nursing. It is an available and easy way to create a bridge from nursing to the public, the media and politicians, and young nurses who are just now qualifying will already be engaged and familiar with it.

THINK BOX 11.5

- Do you know how many people use social media in your country/location?
- Is it available?
- What do you think it could be used for?
- What are the challenges with social media?

Nursing is the most trusted profession in many places because nurses are skilled and knowledgeable clinicians and communicators. Using these skills on the media platforms available to us is a strategic way to be more influential as a profession to other professions, health policymakers and the public. This certainly worked during the pandemic when nurses sent out tweets about shortages of PPE or ventilators, but that also resulted in nurses being 'silenced' by their employers in that they were not to talk to the media under pain of being fired. Social media engagement is not without its risks: issues of confidentiality, misinformation, ethical considerations and legal limitations on what is allowed by employers must all be considered (Alsughayr, 2015).

Nursing Now had an experienced communications team to guide the use of social media, and even with them overseeing the work, the campaign occasionally and unwittingly fell foul of our readers. Care is needed about confidentiality, especially if a case study or clinical story is told. Messages spread quickly through social media, and there is less time to think, react and control situations as could be done in traditional media (Alsughayr, 2015), so it is important to consider the content of posts carefully and ask for advice if unsure. But even with the risks, social media offers huge benefits of connection globally, and this is what Nursing Now most valued (Holloway et al., 2021). Web-based connections have offered a chance to build a virtual global social movement (Nursing Now) of nurses who shared the same concerns about the nursing profession and wanted to be able to influence high-level decision-makers in health.

There are also new opportunities for global connectivity for nurses and midwives, meaning that information sharing is possible on a massive scale (Kickbush et al., 2019). The overarching trend globally is that more people are able to get online every year. In 2021, the number of internet users worldwide was estimated to be 4.9 billion, which means that almost two-thirds of the global population is currently connected to the worldwide web. Of course, there are still countries where fewer than 5% are online—these include the poorest countries, including Eritrea, Somalia, Guinea-Bissau, the Central African Republic, Niger and Madagascar—as well as North Korea, where the country's oppressive regime restricts the access to the global internet (Roser et al., 2015; Statista, 2022).

But the overarching trend globally is clear: more people are online every year. The world is changing rapidly, and therefore knowledge is changing, too. While it took 75 years for the telephone to be used by 50 million people, it only took 3.5 years for Facebook to reach the same number (Khayat, 2021). Khayat has also pointed out that the pandemic increased the speed at which many people were willing to adopt change. One striking example is the use of internet- and telephone-based consultations; another is the use of data and analytics, especially in public health, but also in the development of vaccines. What Khayat says is that innovations that would have taken 10 years to get into accepted practice were taking 10 days, driven by the urgency of the pandemic.

Nursing Now flourished through the pandemic because it used internet connectivity to bring together nurses globally to share their experiences, innovations, knowledge and strategies for success. The campaign was shaped by the urgent demands of the pandemic; for example, stress and mental health became a great concern for nurses, and so, Nursing Now was able collaborate with partners to offer special webinars to nurses on how to manage stress (Holloway et al., 2021).

Of course, a pandemic is not a desirable driver of change, but the lessons learned from what happened as a result of the pandemic are valuable. For Nursing Now (and for all of us), the value of connectivity through the internet in health care and in nursing was highlighted. Its potential to continue to connect us globally is clear. Nursing as a global profession has exciting opportunities to embrace and manage in this century as the use of digital health technology grows.

USING THE GLOBAL NURSING NARRATIVE

Nursing stories are powerful. During the Nursing Now campaign, nurses often wrote to us with remarkable stories that described their roles and interactions with people. The stories are compelling because nurses interact with people at their most vulnerable and have to respond to fear, helplessness and sometimes death. But in the culture of health care, stories are seen as weak scientific evidence compared with statistical data collected in controlled trials (Guyatt et al., 2008). Nursing stories may therefore be ignored as evidence and do not give credibility to nursing as a science, even though they may be important as an account of patient and nurse experience.

Ganz (2011) has a perspective on a narrative that reframes it and is relevant to the new opportunities given to nurses through bridging networks created by the Nursing Now campaign and social movement. Ganz describes public narrative as bringing together personal narratives (story of self) into a collective narrative (story of us), which addresses a current problem (story of now). Ganz says that a personal story invites listeners to connect with the teller; this is indeed what happens when nurses tell stories about their work. Through Nursing Now, nurses shared personal stories globally, and other nurses were able to see their own experiences through these stories, so they became the 'story of us'—a collective narrative. The problem which the nurses were addressing in their stories—or in Ganz's terms, the story of now—was the goal of the campaign to raise the profile and status of nursing. Stories have been found to be a powerful tool in communicating values and developing trust. Ganz (2011) suggests that stories show how our values are embedded in experience rather than abstraction, and they show not only meaning but where values come from. Thus the nursing narrative is a powerful one and can engage a listener (Stilwell, 2021).

Giving nurses opportunities to speak in powerful arenas during the Nursing Now campaign brought nursing narratives to the attention of high-level leaders and then could be followed up with relevant statistical evidence. Nursing as a profession has accrued much research-based evidence of its efficiency and effectiveness, but it appears that nursing evidence is not yet taken seriously on the global stage, even though it has important contributions to make to policy discussions and media stories. Nursing Now began to change these negative perceptions by showing the valuable contributions nurses could make at the highest international levels. Towards the end of the campaign, Nursing Now was frequently asked for nurse representatives to be interviewed or join panels; in other words, demand for nurses' contributions increased greatly. Of course, the pandemic also influenced this, as there was a new global awareness of the importance of nurses, though it was also noticeable that nurses were featured so often in the media as heroic carers but hardly ever as scientists.

The 2019 global survey of nurse leadership, in which Nursing Now was a partner, found that the majority of nurse respondents felt unable to speak out in a large meeting or in a group of senior managers, as they lacked self-confidence; they also felt they needed skills to be effective advocates (Newman et al., 2019). One reason for nurses' lack of confidence and the uneasy relationship between nurses and the media may be that nurses do not routinely have training in communications and media skills.

THINK BOX 11.6

- Are you a confident public speaker?
- Can you identify a mentor or coach who can help you improve your speaking skills and confidence?

The ability to frame an argument for change is a critical component of communication. The Nursing Now campaign offered some online training to nurses on how to write a press briefing and how to interact with reporters. Offering nurses the opportunity for media training skills on leadership programmes and, indeed, in postqualification management training would be one way of raising the profile of nurses, as they could work with the media more effectively. Getting a mentor and coach who you respect as a credible speaker is another way to improve your skills.

THE NEXT GENERATION OF NURSE LEADERS

The context of health care, and, indeed, our lives, is constantly changing, especially with the immediacy of global communications and information sharing, but also with increasingly precarious jobs following the global recession (Berry & McDaniel, 2022). There is now significant research that supports the popular notion that 'millennial' or 'Generation Y' workers (born between the early 1980s and the late 1990s) are individualistic, uncommitted to their jobs and have unreasonably high expectations from their employers (Berry & McDaniel, 2022). Younger people seem to want greater flexibility in working hours plus higher salaries. This does not bode well for recruiting nursing students and retaining nurses, and as already discussed in this chapter, the looming shortfall of millions of nurses by 2030

means that recruiting young nurses into the profession is mission critical if there is to be an adequate health workforce. To do so will require new ways of thinking and codesigning work with young people so that there is a nursing workforce that can offer what they are seeking: decent work which is engaging and worthwhile with flexibility and adequate pay.

The Nursing Now campaign appeared to motivate young nurses to be engaged in raising the status and profile of nursing and to progress their careers, and it may be that young nurses were particularly attracted by the global social movement offering links worldwide. The contribution of young people to social change in the 21st century is more noticeable than in previous generations. One example is the support for climate and environmental concerns: in 2019, in what may be the largest youth-led protest in history, millions of students in 300 cities around the world walked out of school to march for climate action.

Nursing Now offered young nurses a global platform to advocate both for their profession and for themselves, and young nurses enthusiastically embraced this opportunity to participate, engage and network. Through local group and by engaging in global social media platforms, young nurses took the opportunity to interact with leaders, in the nursing profession and the broader international health community, in ways they could not have done before the campaign or, indeed, without global connectivity. Young nurses participated as speakers in special webinars that Nursing Now held on difficult subjects, such as racism in the health sector and social inequalities, showing a willingness to engage in these subjects.

The Nursing Now campaign showed how it is possible to engage with young nurses, but the challenge now is to find ways to continue this engagement and to recruit and keep them in the profession. The Nursing Now Challenge continues and aims to link young nurses to each other. Investing in young nurses by codesigning systems that they want to work in, by investing in their learning and harnessing the new thinking they bring, is essential if nursing is to continue to grow and thrive in the 21st century.

LOOKING TO THE FUTURE

There is not one story about the future. Anything is possible, and we need lots of stories to explore all possibilities, and yet, we spend little time considering what the future will be like (Thimbleby, 2013). Thimbleby reminds us that when we get to the future, it, too, will have another future—there are many futures ahead that we should be considering in looking at the future of nursing. And Thimbleby (2013, p. 161) reminds us of something else: '… while technology drives changes in healthcare, the fundamental problems of wellbeing, health and happiness, will remain'.

For nursing in particular, the point about well-being, health and happiness always being a desirable goal for people is one that we should mark well as technology advances. The pace of change in technological innovation is accelerating, and new solutions emerge constantly—many of which are highly desirable. such as cancer or dementia treatments, robotic keyhole surgery or the use of computer-generated algorithms that use big data to generate likely diagnoses. Genomics is changing everything, too; eventually we might all be given, at birth, a forecast of our lifetime morbidity profile (National Human Genome Research Institute, 2022).

Where is the place of nurses in this story of the future? It is not easy to predict, of course, but there are some indicators from the Nursing Now campaign about nursing's adaptability and the value nurses perceive in their own profession. Read Chapter 4 on the role of nurses in humanitarian emergencies to see how nursing adapted its skills and approaches from nurses' learning in theatres of war. The Nursing Now final report was called 'Agents of Change' because the stories that nurses shared with us demonstrated that they are constantly looking for ways to improve care and to innovate. The pandemic of 2020 showed this only too well when nurses had to find ways to care for dying people who could not see their families (using technology to connect them face to face) or find a way to create adequate PPE (bin bags in some cases). In looking at the role of nurses in technologically advanced future scenarios, it is to the human aspects of health and well-being that we should turn.

THINK BOX 11.7

Imagine you are transported to a health facility in your current location—but in the year 2123.

- What will it look like?
- Who will be there?
- What will the nurses be doing?

POSSIBLE (AND PROBABLE) FUTURES—A MORE RADICAL PLANNING APPROACH

The Nursing Now campaign was a repository for 'a rich tapestry' of stories of what was happening in nursing around the world (Holloway et al., 2021, p. 59) from 2018 until 2021, so through the pandemic. These stories showed that nurses are innovative and can be change-makers, too. To plan effectively for the future, we need to take a wide view of the context of change into which technological advances will be implemented. Planners who consider the complexity of systems—including health systems planners—often use scenario planning to create a 'storyline' of what might be happening and consider ways of responding to change (Wiles, 2022). As with the stories we collected in Nursing Now, future stories help the ideas to come alive and be more real. Scenario planning, while specialised, is widely available and used in business. With the complexity of future in health, this is a tool that nurses should consider.

Scenarios are imagined descriptions of possible futures—not necessarily the most probable ones, but plausible and different from the present. Though there had been much global planning in the health sector for a pandemic, not much went according to plan. This shows how critical it is to prepare for even the most unlikely scenarios. Here are six possible future scenarios and some ideas for responding to them. The scenarios are built on the vision of Khayat (2021) and are those that seem most relevant to nursing in the future.

Scenario 1: Proactive, Preventive, Predictive Health Care

Khayat (2021) predicts that instead of being reactive to the needs of the sick, health care in the future will be proactive, preventive and predictive, taking what can be predicted about a person's health life course and planning good health management for maximum well-being. Most people—especially young people—now know where to look for health-related information (Topol, 2015). In many areas of our lives, we have taken control of our own behaviour—booking our own travel, banking online, watching programmes on our TVs when we want to; health is not far behind.

Soon, says Topol, patients will have instant access on smartphones to their own health care data combined with information from huge central databases that will explain risk and best management options. It will be in the power of the patient to share information with their medical team—hence the title of his recent book: *The Patient will See You Now* (Topol, 2015). This is a huge power shift from medical system–centred care delivery, and it opens up new opportunities for nurses who can become interpreters for people of the information they find and receive. How does someone deal with all their health information? How does it affect their physical and mental being? In the future, being the most trusted profession will become even more significant as people have to make sense of predictive information.

Scenario 2: Precise, Personalised Care

Because of advances in genomics, it will be possible to tailor treatments to each person based on many individual factors—but will it be acceptable to the person? Will it be what they want as well as what the science suggests they should have? Who will advocate for the individual? This is where the 'what matters to you' movement, which has taken off in recent years, will come into its own. Maureen Bisognano, who was a board member for Nursing Now, advocates for nurses—and all health workers—to ask not only 'what is the matter with you?' but 'what matters to you?'. As we can each get a treatment tailored for us by science and statistics, how vital it will be to have a nurse by our side who will ask this important question as choices are made.

Scenario 3: Care Anywhere

The pandemic has accelerated what was coming; we had Covid tests in our cars and village halls and immunisations in pharmacies and community centres. Already, pharmacies have consultation rooms for minor illnesses. End-of-life care is delivered at home. Community nurses care for mental and physical health outside of institutions. If you can imagine places for health care to be delivered, then it will probably be so. Nurses excel at this, for nurses have always led care in the community and are to be found in many community locations, from stores to schools to homes to prisons. Technology is again driving

these changes. Clinical decisions will be supported by long-distance virtual consultations with a team. We will all be able to look for evidence in real time on our smartphones to give the best care. Big data will be collected routinely and—this is even more exciting—analysed and fed back to all of us so that we can talk about the science behind our health outcomes: how nursing care changes the course and outcome of a disease or how costs are changed through more efficient care. The possibilities are huge, and we should be excited and involved and learning the languages of economics and policy.

Scenario 4: Continuous, Team Based

Nurses have always worked as part of a team—this mode of working will not be new. But we need new attitudes to teamwork, where we learn to be consulted as part of a team and be able to speak up with our science so that we are properly heard, and we can advocate for patients if we need to. Nursing Now showed that many nurses remain intimidated by speaking in a large group (Newman et al., 2019), and for nurses to be truly effective team members contributing fully, our voices have to be heard. How will this happen? Learning the skills of communication—discussed already in this chapter—is a vital first step and must be in every nurse's curriculum.

We have to learn to be more nimble, agile and consultative in the interests of those we will be caring for, rather in the way nurses showed they could do during the pandemic. Our teams will be far more dynamic—a matrix of many teams that we belong to that come together to support people along their care pathways. Team members will vary, team leaders will change and decisions will be taken in consultation with each other and with the person whose care we discuss. This is a different way of working, currently seen in some technology industries but not so much in health care.

Continuous care will focus on human flourishing rather than health alone. There are many nurses who already support people to be living their best lives (Crisp, 2020). They make it their business to be part of their communities, available to be consulted and innovating so that communities really do flourish. Take a look at Chapter 2 in this book on planetary health: another area where nurses must be involved far more than presently. Chapter 1 on the Sustainable Development Goals (SDGs) points us to what we as nurses can do to influence policies for a fairer society and to reduce the health gaps between rich and poor. That is our business, too, and together we should be involved activists—another example of where we can use social media to bring our messages to a wide public.

Scenario 5: People Powered

The traditional relationship between patient and provider has been viewed as paternalistic, with the provider really holding all the power to be the authority on treatment. In those relationships, the patient took a subordinate role and was often glad to. After all, the provider was the expert with years of clinical training and 'knew best'. But society as a whole, as well as health care professionals, are now calling these power hierarchies into question, saying that they do not align with patient-centred and value-based health care models.

A 2018 survey of over 1000 current or past intensive care unit patients showed that very few patients or family members are raising their worries during care encounters (Heath, 2018). Between 50% and 70% of respondents reported hesitation when voicing concerns about possible mistakes, mismatched care goals, confusing or conflicting information or inadequate clinician hand hygiene. About half of respondents said they did not want to be perceived as a 'troublemaker' or that the team appeared too busy to hear a concern. Patients also said they did not know how to report a health care concern in this setting. This should be of huge importance to nurses everywhere and points to how far we have yet to travel to really change power dynamics in health care.

With health care priorities trending toward overall patient wellness, a more balanced partnership between patients and providers will be key so that people can speak up as equals and truly participate in their own health care decisions. Nurses will be able to facilitate this power shift as ambassadors of health teams, learning to listen deeply to what is being said.

Scenario 6: Focusing on Health Outcomes

Health care is expensive everywhere, but what gets paid for is, in fact, curing sickness rather than creating healthy and resilient communities, families and individuals. It is important, of course, that a society can offer treatment for illness, but there is so much that could be invested in health: good housing, green spaces, a healthier environment, food that keeps us active, safe exercise like walking and biking, access to a gym, early education opportunities—the list is long and essentially addresses the social determinants of health (Marmot et al., 2020; Rosa & Mason, this book [Chapter 1]).

This list is as much our business as is the use of evidence-based treatments. Nurses can be pivotal in helping people have a lifestyle of remaining active, lessening their stress, boosting their mental health and living safely. Yet we know that the budget for health care goes mainly to fund hospitals and high-tech care. To be all that we should be in the future of health care, nurses have to learn about health economics and the cost savings inherent in having a healthier, happier society and advocate for different investments in community health.

As people become more health literate, we will all be called to account for the outcomes of what we are doing.

THINK BOX 11.8

- Having considered these future scenarios, have you changed any ideas about the future of nursing?
- If you teach or mentor others, why not ask them about their ideas too and then present these scenarios—or carry out your own scenario building exercise where you are working?

CONCLUSION

The world is currently facing a new reality in its health care landscape: health care demands are changing, with noncommunicable diseases on the rise everywhere and requiring both prevention and long-term care strategies. There is a call for universal health coverage—health care for everyone, everywhere; people want care at home, not in hospital, until the end of their lives, and technology is advancing quickly to make the care on offer unrecognisable. Nurses are needed to help shape future health systems, yet they struggle to participate in health policy decision-making (Hajiza-deh et al., 2021).

The Nursing Now campaign aimed to raise the status and profile of nurses, recognising that nurses alone could not do this, so the campaign relied on creating bridging networks and coalitions with more powerful players in the health arena. This was possible because of the origins of the Nursing Now campaign with enthusiastic backing from a senior British politician and his networks that linked the campaign to high levels of decision making. In addition, the Nursing Now campaign became a successful global social movement which gave nurses a new sense of power and cohesion through working together. Nationally and internationally, nurses were united around the common mission of improving their working lives and thus maximising the benefits of nursing to health. The connectedness and new thinking of young nurses was valued and developed.

The campaign has created a new global solidarity, allowing greater interchange of partnerships, ideas and mutual support. Its legacy is that many Nursing Now groups, with their ability to bring together diverse organisations—nursing and nonnursing—for a common purposewill continue to operate into the future and that the Nursing Now Challenge has convened a remarkable network of young professionals who can work together to influence the future.

The COVID-19 pandemic dominated our world for 2 years and will influence its shape for the future. It has made the work that nurses do—from work in the community to the most intensive of care—visible to the wider public, and there is some evidence that nurses have become more respected and valued. It has also revealed the dangerous and difficult situations in which so many nurses work and demonstrated beyond doubt how important their role is to us all. The final report of the Nursing Now campaign, 'Agents of Change' (Holloway et al., 2021), tells the stories of how nurses and their allies created a powerful platform from which to improve health and develop nursing. It has been a step change in what will necessarily be a long journey to address the major cultural and social shifts that are necessary to match societal changes and transform nursing for a dynamic future.

REFERENCES

All-Party Parliamentary Group on Global Health. (2016). *Triple Impact: How developing nursing will improve health, promote gender equality and support economic growth.* APPG on Global Health. https://globalhealth.inparliament.uk/news/triple-impact-how-investing-nursing-will-improve-health-improve-gender-equality-and-support. (Last accessed February 2024).

Alsughayr, A. (2015). Social media in health care: Uses, risks and barriers. *Saudi Journal of Medicine and Medical Sciences, 3*(2), 105–111.

Battilana, J., & Casciaro, T. (2013). The network secrets of great change agents. *Harvard Business Review.* https://hbr.org/2013/07/the-network-secrets-of-great-change-agents. (Access February 2024.)

Beard, M. (2017). *Women and power: A manifesto.* Profile Books.

Berry, C., & McDaniel, S. (2022). Post-crisis precarity: Understanding attitudes to work and industrial relations among young people in the UK. *Economic and Industrial Democracy, 43*(1), 322–343. doi:10.1177/0143831X19894380.

Black Lives Matter (2024). https://blacklivesmatter.com/about/.

Brown, P., & Zavetoski, S. (2005). *Social movements in health.* Wiley Blackwell.

Buchan, J., Catton, H., & Schaffer, F. (2022). *Sustain and retain in 2022 and beyond. International council of nurses commissioned papers—International centre on nurse migration (intlnursemigration.org).* Retrieved, Februrary 2024, from https://www.intlnursemigration.org/commissioned-papers/. (Accessed February 2024).

Crisp, N. (2020). *Health is made at home. Hospitals are for repairs.* Salus.

Della, P. D., & Diani, M. (2020). *Social movements an introduction.* Wiley Blackwell.

Eisler, R. (2015). Human possibilities: The interaction of biology and culture. *Interdisciplinary Journal of Partnership Studies, 1*(1), 3.

Ghana Registered Nurses and Midwives Association. (2020). *One million PPE for frontline health workers campaign* [Video]. YouTube. https://www.youtube.com/watch?v=TiI7K_pF_xA.

Girvin, J., Jackson, D., & Hutchinson, M. (2016). Contemporary public perceptions of nursing: A systematic review and narrative synthesis of the international research evidence. *Journal of Nursing Management, 24*(8), 994–1006. doi:10.1111/jonm.12413.

Glasdam, S., Sandberg, H., Stjernswärd, S., Jacobsen, F., Grønning, A., & Hybholt, L. (2022). Nurses' use of social media during the COVID-19 pandemic—A scoping review. *PLoS One, 22.* https://www.ncbi.nlm.nih.gov/pmc/articles/PMC8856556/. (Last accessed February 2024).

Godsey, J. A., Houghton, D. M., & Hayes, T. (2020). Registered nurse perceptions of factors contributing to the inconsistent brand image of the nursing profession. *Nursing Outlook, 68*(6), 808821. doi:10.1016/j.outlook.2020.06.005.

Guyatt, G. H., Oxman, A. D., Vist, G. E., Kunz, R., Falck-Ytter, Y., Alonso-Coello, P., & Schünemann, H. J.; GRADE Working Group. (2008). GRADE: an emerging consensus on rating quality of evidence and strength of recommendations. *British Medical Journal, 336*(7650), 924–926. doi: 10.1136/bmj.39489.470347.AD. PMID: 18436948; PMCID: PMC2335261.

Hajizadeh, A., Zamanzadeh, V., Kakemam, E., Bahreini, R., & Khodayari-Zarnaqet, R. (2021). Factors influencing nurses participation in the health policy-making process: A systematic review. *BMC Nursing, 20*, 128. doi:10.1186/s12912-021-00648-6.

Heath, S. (2018). *Understanding the power hierarchy in patient-provider relationships*. Patient Engagement. https://patientengagementhit.com/news/understanding-the-power-hierarchy-in-patient-provider-relationships.

Holloway, A., Thomson, A., Stilwell, B., Finch, H., Irwin, K., & Crisp, N. (2021). Agents of change: The story of the Nursing Now Campaign. *Nursing Now/Burdett Trust for Nursing*. https://www.nursingnow.org/wp-content/uploads/2021/05/Nursing-Now-Final-Report.pdf. (Last accessed February 2024).

Khayat, Z. (2021). *Future of NP/APN: Innovation*. Rotman School, University of Toronto Faculty, Singularity University, Canada. Singularity University ICN NP/APN Virtual Conference 2021. www.icn.ch.

Kickbush, I., Agrawa, A., Jack, A., Lee, N., & Horton, R. (2019). Governing health futures 2030: Growing up in a digital world—a joint The Lancet and Financial Times Commission. *The Lancet, 394*(10206), 1297–1386. The Lancet and Financial Times Commission on governing health futures 2030: growing up in a digital world.

Levin, S., & Bekiempis, V. (2022). "'It's important to fight": US cities erupt in protest as Roe v Wade falls. *The Guardian*. https://www.theguardian.com/us-news/2022/jun/24/us-cities-protest-roe-v-wade-abortion-rights.

Marshall, G. (2011). Public narrative, collective action, and power. In Odugbemi, S., & Lee, T. (Eds.), *Accountability through public opinion: From inertia to public action* (pp. 273–289). The World Bank. https://dash.harvard.edu/handle/1/29314925.

Marmot, M., Allen, J., Boyce, T., Goldblatt, P., & Morrison, J. (2020). *Health equity in England: The marmot review 10 years on*. Institute of Health Equity. www.health.org.uk/publications/reports/the-marmot-review-10-years-on.

Mason, D., Nixon, L., Glickstein, B., Han, S., Westphaln, K., & Carter, L. (2018). The woodhull study revisited: Nurses' representation on in health news media 20 years later. *Journal of Nursing Scholarship, 50*(6), 695–704.

Mason, D. (2020). Nurses lack representation in media: Recognize them for the leaders that they are. *Opinion USA Today*. https://eu.usatoday.com/story/opinion/2020/06/26/nurses-leaders-medicine-but-overshadowed-media-column/3223242001/. (Last accessed February 2024).

National Human Genome Research Institute. (2022). *A brief guide to genomics*. https://www.genome.gov/about-genomics/fact-sheets/A-Brief-Guide-to-Genomics.

Newman, C., Stilwell, B., Rick, S., & Peterson, K. (2019). *Investing in the power of nurse leadership: What will it take?* IntraHealth International. https://www.intrahealth.org/resources/investing-power-nurse-leadership-what-will-it-take.

RCN Bulletin. (2022). History shows that when members act they are formidable. https://www.rcn.org.uk/magazines/History/2022/Oct/History-shows-that-when-members-act-they-are-formidable.

RCN News. (2022). We strike for the future of the NHS. Retrieved, December 15, 2022 from https://www.rcn.org.uk/news-and-events/news/uk-rcn-nhs-nursing-strikes-2022-first-day-151222.

Roser, M., Ritchie, H., & Ortiz-Ospina, E. (2015). "Internet." Published online at *OurWorldInData.org*. https://ourworldindata.org/internet.

Salvage, J., & Stilwell, B. (2018). Breaking the silence: A new story of nursing. *Journal of Clinical Nursing, 27*(7–8), 1301–1303.

Salvage, J., & White, J. (2019). Nursing leadership and health policy: Everybody's business. *International Nursing Review, 66*(2), 147–150. doi:10.1111/inr.12523.

Statista Internet Usage Worldwide. (2022). Internet usage Worldwide: statistics and facts. https://www.statista.com/topics/1145/internet-usage-worldwide/#topicOverview. (Last accessed February 2024.)

Stilwell, B. (2021). *The power of the nursing narrative. Lisbeth hockey memorial lecture*. International Collaboration on Community Health Nursing Research. https://www.icchnr.org/lisbeth-hockey-memorial-lectures/.

Stilwell, B., & Newman, C. (2022). Nurses learning to be powerful leaders: What will it take? *Creative Nursing, 28*(1), 23–28. doi:10.1891/cn-2021-0062. PMID: 35173058.

Ten Hoeve, Y., Jansen, G., & Roodbol, P. (2014). The nursing profession: Public image, self-concept and professional identity. A discussion paper. *Journal of Advanced Nursing, 70*(2), 295–309.

Thimbleby, H. (2013). Technology and the future of healthcare. *Journal of Public Health Research, 2*(3), 160–167.e28. doi: 10.4081/jphr.2013.e28. PMID: 25170499; PMCID: PMC4147743. (Last accessed February 2024).

Topol, E. (2015). *The patient will see you now*. Basic Books.

Waithaka, D., Kagwanja, N., Nzinga, J., Tsofa, B., Leli H., Mataza, C., Nyaguara, A., Bejon, P., Gilson, L., Barasa, E., & Molyneux, S. (2020). Prolonged health worker strikes in Kenya- perspectives and experiences of frontline health managers and local communities in Kilifi County. *International Journal for Equity in Health, 19*, 23. doi:10.1186/s12939-020-1131-y. (Last accessed February 2024).

Wiles, J. (2022). *What functional leaders should know about scenario planning*. Gartner Insights. https://www.gartner.com/smarterwithgartner/what-functional-leaders-should-know-about-scenario-planning.

Wilson, D. M., Underwood, L., Kim, S., Olukotun, M., & Errasti-Ibarrondo, B. (2022). How and why nurses became involved in politics or political action, and the outcomes or impacts of this involvement. *Nursing Outlook, 70*(1), 5563. doi:10.1016/j.outlook.2021.07.008.

World Health Organization, Global Health Workforce Network and Women in Global Health. (2019). *Global health: Delivered by women, led by men: A gender and equity analysis of the global health workforce* (p. 76). World Health Organization. https://www.who.int/hrh/resources/health-observer24/en/.

World Health Organization. (2020). *State of the world's nursing 2020*. World Health Organization. https://www.who.int/publications/i/item/9789240003279.

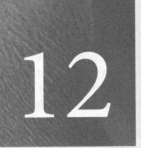

12

THE FUTURE OF NURSING IN THE 21ST CENTURY

HOWARD CATTON
■ with contributions from JUDY KHANYOLA ■ AISHA
HOLLOWAY ■ ELIZABETH MADIGAN ■ PANDORA
HARDTMAN ■ ZIPPORAH IREGI ■ BARBARA STILWELL

'Prediction is difficult – particularly when it involves the future'.
Mark Twain

In this chapter, we describe the problems of predicting the future and then dabble in doing exactly that. We conclude by stating that despite the impossibility of knowing exactly what will happen in the future, a well-funded, -supported and -protected nursing workforce will be ready for whatever is going to come over the horizon. And the reason that is true is because what nurses are doing, at the cutting edge of practice all around the world, is happening as the present becomes the future: the future is effectively already here.

Predicting the future is fraught with difficulty, and predicting the future of nursing is no different. If we think about what nurses in the 1950s would have said about nursing in the first three decades of this century, it is clear that there have been many societal, medical and technological developments that could not have been foreseen.

An experienced nurse in the 1950s could not have predicted the enormous growth in noncommunicable diseases and the advances in nursing, medical, surgical, psychiatric, psychological and pharmacological interventions, or the incredible impact that computers, and especially the internet, have had on nursing practice and nurses' lives.

By the same token, a nurse from the 1950s could not have predicted how much societies have changed or how far nursing has come in terms of its autonomy and influence and how it has become a largely graduate entry profession and an academic discipline in its own right.

And of course, they could not have foreseen the devastating effects of the climate crisis which are overshadowing human civilisation at this time and threatening the very survival of our species on Planet Earth. This book has dealt with the global issues that affect nursing, health systems and health; looking at the future for nursing highlights how important it is for nurses to be aware of the state of the world, who holds the power and how all of that plays out in our lives, professional and personal.

THINK BOX 12.1

Why is it so difficult to predict the future?
List the specific things you can think of that making predicting the future of nursing so complex.

The reason predictions about nursing are so hard to get right are manifold, including:

- The future is inherently uncertain, and random events, chance discoveries or unpredictable changes in circumstances can have significant impacts on outcomes. For example, transplant surgery is more or less routine in many countries, but it was almost nonexistent in the 1950s (Barker & Markmann, 2013).
- The systems that nurses work in are increasingly complex, making it difficult to foresee all the possible outcomes accurately.
- Despite advances in information technology and its use in health care settings, our knowledge of the world is limited, and without comprehensive data, predictions will inevitably be incomplete or inaccurate.

- Technological advances and innovations can lead to disruptive changes, creating unforeseen opportunities and challenges. For example, it is now possible to buy a watch that includes an electrocardiograph monitor that can alert the wearer to abnormal heart rhythms.
- Today's interconnected world makes it difficult to predict the consequences of complex global interactions, evidenced by the COVID-19 pandemic which, despite pandemics having been anticipated and prepared for at the very highest level, spread uncontrollably around the globe within weeks (Independent Panel for Pandemic Preparedness and Response, 2021).
- Societal and cultural changes can have a significant impact on the future, and these are often difficult to predict due to their complex and dynamic nature. For example, the first-wave feminists changed many societies forever and influenced the creation of the International Council of Nurses (ICN) at the start of the 20th century (Brush & Lynaugh, 1999). The second-wave feminists of the 1960s and 1970s had a huge influence on nursing and its status within health care (Roberts & Group, 1995).
- Unforeseen events and challenges can have a profound effect on the future. In the case of nursing, these include emerging infectious diseases, noncommunicable diseases and increased mental health problems; the global climate crisis and increased political instability, including wars, disasters and unexpected mass migrations; the recent challenges of the ageing nursing workforce, and global shortages and the medium- and long-term effects of the COVID-19 pandemic on the health of patients and nurses.

All of these can seem daunting, but what we know is that when these changes take place, nurses are not overwhelmed or paralysed by them. Instead, they respond immediately; they adapt, adopt and evolve in dynamic ways to the new situations that confront them. They move with the present, and that is what ultimately defines the future, not just keeping pace with change but anticipating, innovating and boldly moving ahead of the status quo and, by so doing, changing the game.

What is striking about nursing's influence is that it happens without nurses necessarily being among the key decision-makers in health care policy and planning. Political and health system leaders, and arguably the public as well, do not appreciate that nursing is the engine room of health systems' responses, and because of that, our contribution is often overlooked when it comes to investment in nursing education, jobs, leadership and practice. The potential of nursing and nurses is consistently overlooked, to the detriment of the development of health services and health care outcomes, and part of the blame for that lies with deference within the nursing profession itself.

THINK BOX 12.2

- How has nursing from the past influenced the nursing practice of today?
- Can you think of practices that you have seen that should be consigned to history?
- How does that process happen?

THE INFLUENCE OF THE PAST

In looking to the future, nursing needs to acknowledge its past. The fundamentals of nursing, including those laid out by its founders and definers, such as Florence Nightingale in the 19th century (Nightingale, 1860) and Ethel Gordon Fenwick and Virginia Henderson in the 20th century (Brush & Lynaugh, 1999), have not really changed. They argued that nursing should be an independent profession, they acknowledged the science and art of nursing and they placed health within its broad social and environmental contexts.

Few nurses would argue that they are not as relevant today as they have ever been and that they are likely to remain so for the foreseeable and, indeed, the unforeseeable future.

In terms of the nursing profession, Florence Nightingale suggested (Nightingale Society, 2020):

- That nursing should remain an independent profession in its own right.
- That it should have a career path with excellent training, working conditions, salaries and pensions.
- That nurses' health and safety are important and that they should be involved with other professions in making decisions about health care and the facilities within which it is carried out.

■ That nursing care should be available to all, regardless of their financial situation and their ability to pay.

So, while it is extremely challenging to accurately predict aspects of the future, understanding potential trends and preparing for multiple scenarios can help us navigate the uncertainties ahead. Indeed, we would suggest that nurses have done exactly that and that 'the future' should not be looked on as a challenge but merely as something that nurses have always, and will always, adapted to and coped with.

THINK BOX 12.3

Can you make any predictions about how nursing will change during your career?
Make a list of changes you think will happen in the next 10, 20 or 30 years.

Having said that it is very challenging to predict the future, it is nevertheless possible to suggest some trends, including:

■ Nursing is likely to see the adoption of advanced technologies in patient care, including the widespread use of artificial intelligence (AI) and robotics to assist with nurse education and various tasks, such as patient monitoring, medication administration and repetitive procedures.
■ Telemedicine and remote patient care, which grew extensively during the COVID-19 pandemic, will likely become more common, allowing nurses to provide more personalised care to patients in their homes and in otherwise inaccessible remote areas.
■ Advances in genomics will lead to more personalised medicine, which nurses may be involved in, for example, through testing and administration of tailored medicines for individual patients.
■ Collaboration between various health care disciplines will be essential in providing comprehensive patient care, with nurses working even more closely with doctors, pharmacists, therapists and social workers to address patients' holistic needs.
■ Nurses may become increasingly specialised to maximise their impact on patient care. This will result in the emergence of new roles and specialties, for example, to further address the needs of an ageing population and the management of chronic diseases.
■ Simulation and the use of virtual and augmented reality equipment will increase in pre- and post-registration nurse education, improving learning outcomes and refining skills.
■ The increased focus on primary health care, health promotion, disease prevention and patient education will continue to address burgeoning noncommunicable diseases and other lifestyle-related problems.
■ In an increasingly globalised world, nurses will be responding even more to global health problems, including pandemics, disaster relief efforts and addressing health care inequalities worldwide.
■ Technological advances may create new ethical and legal dilemmas concerning patient privacy, data management and the use of new technology such as AI.
■ Nursing shortages will have to be addressed if the health-related aspects of the Sustainable Development Goals are to be met alongside the inevitable increase in demand for health care services.
■ Efforts to promote diversity and inclusion in the nursing workforce will continue, fostering a larger, more representative and culturally competent health care workforce that will be better able to meet patients' needs.
■ Universal health coverage will not be achieved unless investment is made in the health workforce in order to strengthen health systems.

THINK BOX 12.4

● Can you add anything to the list?
● Which items in the list do you think are most likely to be influential?

In all of these, nurses will have a major focus on prevention, perhaps more so than any other professional group. They will be working alongside people and patients in partnership, helping them manage the complexity of their conditions and coordinating their care to achieve positive health outcomes, overwhelmingly in people's homes and communities.

All too often, the importance of this move to the community is overlooked. It seems to be invisible, yet being cared for at home is very popular with patients, and with the continuing growth in the world's population and the changes in the world's demographics, it is the only approach that is going to be affordable and sustainable in the long term. Universal health coverage will not necessarily be achieved by building new hospitals or clinics: it is more likely to come about by nurses going to where people live and work.

The ICN has always been concerned about the future of the profession. In its early years, it was determined to influence nursing education and regulation to create a globally coherent profession based on a standardised curriculum.

In recent years, the ICN has continued to influence the development and unity of the profession through its many publications and participation in high-level decision-making fora and to urge governments to value, protect, respect and invest in the nursing profession. The ICN's International Nurse Day publications (ICN, 2017–2023) have been closely linked to global health goals, including the Sustainable Development Goals (United Nations, 2015), universal health coverage (World Health Organization, 2019) and health as a human right (World Health Organization, 2017). All of these efforts are intended to secure the relevance and the future of the profession in the long term.

'THE STATE OF THE WORLD'S NURSING' REPORT

In 2020, the World Health Organization (WHO), Nursing Now and the ICN published the first-ever 'State of the World's Nursing' report (World Health Organization, Nursing Now and ICN, 2020), which provided a snapshot of the global nursing workforce. Among other data, it included:

- Data from 191 WHO member states revealed a prepandemic shortfall of nearly 6 million nurses, with lower nurse-to-population ratios in middle- and low-income countries.
- Ninety percent of the global nursing workforce is female.
- The maldistribution of nurses is exacerbated by international recruitment from low- to high-income countries.

Its main recommendations were that governments should:

- Invest in the massive acceleration of nursing education—faculty, infrastructure and students—to address global needs, meet domestic demand and respond to changing technologies and advancing models of integrated health and social care.
- Create at least 6 million new nursing jobs by 2030, primarily in low- and middle-income countries, to offset the projected shortages and redress the inequitable distribution of nurses across the world.
- Strengthen nurse leadership—both current and future leaders—to ensure that nurses have an influential role in health policy formulation and decision-making and contribute to the effectiveness of health and social care systems.

The ICN lobbied the WHO for a second 'State of the World's Nursing' report, and that is due to be published in 2025. It will, for the first time, be able to demonstrate a trend in the size, distribution and component parts of the global nursing workforce and show the differences between before and after the pandemic.

'SUSTAIN AND RETAIN IN 2022 AND BEYOND'

In 2022, the ICN's 'Sustain and Retain in 2022 and Beyond' report, published jointly with the Commission on Graduates of Foreign Nursing Schools (CGFNS) and the ICN International Centre for Nurse Migration, revealed how the COVID-19 pandemic had a dramatic effect on individual nurses, worsening their physical and mental health and making the fragile state of the global nursing workforce much worse. Its conclusions, which concluded that up to 13 million more nurses would be required over the next decade, showed that the ambition of achieving universal health coverage is at serious risk.

The 'Sustain and Retain' report concluded that:

- There is persistent underfunding of the nursing profession worldwide.
- Countries provide safe staffing levels to protect patients and nurses.
- Countries must expand their domestic nurse education systems so that they can become

self-sufficient and end damaging international recruitment drives.

- Governments must adhere to ethical international recruitment standards.
- Improving retention and the attractiveness of nursing careers for females and males will help address the global nursing shortage.
- This is a global health crisis that requires a fully funded and actionable 10-year plan to support and strengthen nurses and the health and care workforce to deliver health for all.

The recommendations in 'Sustain and Retain' were further developed in ICN's next publication, 'Recover to Rebuild'.

'RECOVER TO REBUILD'

In its 2023 report, 'Recover to Rebuild: Investing in the Nursing Workforce for Health System Effectiveness' (International Council of Nurses, 2023), the ICN stated that the worldwide shortage of nurses should be treated as a global health emergency and that health systems around the world would only start to recover from the effects of the pandemic and be rebuilt when there was sufficient investment in a well-supported global nursing workforce.

'Recover to Rebuild':

- Built on the analysis of the 'Sustain and Retain' report;
- Acknowledged the toll the pandemic had on nurses who were on the front lines, and often in the firing line;
- Cited more than 100 studies showing 40%–80% of nurses reported experiencing symptoms of psychological distress, that nurses' intention to leave rates had risen to 20% or more and annual hospital turnover rates increased to 10% and even higher;
- Recounted the vital and often dangerous role nurses played during the pandemic and provided evidence from studies of nurses from 24 countries around the globe;
- Showed how the COVID effect compounded already fragile health systems and the unequivocal need for substantial and sustained investment in nursing education, jobs, leadership and practice;
- Detailed the effects of stress, burnout, absences from work and strikes on the nursing workforce, all of which are symptoms of the perilous state of health care; and
- Declared the postpandemic situation as a direct result of a lack of action and the absence of a long-term vision and a plan for the future of the global nursing workforce.

'Recover to Rebuild' included an action agenda for protecting and supporting the nursing workforce in the future so that health systems could be rebuilt after the pandemic. It included:

Nationally:

- Nurse workforce impact assessments
- Commitment to invest and support for safe staffing levels
- Commitment to support early access to full vaccinations programmes for all nurses
- Reviewing/expanding the capacity of the domestic nurse education systems
- Investing in the retention of nurses and the attractiveness of nursing as a career
- Implementing policies for improved career structures and optimising the workforce through advanced practice roles and appropriate technological support
- Monitoring and tracking nurse self-sufficiency

Internationally:

- Securing an immediate update of the 'State of the World's Nursing' analysis
- Commitment to support for early access to full vaccination programmes for all nurses in all countries
- Commitment to implementing and evaluating effective and ethical approaches to managing the international supply of nurses
- Commitment to supporting regular and systematic nurse workforce impact assessments, particularly in resource-constrained countries
- Commitment to investing in nurse workforce sustainability in small states, lower-income states and fragile states, which are the most vulnerable to nurse outflow and the most severely affected by the pandemic

THINK BOX 12.5

- Take the time out to read the reports given.
- Consider how the global view of ICN can be influential in day-to-day nursing care around the world.

The theme of ICN's 2023 International Nurses Day resources was 'Our Nurses, Our Future'. It included the ICN's Charter for Change (International Council of Nurses, 2023), which was an urgent call to action for governments to start to address the many issues facing the nursing profession and secure its future.

To come to fruition, the charter requires long-term commitments from governments to invest in nursing education, jobs, leadership and practice so that universal health coverage can become a reality.

The Charter for Change's 10 policy actions:

1. Protect and invest in the nursing profession to rebuild health systems that can deliver the Sustainable Development Goals and universal health coverage to improve global health. Recognise and value health and health care as an investment, not a cost. Secure commitments for investment to maintain equitable and people-centred care.
2. Urgently address and improve support for nurses' health and well-being by ensuring safe and healthy working conditions and respecting their rights. Put in place systems to ensure safe staffing levels. Ensure protections against violence and hazards in the workplace and implement and enforce international labour standards on the rights of nurses to work in safe and healthy supportive environments, ensuring physical as well as mental health protections.
3. Advance strategies to recruit and retain nurses to address workforce shortages. Improve compensation for nurses to ensure fair and decent pay and benefits and uphold positive practice environments that listen to nurses and provide them with the resources they need to do their jobs safely, effectively and efficiently. Fund professional governance, recognition and development activities across career trajectories.
4. Develop, implement and finance national nursing workforce plans with the objective of self-sufficiency in the supply of future nurses. Align resources to support a robust workforce to deliver essential health services, reverse unemployment and retain talent. When international migration takes place, ensure it is ethical, transparent, monitored and delivers equal mutual benefits for sending and receiving countries as well as respecting the rights of individual nurses. Undertake system workforce planning and monitoring across the care continuum.
5. Invest in high-quality, accredited nursing education programmes to prepare more new nurses and advance career development for existing nurses. Design curricula so that nurses graduate with the right skills, competencies and confidence to respond to the changing and evolving health needs of communities and support career progression from generalist to specialist and advanced practice.
6. Enable nurses to work to their full scope of nursing practice by strengthening and modernising regulation and investing in advanced nursing practice and nurse-led models of care. Reorientate and integrate health systems to public health, primary care health promotion and prevention, and community, home-based and patient-centred care.
7. Recognise and value nurses' skills, knowledge, attributes and expertise. Respect and promote nurses' roles as health professionals, scientists, researchers, educators and leaders. Involve nurses in decision-making affecting health care at all levels. Promote and invest in an equitable culture that respects nurses as leading contributors to high-quality health systems.
8. Actively and meaningfully engage national nursing associations as critical professional partners in all aspects of health and social care policy, delivery and leadership as the experienced and trusted voice of nursing. Build local, national and global multilateral partnerships.
9. Protect vulnerable populations and uphold and respect human rights, gender equity and social justice. Place and uphold nursing ethics at the centre of health systems' design and delivery so that all people can access health care that is equitable, nondiscriminatory, people centred, rights based and without the risk of financial hardship.

10. Appoint nurse leaders to executive positions of all health care organisations and government policy–making bodies. Strengthen nursing leadership throughout health systems, and create and sustain nursing leadership roles where they are most needed.

THINK BOX 12.6

- How could you use your personal influence to convince policymakers to make the changes suggested in the ICN Charter for Change?
- How can you best ensure that your efforts, combined with those of your colleagues, will be fruitful?

It is clear from all the 10 actions that the ICN has been using the data and evidence it has collected to inform and develop its policy positions and solutions. Such evidence is important, but it needs to be translated into policies that actually change our health care systems.

To create the future we want, nursing as a profession needs to demonstrate the connection and relationship between nursing's contribution and health benefits and outcomes. By so doing, we will open up access to the decision-making forums that matter locally, nationally and globally.

We need to be more than the leaders of nursing: we need to be the leaders of health systems, with our hands firmly on the wheel, designing the health care systems of the future.

Nursing in the future needs to take the many wonderful examples of nursing innovations and disseminate and implement them around the globe. We should not accept the dominance of the medical model, which is simply no longer fit for purpose for the future we face, and instead work holistically with our multiprofessional colleagues to build the best health systems possible, a position echoed by the National Academy of Medicine (2021).

NURSING IS THE VITAL KEY TO A HEALTHY FUTURE FOR ALL

Having the right number of nurses with the right skills in the right place globally is the vital key to solving many of the world's most enduring health problems. Solutions to the global health agenda, including caring for vulnerable and ageing populations, noncommunicable diseases, and health promotion and prevention, lie in the everyday work of nurses.

Nurses are working on these issues and creating solutions, new approaches, new models of care and advanced and specialist practice. But these novel approaches need to be integrated, embedded and aligned with the mainstream of health care system. Not enough nurses are being trained, but there is also a need to fund postgraduate advanced nursing courses to support nurses in developing their roles and having attractive career structures.

There needs to be an alignment between the planning and development of nursing roles, nursing education and how we fund service models to maximise the impact that nursing can have. Worldwide nursing shortages continue, and while the supply and demand gap for nurses is increasing, we are not seeing any significant increases in the education of nurses around the world. It is somewhat ironic that the countries that recruit the most international migrant nurses are the countries that have some of the best health education systems in the world. International recruitment needs to be a two-way process, and there needs to be tangible mutual benefits between source and receiving countries.

More nurses are needed in very senior government positions to push this whole agenda so that governments hear directly from nurses and realise the benefits of investing in nursing. The danger is that governments and health care organisations will dilute the nursing workforce and replace registered nurses with untrained staff. But registered nurses are the professionals who make the biggest difference in health outcomes.

Around the world, there has been an increase in strikes and disputes. Many of these are about pay and decent working conditions, but they are also about nurses' concerns around safe staffing levels and patient safety. Lack of investment in health care affects every part of our societies and every aspect of our lives. Investing in nursing and health is a driver for economic growth, not a drain on resources. The health of a nation should be as important as its economic and national security; government budgets should reflect that fact by funding health care accordingly.

The right investments by governments will enable us to make enormous strides toward the global goals we all want to achieve, and if we get this right for nursing, it will make significant improvements in gender equality and female lives everywhere.

THINK BOX 12.7

How do you think nurses have adapted to changes in the past, especially when the rate of change is especially rapid?

A POSITIVE FUTURE

Notwithstanding all of the challenges mentioned, we believe 'the future' is not some dreadful thing that will suddenly descend upon nursing and nurses. Change and innovation actually come towards us at a pace that, thus far, nurses have always been able to adjust to and cope with.

The truth is, what nurses are doing is the future in practice now. The idea that in the future, nurses will need to be digitally enabled, flexible or providing one-stop shops is wrong because that is the reality of today's nursing in many places already. Examples from the BBC StoryWorks for ICN, *Caring with Courage* (BBC StoryWorks, 2022) films show exactly that.

Looking at what nurses are doing now gives us a window into the future. These are not pipe dreams or fantasies that are shrouded in unknowns about what we can and cannot do; they are practical examples of nurses who are working in a way that will, in time, become the norm. Forty years ago, people were hospitalised for weeks with conditions that are nowadays treated in the person's home. Hospital care has become much more acute, and people in hospital beds are generally sicker than they have ever been. Nursing has adapted to that as the change has taken place over the years.

The ways in which nursing has continually evolved and developed in response to people's needs, new technologies and innovations by finding pragmatic solutions and putting them seamlessly into place are evidence of the profession's ability to evolve to meet the requirements of the populations it serves.

Nurses have been living the future in responding to people's immediate needs and becoming skilled with new technologies. They have, as always, been instrumental in making things work because they have a skillset, adaptability and dynamism necessary to do so.

Nurses make the complexities of health care look simple—they present the complex world of health care in an accessible way. But often, it is only the simple that is seen by the outside world, not the compassion, the intricate problem-solving and decision-making, the way they manage relationships, their technical and organisational skills and the intellectual and emotional work that goes into making things seem so simple.

Patients who are unwell and undergoing treatment and are worried, confused and upset about their illness say only that the nurse 'helped me through it all'. They do not understand the breadth of skills that it takes to 'help them through', nor do nurses talk about nursing in a way that explains that complexity. Much of the time, nurses do not take a ready-made solution 'off the shelf' in response to people's conditions and demands; they are continually creating answers from their huge array of skills to meet the unique needs of individual patients. It is almost as if nurses are creating and living a new future in every decision they make.

The future is not a distant concept for nurses; it is responding to the individual set of health problems or needs that they see in the patient in front of them. Rather than think about the future as some far-off time in 20 years or so, nurses respond in a way that produces a state of improved health for an individual by creating a better future for that person out of the current situation. Nurses should recognise just how remarkable nursing is in turning the world around for people in need, and they should be bolder and speak more confidently about their contributions because, for many people, without the input of nurses in making a new future for them, there would be no future.

Having said all that, nurses cannot secure the best future possible on their own. The ICN has been saying for years that governments need to approach health spending needs in a different way, not as a cost but as an investment. The pandemic showed that inadequate health spending results in long-term problems for societies. We need governments to completely change their attitudes to health care spending to ensure that there are enough nurses to make healthy societies the norm, rather than the exception.

Nurses know only too well the social determinants of health and how policymaking outside of health care has a dramatic effect on the potential health, including the mental health of societies. To ensure a positive future for health care, we need to reorientate health care systems away from hospitals, and let's be honest here, that transition is not going to be led by hospitals. The health policymakers who write endlessly about different models of health care, markets and payment systems are not concentrating on what really matters, which is the assessment of health needs and developing a package of care to respond to those needs.

When we talk about prevention of health care problems, it can be reasonably straightforward when we address physical needs: do not smoke, get exercise, lose weight and eat a balanced diet. But when it comes to mental health, preventative measures are less clear-cut.

All of the debate about investment in health care shows us we are missing out on something important: the value of health care to societies is not acknowledged in many societies, and that is holding back the development of alternative services that will pay dividends in terms of societal and global health, economic prosperity, happiness and overall well-being.

We believe nurses are ready for the future because they live it every day in their practice. No one can predict what will happen, but we are confident that nurses will be ready, willing and able to deal with whatever the future holds, provided the necessary investment and support that they need is put in place. Nurses have always been highly responsive, adaptable and dynamic in responding to people's needs and health system changes, and that is the reason for our realistic optimism for the future.

THINK BOX 12.8

- Do you think there is room for optimism for the future of nursing?
- What will you do to ensure that nursing continues to be the most important profession for the future well-being of the world and all the people in it?

SOME MORE IDEAS ABOUT THE FUTURE

We asked nurse leaders at all stages of their careers and in different parts of the world for their views on what the nurse of 2050 will be doing. As this chapter points out, predicting the future is far from an exact science, but if we can imagine it, perhaps we can do it.

A colleague suggested—maybe in jest—that we ask ChatGPT. This is a section focused on the future, so we did, and what ChatGPT figured out follows. This is useful information in a way, as it tells us what is currently being written about regarding the future of nursing—obviously, ChatGPT takes its information from the articles that the search engine could find, so someone somewhere has already suggested ChatGPT's predications.

What our nursing colleagues told us is more visionary. We asked both new and more experienced leaders for their views, and in all who responded, we found vision and confidence in what nursing and midwifery will be contributing to global health in the decades ahead. We hope these contributions will inspire you.

PREDICTIONS FROM CHATGPT

Request made August 2023:

While we can't predict the future with certainty, we can offer some educated guesses about what nurses might be doing in 2025 based on current trends and emerging health care practices as of our last knowledge update in September 2021. Please keep in mind that health care is a dynamic field, and the roles and responsibilities of nurses can evolve over time. Here are some potential changes and developments in nursing practice by 2025:

Increased use of technology: Nurses are likely to continue using advanced technologies in patient care. This may include electronic health records, telehealth platforms, wearable health monitoring devices and robotics for tasks like medication delivery and patient assistance.

Telehealth and remote monitoring: The COVID-19 pandemic accelerated the adoption of telehealth, and this trend may continue to expand. Nurses may play a significant role in providing virtual care, monitoring patients remotely and conducting virtual health assessments.

Data analysis and informatics: Nurses are expected to become more involved in data analysis and health care informatics. They may use data to identify trends, improve patient outcomes and make informed decisions about care delivery.

Preventive care and health promotion: Nurses will likely continue to focus on preventive care and health promotion to reduce the burden of chronic diseases. This could involve community outreach, education and helping patients adopt healthier lifestyles.

1. Advanced practice roles: Advanced practice nurses, such as nurse practitioners and nurse anaesthetists, may have an expanded scope of practice, allowing them to provide more comprehensive care independently.
2. Genomic nursing: With advancements in genomics, nurses may play a larger role in integrating genetic information into patient care plans, including identifying genetic risk factors and tailoring treatments based on an individual's genetic makeup.
3. Collaborative care models: Interprofessional collaboration will continue to be emphasised in health care. Nurses may work closely with physicians, pharmacists, social workers and other health care professionals to provide holistic care.
4. Mental health care: Given the growing awareness of mental health issues, nurses may have an increased role in providing mental health care, including screening, assessment and support for patients with mental health disorders.
5. Crisis response and disaster nursing: Nurses may be involved in responding to public health crises, natural disasters and pandemics, providing essential health care services in emergency situations.
6. Cultural competence and diversity: Nurses will likely receive training to be culturally competent and provide care that is sensitive to the diverse backgrounds and needs of patients.
7. Education and training: Nursing education may evolve to incorporate more simulation-based training, virtual reality and online learning to prepare nurses for the challenges of modern health care.
8. Ethical dilemmas and advocacy: Nurses will continue to face ethical dilemmas in health care. They may also play a significant role in advocating for patients' rights and addressing health care disparities.

It's important to note that the specific roles and responsibilities of nurses can vary by region, health care setting and individual specialisation. The health care landscape is continually changing, influenced by factors such as technological advancements, health care policies and societal needs. Therefore, nurses in 2025 will likely adapt to new challenges and opportunities as they arise.

Predictions from Dr Pandora Hardtman

Chief Nursing and Midwifery Officer
Technical Leadership & Innovations Office
JHPIEGO, Baltimore, Maryland, United States

Step into the future of birthing—a realm where newborns arrive as they always have, cradled by the ageless embrace of the rotations inherent in the mechanisms of labour. A paradox unfolds: amid this familiar dance of life, the very air whispers of change, of progress weaving itself into the fabric of time.

The anatomy of reproduction persists, the gynecoid pelvis unyielding to the tides of transformation. Yet words reshape their contours, narratives reshuffle their hues and the intimate dialogue between birth and language takes on new shades.

In lands kissed by abundance, conversations are embarked upon with respect's compass: 'Born or assigned as female? Welcoming a boy, girl or an identity yet to be revealed? What might I call you?' A harmony of names, an orchestra of identities unfurl.

Conversely, in the realms unyielding to outside influences, names echo with the resonance of heritage and deep formality and respect in terms of address— Mama X, Madam Y, Mrs Z. A tapestry woven of familiarity, roots planted deep.

Amid this mosaic stands the sentinel of care, the nurse-midwife, a bridge between yesteryears and tomorrows. A beacon of continuity in an ever-evolving world, a guardian of ageless traditions.

And amidst the symphony of change, the nurse-midwife's stage transforms. With a digital caress, histories unfurl; biometrics illuminate. Technology paints a backdrop of enriched connections.

Machine-enabled marvels whisk resources to her side as she orchestrates a ballet of health data, choreographing entries into national health archives. Meanwhile, virtual forecasts unfurl, whispering the potential for obstetric turbulence, a microlearning interlude unfolds, a ballet of integrated insights.

Yet at the core, the heartbeat of the fetus remains steadfast, undaunted by the ebbs of time. Midwifery's essence remains unchanged. The vocation, a calling heard in the whispers of compassion or perhaps charted by the algorithms of aptitude and standardised testing.

A new era has dawned, casting the shadows of disrespect and abuse to the annals of history. The notable contributions to health care will remain embedded in the memories of the clients served.

Across continents and horizons, connectivity knows no bounds. A telephonic touch spans borders, healing hands bridging gaps, cradling lives amidst crises.

In this new, youth's chorus echoes. Comprehensive reproductive health steps into the spotlight, steering nurse-midwives away from the birth's body and into the embrace of holistic care. A symphony of transformation, a recalibration of competence and curricula.

Dreams alight upon intercontinental licensure boards, a mosaic of accountability and unity. Clients will still be confused about all of the pathways to practice, but in their moment of need, not really care, so long as someone is there to care for them.

Bound by the fusion of the path to midwifery 2030, female health, human rights and economic empowerment converge. Progress shrouded by familiar strife—hierarchies, models, autonomy. A tale as old as time, cast in the echoes of evolution.

The future beckons, a progress made in incremental strides, demanding more than a generation's journey. Nurse-midwifery—'ancient as wisdom, modern as time'.

The Future of Nursing in Africa by Judy Khanyola
Chair: Center for Nursing and Midwifery
University of Global Health Equity, Kigali, Rwanda

Africa is the second-largest continent, after Asia, and covers one-fifth of the Earth's total land surface (World Population Review, 2024). It also holds the unique position of being the only continent with fossil evidence of human evolution through each key evolutionary phase, earning it the autograph 'cradle of humankind' (National Geographic Education, 2024).

Despite this unique and advantageous locus, Africa remains the poorest continent on Earth, following centuries of degradation and depredations.

I will share my thoughts, musings and ruminations on the future of nursing in Africa, adding my voice to esteemed and honourable colleagues in the profession, writing this important chapter, so very important to nursing at this time.

I am an African nurse, proud of my African heritage, passionate about my chosen profession, but greatly disappointed by the current trajectory that nursing in Africa is taking. Nursing in Africa was born out of the colonial system put in place by Europeans who scrambled in the 1880s and partitioned Africa for their imperialistic gain. As such, the education systems, scope of practice, prestige and value in society of the profession, salary structure, role in the health system, career progression, entry into practice and related support structures were put in place by external people who did not understand Africa. The resultant effect of this is the weak, fragmented nursing system we see in Africa today.

One personal outcome of colonialism for me has been the love of reading and all things English literature. One of my favourite authors is England's Charles Dickens, and I have read his books over and over again. I would like to refer to his book, *A Tale of Two Cities*, and use it to set the stage for my thoughts on the future of nursing in Africa (Dickens, 1859):

In the book, Sydney Carton has exchanged his life for Charles Darnay and is guillotined in the madness that was the 1789 French Revolution. Dickens captures the thoughts of Sydney Carton in words I love so well and that I will take the utmost liberty to paraphrase and use to share my thoughts of nursing's future in Africa.

'...long ranks of the new oppressors...perishing...'

Nursing in Africa postcolonialism exchanged the old colonial oppressors with new African ones. Nursing in many African countries is oppressed by selfish, tribal and nepotistic structures found everywhere from academia to associations, unions and even at the ministries of health. I see these 'new oppressors... perishing'

'...a beautiful city and a brilliant people rising from this abyss...'

Following the perishing of tribal and selfish agendas will arise a new nursing dawn in Africa. I see:

- One Africa Nursing that goes beyond the colonial country boundaries of Africa, allowing for:
  - Harmonised entry into practice
  - Harmonised career progression
  - Harmonised nomenclature for the different nursing qualifications
  - Harmonised licensure and examinations and continuous professional development
  - National office at the ministry of health for a chief nurse
  - Removal of all restrictions for nurse migration, allowing nurses to work anywhere in Africa
  - Expansion of the profession to include new and emerging technologies such as AI and virtual reality and new roles like forensics, space exploration, climate and planetary health
- It has the following as its foundation:
  - Scientific underpinnings that not only use nursing science but all other physical-, biological-, social-, economic- and population-related sciences
  - Leadership based on merit and equity
  - Dedicated national nursing budgets
- And I see the future nurse in Africa that will come out of the above will be:

'...a far, far, better...' one:

i. Using the 'ubuntu' spirit of Africa—caring not for patients, but for families and utilising both African and Western knowledge
ii. Focusing on disease prevention instead of disease management and, instead of being stationed in hospitals, health centres and clinics, will be integrated as a family nurse practitioner attached to families and living and working in the community. Entering homes, doing their work, respected and cherished.
iii. Using technology to improve population health
iv. Keeping to the core ethos of nursing which is the 'human being'

As long as we have human beings, nurses will always have a place. The only difference is that this 'place' continually shifts and changes. The future nurse only needs to adapt and adjust.

From a young nurse leader, Zipporah Iregi
AU Bingwa, African Union, based in Kenya
SwitchPoint Future League Leader
Intrahealth International Nursing Now Challenge Champion

As an early career nurse, I have seen the nursing workforce adapt to ensure that communities are cared for even as situations change. An example, some student and novice nurses in Kenya saw the need for mentorship and collaborated to start a mentorship program for student nurses. They organised leadership training sessions with nursing and other global health leaders and coordinated community outreach programs. COVID-19 also showed the contributions of nurses around the world to ensure that each one was cared for. This is nursing at its very core, and governments and other leaders are slowly beginning to appreciate nursing as a profession.

The future of nursing is very bright, and this future lies in the hands of the early-career nurses. We must include them in the conversation about the future. These young nurses not only understand the health care system but also have the technological know-how, and after school and their internships, they move on to occupy every level of health care.

Post-COVID, there has been a great discussion on the role of technology in achieving health for all and the need to shift to primary health care with a focus on health promotion and prevention. These early-career nurses are at the forefront of helping their families and communities through this transition.

The fact that nurses make up 59% of the health care workforce speaks to this fact, with a significant percentage being young nurses. Nurses are pivotal to the achievement of universal health coverage. They ought to be driving that conversation forward.

When I think about 2050, I see nurses contributing to global health at the highest level of decision-making and policy development. I see them leading teams and helping their countries adapt to the rising concerns of the aging population and noncommunicable diseases. I see them at the heart of the health digital transformation journey, not just helping with the transition but also contributing to the development of need-specific solutions for their communities. I see nurses leading research teams to ensure that data inform the decisions in building better health systems for all. Besides that, I also see nurses working in their communities, ensuring that no one is left behind. I see nurses practicing at the very top of their profession, driving positive change at every level of health care.

We cannot wait 10 years to start the journey to this future. It starts now; better yet, this future has already begun, as I have seen early career nurses stepping up to be leaders of influence. As early as now, they need to be supported and encouraged to build the kind of future they want by ensuring that the training is adaptive to the needs of the communities, the working environment is safe and healthy, they are equipped with the necessary leadership skills and provided with opportunities to lead teams, and they are allowed the freedom to practice at the top of the profession.

We can genuinely achieve Health for All.

The Future of Community Nursing by Dr Liz Madigan
CEO Sigma Theta Tau, USA

The nurse of 2050 will be an expert in care in the home and community. Nursing students in 2050 will be educated to provide basic care in the home and community along the entire spectrum from health promotion/disease prevention, care of those with noncommunicable diseases, care of those with communicable diseases, those who need rehabilitation, palliative care and end-of-life care. Specialty nurses within each of these areas will have postgraduate specialty training and serve as mentors and preceptors for nurses who have the basic preparation for home- and community-based care. The care provided in the home and community will be team based, with the nurses with basic preparation providing most of the care, while the specialty nurses will be involved in care that is particularly challenging or complex or requires advanced skills. Nurses are the primary sources of care working with community health workers, physiotherapists, psychologists, social workers and others to provide the wraparound care needed.

All care will be technologically supported, but nothing replaces the actual presence of the nurse and the therapeutic and professional benefits of in-person care. Assistive robots will be routine; sensors in the home for those at risk will be ubiquitous, all care informed by AI. However, the human component of the care will be paramount, as the individual trajectories and life experiences require human insight and interaction.

'Hospitals' will be locations where there is critical care and intensive surgery and staffed by nurses who have done postgraduate education in acute care, unlike the present, where all nurses receive acute care education and clinical experience.

"Neighbourhood" nurses are nurses who serve a specific geographic area, understand deeply the issues of that neighbourhood, are influential in promoting change, working with other groups and organisations, and providing health education, referrals to other nurses and services, and recognising and building upon the strengths of that community.

The Future of Community Nursing by Professor Aisha Holloway
Professor of Nursing Studies
Codirector, Edinburgh Global Nursing Initiative
University of Edinburgh, Scotland

People, power and politics. To survive, nurses in 2050 must be at the heart of all three.

Whilst I sit here, as a nurse considering the prospect of 2050, I do so with a sense of uneasiness and fear. Fear for the future of our profession. Fear for the future of the communities we serve, in response to the impact of the global burden of disease, alongside the escalating ravages of conflict. Fear for our planet, already facing the unimaginable consequences of climate change.

The geopolitics of health and well-being; the proposition of a well-being economy; the global One Health paradigm, where societies, sectors, disciplines and ecosystems come together in harmony; the emergence of a digital and data driven world, where AI is a juggernaut. These may all seem far away from the minds of the nursing profession. They should not be. Our literacy in associated areas of health and well-being requires a seismic shift to optimise our impact. This is where nurses in 2050 should be, as scientists and curators of care.

Of course, we must protect our unique nursing contribution, but we must also understand the power of collaboration and partnership, the power of the collective. As the very fabric of society, we must position ourselves across and within communities, disciplines and multiple sectors. Fostering relationships in prevention and protection, as well as taking action against emerging and current global threats.

My final thoughts lead me to consider what we must change immediately to set us on a new path towards 2050. Whilst we may prophecise and envision solely a panacea of wonder of what our clinical contribution to disease prevention, care and treatment and scope of practice will be, we do so at our peril. We must become the powerhouse. We must politic, we must command, we must be sagacious in our ability to engage effectively in our own professional narrative and worth. Not as a chosen few, but as a unified and mobilised global nursing movement. This should and must be at the hands of the youth and early career nurses. No longer can those of us who hold positions of authority and power as a result of our 'time at the helm' be leading the charge. It is time to let go. It is time to hand over the mantle. Our role? We must support, we must lift up and we must provide opportunity after opportunity. It is time. *To articulate, to effect, to influence* were key to the thesis of the politics of nursing (Salvage, 1985). We must hold ourselves to account on progress. The status quo is no longer viable.

We are the nurses of the people, by the people and for the people.

A LAST WORD

As it says at the beginning of this chapter, predicting the future is, at best, an uncertain science. So why, ask our colleagues, try to do so?

Imagining all that may be possible is one way to open our minds to exactly that—a vision of what is possible. All of the reflections on the future of our profession show us the potential of what we might achieve in the future but also the complexity of the art and science of nursing—and indeed, as highlighted so lyrically by Pandora Hardtman, of midwifery. Our profession is broad and deep, and sometimes we are lost for words to describe it accurately. Nurses are with people everywhere—homes, shopping centres, schools, prisons, refugee camps and, of course, in health facilities of all kinds. It is nurses and midwives who are there at the beginning and the end of life. This is the wonderful art of nursing and midwifery. Both of these sciences need sophisticated problem-solving skills to function well, with facets of many health sciences underpinning it; it is applied through the wonderful art of nursing, and that is the magic of our profession at its best.

All of the contributors on the future of nursing point this out in different ways. Hardtman points out how connected the elements of globalisation are and how closely woven with the work of nursing: 'Bound by the fusion of the path to Midwifery 2030, women's health, human rights, economic empowerment converge. Nurse-Midwifery—"ancient as wisdom, modern as time"'.

Judy Khanyola gives a powerful reminder that there could be a new dawn for nursing in Africa, 'One Africa Nursing that goes beyond the colonial country boundaries of Africa'. This is the message in Chapter 6 of this book, and if you have started the book at the back, you can head to that chapter for much more on decolonising nursing in the future.

A talented young nurse leader, Zipporah Iregi, give us so much hope for our future profession: 'When I think about 2050, I see nurses contributing to global health at the highest level of decision-making and policy development. I see them leading teams and helping their countries adapt to the rising concerns of the aging population and noncommunicable diseases'.

This theme of the breadth of practice of nursing continues when Dr Madigan shares a vision for nursing in the community, echoing the significance of place of practice. Our ageing population will want to choose where they live out their years and where they can be cared for; we will all need the best of nursing in our homes and communities.

Professor Aisha Holloway closes this section by reminding us that the reason for reading this book is to be effective advocates for nursing, health and the people we care for by understanding how we 'join the dots' between all the global systems within which we live and work. Holloway says this: 'We must become the powerhouse. We must politic, we must command, we must be sagacious in our ability to engage effectively in our own professional narrative and worth. Not as a chosen few, but as a unified and mobilised global nursing movement'.

That is the message with which this book should close. We can power together as nurses, and modern technology gives us the opportunity to remain connected and mobilise our strengths together to be key influencers of future health systems.

If we can seize it now, the future can be ours.

REFERENCES

Barker, C. F., & Markmann, J. F. (2013). Historical overview of transplantation. *Cold Spring Harbor Perspectives in Medicine, 3*(4), a014977. doi: 10.1101/cshperspect.a014977.

BBC StoryWorks. (2022). *Caring with courage.* BBC StoryWorks. Retrieved, August 8, 2023, from. https://www.icn.ch/how-we-do-it/projects/caring-courage.

Brush, L., & Lynaugh, J. (1999). *Nurses of all nations: A history of the International Council of Nurses, 1899–1999.* Lippincott.

Dickens, C. (1859). *A Tale of Two Cities. Historical Novel.* Chapman.

Independent Panel for Pandemic Preparedness and Response. (2021). *COVID-19: Make it the Last Pandemic.* IPPPR.

International Council of Nurses. (2017–2023). *International nurses day (portal).* Retrieved, August 8, 2023, from https://www.icn.ch/how-we-do-it/campaigns/international-nurses-day.

International Council of Nurses. (2022). *Sustain and retain in 2022 and beyond.* ICN. Retrieved, August 8, 2023, from. https://www.icn.ch/node/1463.

International Council of Nurses. (2023). *Charter for change.* ICN. Retrieved, August 8, 2023, from. https://www.icn.ch/sites/default/files/2023-05/IND_2023_Charter_EN.pdf.

International Council of Nurses. (2023). *International nurses day report 2023.* ICN. Retrieved, August 8, 2023, from. https://www.icn.ch/sites/default/files/2023-05/ICN_IND_2023_Report_EN_web.pdf.

International Council of Nurses. (2023). *Recover to rebuild: Investing in the nursing workforce for health system effectiveness.* ICN. Retrieved, August 8, 2023, from. https://www.icn.ch/resources/publications-and-reports/recover-rebuild-0.

National Academy of Medicine. (2021). *The future of nursing 2020–2030: Charting a path to achieve health equity.* National Academy of Medicine.

National Geographic Education. (2024). *Africa: Human geography.* Retrieved, March, 2024, from. https://education.nationalgeographic.org/resource/africa-human-geography/

Nightingale, F. (1860). *Notes on nursing: What it is and what it is not.* Appleton and Company.

Nightingale Society. (2020). *Who was Florence Nightingale and why does she matter now?* Retrieved, August 8, 2023, from https://nightingalesociety.com/papers/who-was-florence-nightingale-and-why-does-she-matter-now/.

Roberts, J., & Group, T. (1995). *Feminism and nursing: An historical perspective on power, status and political activism in the nursing profession.* Praeger Publishers.

United Nations. (2015). *Sustainable development goals.* United Nations.

World Health Organization. (2017). *Health as a fundamental human right.* World Health Organization. Retrieved, August 14, 2023, from. https://www.who.int/news-room/commentaries/detail/health-is-a-fundamental-human-right.

World Health Organization. (2019). *Universal health coverage.* WHO. Retrieved, August 23, 2023, from https://www.who.int/news-room/fact-sheets/detail/universal-health-coverage-(uhc)

World Health Organization, Nursing Now and ICN. (2020). *State of the world's nursing report: Investing in education, jobs and leadership.* WHO. Retrieved, August 8, 2023, from. https://www.who.int/publications/i/item/9789240003279.

World Population Review. (2024). Countries in Africa. https://worldpopulationreview.com/country-rankings/countries-in-africa. (Last accessed March 2024).

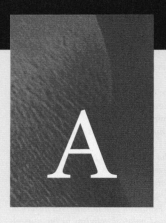

A   NURSE LEADERS' INTERVIEW NARRATIVE

■ ■ ■ ■ ■ ■ ■ ■ ■ ■ ■ ■ ■ ■ ■ ■ ■ ■ ■

Based on transcripts of Nurse Leader Interviews related to the report by Newman, C., Stilwell, B., Rick, S., & Peterson, K. (2019). Investing in the power of nurse leadership: what will it take? *IntraHealth International, Nursing Now, Johnson & Johnson.*

Six nurse leaders representing policy, research, services and academia from the Middle East and North Africa, sub-Saharan Africa, Latin America and the Caribbean, Europe, Central and South Asia and East Asia and the Pacific were interviewed on topics such as the impact of gender on the nursing profession, career progression and leadership achievements. The following narrative weaves together quotes illustrating nurse leaders' experiences of gender stereotyping and constraints, work–life conflict, child care and time poverty, barriers to career progression, the need to 'prove it again', male preference and the glass elevator at work in their careers and what cultural changes are needed in the future.

We particularly wanted to offer a chance to 'hear' the voices of nurses who have contributed so much to our work on gender and nursing.

I think to the highest level, if I can say that. I think gender is still acting is the one thing that limits progress and limits women to move in their life. …I have been here for five years now, and in those five years I have seen two male deans. I don't even think they are thinking of having a female dean. So those are the things that you can see that the society still sees us as inferior despite being in education or academia … And then another thing talking about that is in

research. Usually, we do an application to apply for research funding and basically when we look at the funding outcomes in most cases they will say that men get it. And in our case here we are in the department of health sciences - those that are always trying to say those in medicine, they are always trying to say that we are the soft sciences, the males that are in medicine. So those are you see, the system - so that is why I think it is the system and the structure that still perpetuate this issue for women.

I cannot be associate professor being a woman within my appointment, so I need to work harder and prove to them, to the management of the university, that being a woman doesn't mean that I don't work hard. I worked hard for those past four years and then within that period which is a long period for some, I obtained it. Because I think that if it was a man, for sure he could have just been given the position straight away, but because of my gender that is why I was given another year, another two, three, four years, to prove to these people that I can have a leadership position.

I think the policies are needed to facilitate that. Like for example, you gave two examples of sexual bias, especially the equity one - or affirmative action policies. They work to our advantage and to our disadvantage, because when we are in this space, people think we are just here because of affirmative action, despite being qualified, despite having those qualifications and earning those skills and competencies to work the same way as men. So those policies are there - sometimes they facilitate us, and sometimes you are just seen as a body, just a warm body who was put there because of this policy.

I think gender is still acting as the one thing that limits progress and limits women to move in their life....And for me I can't say I blame gender or whatever, I blame the system as a whole. Because the department here are run by women, but the dean who takes a decision - I have been here for five years now, and in those five years I have seen two male deans. I don't even think they are thinking of having a female dean. So those are the things that you can see that the society still sees us as inferior despite being in education or academic... And then another thing talking about that, is in research, usually we do an application to apply for research funding and basically when we look at the funding outcomes in most cases they will say that men get it. And in our case here we are in the department of health sciences - those that are always trying to say those in medicine, they are always trying to say that we are the soft sciences, the males that are in medicine. So that is why I think it is the system and the structure that still perpetuate this issue for women.

They believe their role is just support medical doctoring... And the second point, the medical doctor, they don't want nurse to be independent. Because the field, nurses [are] to be independent, they may not control nurse strictly. So, they want to control nurses.

You know as a profession they think, the nursing profession is just an assistant to medical doctors. I talked to one of the key person from WHO, and they ask medical doctors to check what to do about nursing workforce in [country] in the health center. They think because the doctor is involved, so I said if you let the medical doctor to evaluate this kind of nursing workforce in the health center, it doesn't work well because they don't understand the meaning... they don't understand the concept of the nursing profession. They don't understand the standard of nursing practice, so how could they check—how can they evaluate effectively?

...in the hospitals there are many women, it comes to the other side of the coin where if you are a male in the hospital, you are a minority. So, there are women in nursing, however when you move to the upper rungs, that is where we meet the male counterpart, and then usually given the space that we are coming from as women, we don't usually meet the required standard because these men have been in the higher position more than us and for a longer time.

There is something about nursing that has a stigma of being secondary, tertiary even more towards medicine, towards anything else, it is a serving position.

In the place I am now, I have indicated that the deans are all males. And if I can elaborate more, as part of management now, as part of leadership now, we usually attend the - when they are appointing new people, to go and vote, and when we reach that, I have never seen in the higher positions there was a woman who came to the interview - except that we have a female VC, who left. So, I still think there is this misconception that males are leaders. That is why women in the applications, in the CVs that we are to look at, we find that all the applicants are males. Do women not apply to those positions, or women are not chosen in those positions? That is the question that we need to interrogate.

...when I arrived here I knew directly I would qualify straight away to be a professor. I knew. What I brought, I could have just gone to get oriented to the area. But I was given a [period] just like any other persons. But there are those males who come directly and occupy those positions.

You are seen as someone who is trying to be a male and is not, or someone who is trying to be something they're not, and for me I am considered to be someone that I am not. So, for me I am in a white space now, majority white space ... And another thing is they would tell me "you don't belong to this because you are black, this is a white university... when we go to research meetings, in those meetings, that is where you can find this backlash.

I think that nursing as a profession is discriminated against, because it is women, and so that was, that made it tough I think, quite a bit.

To recognize that nurses need to have university education, and they can make decisions, was a huge challenge… they are not making decisions, it is the doctors.

But I think as nurses we do not get the credit and respect we often deserve and I think that is gender-related.

The organizational culture of the World Health Organization was not supportive to nursing. I made things happen but it was despite the organizational culture. But that goes more to nursing in a basically medical organization. The organizational culture in universities usually doesn't make things easy. It definitely doesn't, the organization culture in most universities makes things difficult, and that is also gender-related but it is also related to nursing per say. But it is also gender-related.

Not many nurses, female nurses who want to lead…So my job, my role, I start from the students, nursing students. I start from them to encourage them to look in the future to be a leader, not to be a follower.

Because in our country, and in most African countries, nursing is a predominantly female profession. So, we've been trying to push forward. Usually where there are more women in the profession, people do not take it seriously. I think it is now, we are doing research, we are professors….and when we published and …we presented our research to the public, then you have all this publications and books, that is when people start taking you seriously.

I must say… the challenges we face in leadership is recognition. I remember what pushed me to do a PhD. I went to a meeting after my masters' degree. I had a colleague of mine with a PhD and every time she spoke, everybody would listen. And me with my masters, I would say the same points, and nobody

would acknowledge me. So, I said to myself: this is a status issue. So, I decided I should get my PhD. I also knew it was because I was a woman. Because men, if they speak even without a PhD, many times they receive recognition. And, also because many positions in our country is held by men.

…men are the ones who are doing the final say, we are bound and we are instructed as women, we are tailoring this act to be what we wish to be, but when it comes to the final realization the men are the one making the decision about this act taking place. However, I still cherish those moments when I was in the political space.

What my recommendation to address the gender-related barriers is, we need the society - and I know it's a hard thing and sometimes it's not doable - but we need the society to recognize that women are as much as talented, as much as competent as males. And secondly, we need to teach our girl child that they see no difference between a male or a female. They need to know whatever this male partner can do, she can do it also. Those are the things we need to talk about continuously. We need to engage about that continuously. And as I teach here, I usually tell my undergraduate nurses that they must know that much they are women, because most of them are women, they must know that they are not in the wrong position… there's no way they should be undermined by the medical students when they are in the ward. Those are the things that I usually talk about in these classes, I recommend some things that there should be a continuous push to say that we are all equal.

But we've got to be able to make sure we know what we contribute. It is not enough to say we are leaders and we want to make policy. I mean, we have got to be clear in able to define what we actually contribute.

For nursing to have a voice in the national public it is very difficult because it is being discounted. And in all of our human resource planning, we would have to sit together with the medical association, and the nursing association and the others and see what *changing healthcare needs with the changing population and make decisions together. But …the docs aren't into it. So that's problematic…as a profession it doesn't have the glory that medicine has.*

So, we have to talk about and produce our voice in terms of nursing professions.

You know, where I was socialized to be a leader to speak up. My father would always say "there is no argument you cannot win, speak up". Even against him, lots of women are taught to be obedient, gentle, women shouldn't, you should always be…so then you meet various people who say "she has a lot of potential, if only she could speak up, if only she could be more assertive in this." So yeah, those roles are especially, how we are socialized. Within the family, within the community.

I used to see the culture where a lot of informal work was done late in the evening in the pub. And that would be physicians and administrations, and men predominantly. And women with or without children would choose to go home. I remember one of my director of nursing colleagues would have a formal management meeting, various things would be agreed, then the men would go off to the pub and she would go home, and the next day she would find half the decisions had been changed. So, I think those sorts of complexes, I think come in.

Women themselves need to be stronger, need to have higher education, need to be not talkative… Some people may not respect that. For example, they talk and talk and talk about bad things in front of men. So, the men will see that and they will disrespect a woman. So, this is kind of status of woman that must be upgraded, respect themselves and respect others.

And, for developing leadership positions, I think that…it is important of course for nurses to have education… it is also very important to communicate with public, to show what nurses can do, to show advancement…even movies about positive roles of nurses are very important. Still there is, I would say such an image, that it's a female profession in the society.

I'm not sure about this question on how to make impact on profile -status on nursing. But in my country, there is a lack of policy support in the nursing profession. Currently, there are some laws or regulations that concern nurses' profession. But there is still a limit when compared to others. This profession in [Country] is a low profession. We have a low image. I think it's better to have policy support to the retirement, support for positioning in the organization, policy to support insurance, policy to talk about how can they leave after retirement.

As some nurse leaders have high competence, when the men listen to them and this is very important that if they have high competency the same as men…

I taught about gender balance, you need to promote them. Not just only woman to follow men to upgrade to high education, not to just follow anyone, but we need to initiate some work to prove to some people that they have the competence enough to work.

I am a nurse leader and my problem comes when we have to apply for funding as I have indicated somewhere in this interview, you will find that the applicants are males. One thing that makes more applicants to be males is that they don't do anything at home. When I leave here, I'm still going to cook, I am still going to attend to the household, but for the man, he can stay here after work and go home and sleep. They go to bed and sleep, eat and sleep. … they will all just continue waiting at work and finish the proposal. For me now, as we are talking, I'm still going to be here the coming hour trying to finalize a grant. Mind you I must go home and cook, and clean, and do whatever. So, this issue you are talking about, my grant will never be perfect like the one of my male counterpart.

…So usually then the review committee also, you will find that the candidates are males. If you are invited to go there, you will find that you are the only woman there, they are all males. So, it's obvious when they see a female application they will just put it aside, regardless of reading the proposal or trying to interrogate the proposal, they will find a male,

and that is a fact. You will find that if we go to this senior management meeting, we reach the outcome of the grant, most of them are given to male. There will be one woman against five males. So, these are the things that you are talking about on the glass ceiling. They are invisible barrier and they derail our promotion to higher levels in nursing leadership roles.

They lost their families because their husband could not cope with their wife being more success than or being too busy with a job. And this is a part of the [Country] culture where husbands think that the role of the wife is to put housing and ...cooking and caring for the family as the priority.

So, for me, that is something that I want to support young women with, is to balance work, family and we live in society where we have extended family members. It can be quite overwhelming. So, all you really need is support... support of your spouse, support of your parents, otherwise, if you don't it can be difficult. My late mother and my-mother- in law came in many times to support and take care of the babies when I was studying and I had to travel overseas.

Or change responsibilities in the family together, for example, so men can take care of the children, or help their wife, or help his wife to do household chores...such as washing clothes or cleaning house, or washing dish is maybe help. The wife, to help her have more time now and is not too tired. And the wife can spend the time in her work.

I was lucky enough to have support, especially when it came to ... motherhood and childbearing. I had support, my mother- in- law was there so I didn't have to be bogged down...I was breastfeeding my child. And you know my husband said, I'm going to pay, you know, they are paying for your ticket, I'm going to pay, ...they paid also for the baby, but he also paid for the keeper so that, you know there were three of us, I had somebody taking care of the baby, so I could do the workshops and all that. So, they facilitated, but you really need the support. Otherwise there can be real barriers.

...because of performance, people respect me. So, they say: Oh, you are a nurse, but you are so good at what you do. So, it's really fighting.

INDEX

Note: Page numbers followed by "*f*" indicate figures, "*t*" indicate tables, and "*b*" indicate boxes.